DENTAL SECRETS
Third Edition

DENTAL SECRETS

Third Edition

STEPHEN T. SONIS, D.M.D., D.M.Sc.

Professor and Chairman
Department of Oral Medicine and
    Diagnostic Sciences
Harvard School of Dental Medicine
Chief, Division of Oral Medicine, Oral and
    Maxillofacial Surgery and Dentistry
Brigham and Women's Hospital
Boston, Massachusetts

HANLEY & BELFUS, INC.
An Affiliate of Elsevier

HANLEY & BELFUS, INC.
An Affiliate of Elsevier

The Curtis Center
Independence Square West
Philadelphia, Pennsylvania 19106

Note to the reader: Although the techniques, ideas, and information in this book have been carefully reviewed for correctness, the authors, editor, and publisher cannot accept any legal responsibility for any errors or omissions that may be made. Neither the publisher nor the editor makes any guarantee, expressed or implied, with respect to the material contained herein.

Library of Congress Control Number: 2003101059

DENTAL SECRETS   ISBN 1-56053-573-3

Printed in the United States

Last digit is the print number: 9   8   7   6   5   4   3   2   1

DEDICATION

To my father, H. Richard Sonis, D.D.S.,

with admiration and gratitude

CONTENTS

CONTRIBUTORS

Helene S. Bednarsh, B.S., R.D.H., M.P.H.
Boston Public Health Commission, Boston, Massachusetts

Walter W. Bond, M.S.
Consulting Microbiologist, RCSA, Inc., Lawrenceville, Georgia

Joseph W. Costa, Jr., D.M.D.
Instructor, Division of Oral Medicine, Infection, and Immunity, Harvard University School of Dental Medicine; Chief of Dentistry, Brigham and Women's Hospital, Boston, Massachusetts

Kathy J. Eklund, B.S., R.D.H., M.H.P.
Assistant Professor, Department of Safety and Occupational Health, The Forsyth Institute, Boston, Massachusetts

Elliot V. Feldbau, D.M.D.
Surgeon, Division of Oral Medicine and Dentistry, Brigham and Women's Hospital; Instructor, Department of Oral Medicine, Infection, and Immunity, Harvard University School of Dental Medicine, Boston, Massachusetts; Private Practice, Hammond Pond Dental Associates, Chestnut Hill, Massachusetts

Joseph P. Fiorellini, D.M.D., D.M.Sc.
Associate Professor, Department of Oral Medicine, Infection, and Immunity, Harvard University School of Dental Medicine, Boston Massachusetts

Bernard Friedland, B.Ch.D., M.Sc., J.D.
Assistant Professor, Department of Oral Medicine, Infection, and Immunity, Harvard University School of Dental Medicine, Boston, Massachusetts

Steven P. Levine, D.M.D.
Diplomate, American Board of Endodontics; Assistant Clinical Instructor, Department of Endodontics, Harvard University School of Dental Medicine, Boston, Massachusetts

Steven A. Migliorini, D.M.D.
Private Practice, Stoneham, Massachusetts

John A. Molinari, Ph.D.
Professor and Chairman, Department of Biomedical Sciences, University of Detroit Mercy School of Dentistry, Detroit, Michigan

Bonnie L. Padwa, D.M.D., M.D.
Assistant Professor of Oral and Maxillofacial Surgery, Harvard School of Dental Medicine; Children's Hospital and Brigham and Women's Hospital, Boston, Massachusetts

Edward S. Peters, D.M.D., M.S.
Department of Oral Medicine and Diagnostic Sciences, Harvard University School of Dental Medicine; Associate Surgeon, Division of Oral Medicine and Dentistry, Brigham and Women's Hospital, Boston, Massachusetts

Dale Potter, D.D.S., M.P.H.
Indian Health Services and Zuni Comprehensive Community Health Center, Zuni, New Mexico

Andrew L. Sonis, D.M.D.
Associate Clinical Professor, Harvard University School of Dental Medicine; Associate in Dentistry, Boston Children's Hospital, Boston, Massachusetts

Stephen T. Sonis, D.M.D., D.M.Sc.
Professor and Chairman, Department of Oral Medicine and Diagnostic Sciences, Harvard University School of Dental Medicine; Chief, Division of Oral Medicine, Oral and Maxillofacial Surgery, and Dentistry, Brigham and Women's Hospital, Boston, Massachusetts

Ralph B. Sozio, D.M.D.
Former Associate Clinical Professor in Prosthetic Dentistry, Harvard University School of Dental Medicine; Consultant, Division of Oral Medicine and Dentistry, Brigham and Women's Hospital, Boston, Massachusetts

Harvey N. Waxman, D.M.D.
Private Practice, Worcester, Massachusetts

Sook-Bin Woo, D.M.D., M.M.Sc.
Assistant Professor, Department of Infection, Immunity, and Oral Medicine, Harvard University School of Dental Medicine; Consultant Pathologist, Brigham and Women's Hospital, Boston, Massachusetts

PREFACE TO THE THIRD EDITION

More than 10 years have elapsed since *Dental Secrets* was first conceived. The response to the question-and-answer format has been enthusiastic. This third edition maintains our original objective of providing important "pearls" of information in a succinct way that is free of the formality of standard texts. A comparison of this edition with the second edition demonstrates changes, in almost every chapter, that respond to recent advances in the science and practice of dentistry. Additionally, two new contributors have joined the group: Bonnie Padwa, an oral and maxillofacial surgeon, and Joe Fiorellini, a periodontist. Like everyone else involved in *Dental Secrets*, they also love to teach those who love to learn.

I wish to thank Stan Ward of Hanley and Belfus for his help in putting this edition together.

Stephen T. Sonis, D.M.D., D.M.Sc.
Boston, Massachusetts

PREFACE TO THE FIRST EDITION

This book was written by people who like to teach for people who like to learn. Its format of questions and short answers lends itself to the dissemination of information as the kinds of "pearls" that teachers are always trying to provide and for which students yearn. The format also permits a lack of formality not available in a standard text. Consequently, the reader will note smatterings of humor throughout the book. Our goal has been to provide a work that readers will enjoy and find useful and stimulating.

This book is not a substitute for the many excellent textbooks available in dentistry. It is our hope that readers will pursue additional readings in areas which they find stimulating. While short answers provide the passage of succinct information, they do not allow for much discussion in the way of background or rationale. We have tried to provide sufficient breadth in the sophistication of questions in each chapter to meet the needs of dental students, residents, and practitioners.

It has been a pleasure working with my colleagues who have contributed to this book. I would like to thank Mike Bokulich for initiating this project. Finally, I am grateful to Linda Belfus, our publisher and editor, for her assistance, attention to detail, and patience.

Stephen T. Sonis, D.M.D., D.M.Sc.
Boston, Massachusetts

1. PATIENT MANAGEMENT:
THE DENTIST-PATIENT RELATIONSHIP

Elliot V. Feldbau, D.M.D.

After you seat the patient, a 42-year-old woman, she turns to you and says glibly, "Doctor, I don't like dentists." How should you respond?

Tip: The patient presents with a gross generalization. Distortions and deletions of information need to be explored. Not liking you, the dentist, whom she has never met before, is not a clear representation of what she is trying to say. Start the interview with questioning surprise in your voice as you cause her to reflect by repeating her phrasing, "You don't like dentists?," with the expectation that she will elaborate. Probably she has had a bad experience, and by proceeding from the generalization to the specific, communication will advance. It is important to do active listening and to allow the patient who is somewhat belligerent to ventilate her thoughts and feelings. You thereby show that you are different perhaps from a previous dentist who may not have developed listening skills and left the patient with a negative view of all dentists. The goals are to enhance communication, to develop trust and rapport, and to start a new chapter in the patient's dental experience.

As you prepare to do a root canal on tooth number 9, a 58-year-old man responds, "The last time I had that dam on, I couldn't catch my breath. It was horrible." How should you respond? What may be the significance of his statement?

Tip: The comment, "I couldn't catch my breath," requires clarification. Did the patient have an impaired airway with past rubber dam experience, or has some long ago experience been generalized to the present? Does the patient have a gagging problem? A therapeutic interview clarifies, reassures, and allows the patient to be more compliant.

A 55-year-old man is referred for periodontal surgery. During the medical history, he states that he had his tonsils out at age 10 years and since then any work on his mouth frightens him. He feels like gagging. How do you respond?

Tip: A remembered traumatic event is generalized to the present situation. Although the feelings of helplessness and fear of the unknown are still experienced, a reassured patient, who knows what is going to happen, can be taught a new set of appropriate coping skills to enable the required dental treatments. The interview fully explores all phases of the events surrounding the past trauma when the fears were first imprinted.

After performing a thorough examination for the chief complaint of recurrent swelling and pain of a lower right first molar, you conclude that, given the 80% bone loss and advanced subosseous furcation decay, the tooth is hopeless. You recommend extraction to prevent further infection and potential involvement of adjacent teeth. Your patient replies, "I don't want to lose any teeth. Save it!" How do you respond?

Tip: The command to save a hopeless tooth at all costs requires an understanding of the denial process, or the clinician may be doomed to perform treatments with no hope of success and face the likely consequences of a disgruntled patient. The interview should clarify the patient's feelings, fears, or interpretations regarding tooth loss. It may be a fear of not knowing that a tooth may be replaced, a fear of pain associated with extractions, a fear of confronting disease and its consequences, or even a fear of guilt due to neglect of dental care. The interview should clarify and inform while creating a sense of concern and compassion.

With each of the above patients, the dentist should be alerted that something is not routine. Each expresses a degree of concern and anxiety. This is clearly the time for the dentist to remove the gloves, lower the mask, and begin a comprehensive interview. Although responses to such situations may vary according to individual style, each clinician should proceed methodically and carefully to gather specific information based on the cues that the patient presents. By understanding each patient's comments and the feelings related to earlier experiences, the dentist can help the patient to see that change is possible and that coping with dental treatment is easily learned. The following questions and answers provide a framework for conducting a therapeutic interview that increases patient compliance and reduces levels of anxiety.

1. What is the basic goal of the initial patient interview?

To establish a therapeutic dentist-patient relationship in which accurate data are collected, presenting problems are assessed, and effective treatment is suggested.

2. What are the major sources of clinical data derived during the interview?

The clinician should be attentive to what the patient verbalizes (i.e., the chief complaint), the manner of speaking (how things are expressed), and the nonverbal cues that may be related through body language (e.g., posture, gait, facial expression, or movements). While listening carefully to the patient, the dentist observes associated gestures, fidgeting movements, excessive perspiration, or patterns of irregular breathing that may hint of underlying anxiety or emotional problems.

3. What are the common determinants of a patient's presenting behavior?

1. The patient's perception and interpretation of the present situation (the reality or view of the present illness)
2. The patient's past experiences or personal history
3. The patient's personality and overall view of life

Patients generally present to the dentist for help and are relieved to share personal information with a knowledgeable professional who can assist them. However, some patients also may feel insecure or emotionally vulnerable because of such disclosures.

4. Discuss the insecurities that patients may encounter while relating their personal histories.

Patients may feel the the fear of rejection, criticism, or even humiliation from the dentist because of their neglect of dental care. Confidential disclosures may threaten the patient's self-esteem. Thus patients may react to the dentist with both rational and irrational comments, and their behavior may be inappropriate and even puzzling to the dentist. In a severely psychologically limited patient (e.g., psychosis, personality disorders), behaviors may approach extremes. Furthermore, patients who perceive the dentist as judgmental or too evaluative are likely to become defensive, uncommunicative, or even hostile. Anxious patients are more observant of any signs of displeasure or negative reactions by the dentist. The role of effective communication is extremely important with such patients.

5. How can one effectively deal with the patient's insecurities?

Probably acknowledgment of the basic concepts of empathy and respect gives the most support to patients. Understanding their point of view (empathy) and recognition of their right to their own opinions and feelings (respect), even if different from the dentist's personal views, help to deal with potential conflicts.

6. Why is it important for dentists to be aware of their own feelings when dealing with patients?

While the dentist tries to maintain an attitude that is attentive, friendly, and even sympathetic toward a patient, he or she needs an appropriate degree of objectivity in relation to patients and their problems. Dentists who find that they are not listening with some degree of emotional neutrality to the patient's information should be aware of personal feelings of anxiety, sadness, indifference, resentment, or even hostility that may be aroused by the patient. Recognition of any aspects of the patient's behavior that arouse such emotions helps dentists to understand their own behavior and to prevent possible conflicts in clinical judgment and treatment plan suggestions.

7. List two strategies for the initial patient interview.
1. During the verbal exchange with the patient all of the elements of the medical and dental history relevant to treating the patient's dental needs are elicited.
2. In the nonverbal exchange between the patient and the dentist, the dentist gathers cues from the patient's mannerisms while conveying an empathic attitude.

8. What are the major elements of the empathic attitude that a dentist tries to relate to the patient during the interview?
- Attentiveness and concern for the patient
- Acceptance of the patient and his or her problems
- Support for the patient
- Involvement with the intent to help

9. How are empathic feelings conveyed to the patient?
Giving full attention while listening demonstrates to the a patient that you are physically present and comprehend what the patient relates. Appropriate *physical attending skills* enhance this process. Careful analysis of what a patient tells you allows you to respond to each statement with clarification and interpretation of the issues presented. The patient hopefully gains some insight into his or her problem, and rapport is further enhanced.

10. What useful physical attending skills comprise the nonverbal component of communication?
The adept use of face, voice, and body facilitates the classic bedside manner, including the following:
Eye contact. Looking at the patient without overt staring establishes rapport.
Facial expression. A smile or nod of the head to affirm shows warmth, concern, and interest.
Vocal characteristics. The voice is modulated to express meaning and to help the patient to understand important issues.
Body orientation. Facing patients as you stand or sit signals attentiveness. Turning away may seem like rejection.
Forward lean and proximity. Leaning forward tells a patient that you are interested and want to hear more, thus facilitating the patient's comments. Proximity infers intimacy, whereas distance signals less attentiveness. In general, 4–6 feet is considered a social, consultative zone.
A verbal message of low empathic value may be altered favorably by maintaining eye contact, forward trunk lean, and appropriate distance and body orientation. However, even a verbal message of high empathic content may be reduced to a lower value when the speaker does not have eye contact, turns away with backward lean, or maintains too far a distance. For example, do not tell the patient that you are concerned while washing your hands with your back to the dental chair.

11. During the interview, what cues alert the dentist to search for more information about a statement made by the patient?
Most people express information that they do not fully understand by using generalizations, deletions, and distortions in their phrasing. For example, the comment, "I am a horrible patient," does not give much insight into the patient's intent. By probing further the dentist may discover specific fears or behaviors that the patient has deleted in the opening generalization. As a matter of routine, the dentist should be alert to such cues and use the interview to clarify and work through the patient's comments. As the interview proceeds, trust and rapport are built as a mutual understanding develops and levels of fear decrease.

12. Why is open-ended questioning useful as an interviewing format?

Questions that do not have specific yes or no answers give patients more latitude to express themselves. More information allows a better understanding of patients and their problems. The dentist is basically saying, "Tell me more about it." Throughout the interview the clinician listens to any cues that indicate the need to pursue further questioning for more information about expressed fears or concerns. Typical questions of the open-ended format include the following: "What brings you here today?," "Are you having any problems?," or "Please tell me more about it."

13. How can the dentist help the patient to relate more information or to talk about a certain issue in greater depth?

A communication technique called *facilitation by reflection* is helpful. One simply repeats the last word or phrase that was spoken in a questioning tone of voice. Thus when a patient says, "I am petrified of dentists," the dentist responds, "Petrified of dentists?" The patient usually elaborates. The goal is to go from generalization to the specific fear to the origin of the fear. The process is therapeutic and allows fears to be reduced or diminished as patients gain insight into their feelings.

14. How should one construct suggestions that help patients to alter their behavior or that influence the outcome of a command?

Negatives should be avoided in commands. Positive commands are more easily experienced, and compliance is usually greater. To experience a negation, the patient first creates the positive image and then somehow negates it. In experience only positive situations can be realized; language forms negation. For example, to experience the command "Do not run!," one may visualize oneself sitting, standing, or walking slowly. A more direct command is "Stop!" or "Walk!" Moreover, a negative command may create more resistance to compliance, whether voluntary or not. If you ask someone not to see elephants, he or she tends to see elephants first. Therefore, it may be best to ask patients to keep their mouth open widely rather than to say, "Don't close," or perhaps to suggest, "Rest open widely, please."

A permissive approach and indirect commands also create less resistance and enhance compliance. One may say, "If you stay open widely, I can do my procedure faster and better," or "By flossing daily, you will experience a fresher breath and a healthier smile." This style of suggestion is usually better received than a direct command.

Linking phrases—for example, "as," "while," or "when"—to join a suggestion with something that is happening in the patient's immediate experience provides an easier pathway for a patient to follow and further enhances compliance. Examples include the following: "As you lie in the chair, allow your mouth to rest open. While you take another deep breath, allow your body to relax further." In each example the patient easily identifies with the first experience and thus experiences the additional suggestion more readily.

Providing pathways to achieve a desired end may help patients to accomplish something that they do not know how to do on their own. Patients may not know how to relax on command; it may be more helpful to suggest that while they take in each breath slowly and see a drop of rain rolling off a leaf, they can let their whole body become loose and at ease. Indirect suggestions, positive images, linking pathways, and guided visualizations play a powerful role in helping patients to achieve desired goals.

15. How do the senses influence communication style?

Most people record experience in the auditory, visual, or kinesthetic modes. They hear, they see, or they feel. Some people use a dominant mode to process information. Language can be chosen to match the modality that best fits the patient. If patients relate their problem in terms of feelings, responses related to how they feel may enhance communication. Similarly, a patient may say, "Doctor, that sounds like a good treatment plan," or "I see that this disorder is relatively common. Things look less frightening now." These comments suggest an auditory mode and a visual mode, respectively Responding in similar terms enhances communication.

16. When is reassurance most valuable in the clinical session?

Positive supportive statements to the patient that he or she is going to do well or be all right are an important part of treatment. Everyone at some point may have doubts or fears about the outcome. Reassurance given too early, such as before a thorough examination of the presenting symptoms, may be interpreted by some patients as insincerity or as trivializing their problem. The best time for reassurance is after the examination, when a tentative diagnosis is reached. The support is best received by the patient at this point.

17. What type of language or phrasing is best avoided in patient communications?

Certain words or descriptions that are routine in the technical terminology of dentistry may be offensive or frightening to patients. Cutting, drilling, bleeding, injecting, or clamping may be anxiety-provoking terms to some patients. Furthermore, being too technical in conversations with patients may result in poor communication and provoke rather than reduce anxiety. It is beneficial to choose terms that are neutral yet informative. One may prepare a tooth rather than cut it or dry the area rather than suction all of the blood. This approach may be especially important during a teaching session when procedural and technical instructions are given as the patient lies helpless, listening to conversation that seems to exclude his or her presence as a person.

18. What common dental-related fears do patients experience?
- Pain
- Drills (e.g., slipping, noise, smell)
- Needles (deep penetration, tissue injury, numbness)
- Loss of teeth
- Surgery

19. List four elements common to all fears.
- Fear of the unknown
- Fear of loss of control
- Fear of physical harm or bodily injury
- Fear of helplessness and dependency

Understanding the above elements of fear allows effective planning for treatment of fearful and anxious patients.

20. During the clinical interview, how may one address such fears?

According to the maxim that fear dissolves in a trusting relationship, establishing good rapport with patients is especially important. Secondly, preparatory explanations may deal effectively with fear of the unknown and thus give a sense of control. Allowing patients to signal when they wish to pause or speak further alleviates fears of loss of control. Finally, well-executed dental technique and clinical practices minimize unpleasantness.

21. How are dental fears learned?

Most commonly dental-related fears are learned directly from a traumatic experience in a dental or medical setting. The experience may be real or perceived by the patient as a threat, but a single event may lead to a lifetime of fear when any element of the traumatic situation is reexperienced. The situation may have occurred many years before, but the intensity of the recalled fear may persist. Associated with the incident is the behavior of the past doctor. Thus, in diffusing learned fear, the behavior of the present doctor is paramount.

Fears also may be learned indirectly as a vicarious experience from family members, friends, or even the media. Cartoons and movies often portray the pain and fear of the dental setting. How many times have dentists seen the negative reaction of patients to the term "root canal," even though they may not have had one?

Past fearful experiences often occur during childhood when perceptions are out of proportion to events, but memories and feelings persist into adulthood with the same distortions. Feelings of helplessness, dependency, and fear of the unknown are coupled with pain and a possible uncaring attitude on the part of the dentist to condition a response of fear when any element of the past event is reexperienced. Indeed, such events may not even be available to conscious awareness.

22. How are the terms *generalization* and *modeling* related to the conditioning aspect of dental fears?

Dental fears may be seen as similar to classic Pavlovian conditioning. Such conditioning may result in **generalization**, by which the effects of the original episode spread to situations with similar elements. For example, the trauma of an injury or the details of an emergency setting, such as sutures or injections, may be generalized to the dental setting. Many adults who had tonsillectomies under ether anesthesia may generalize the childhood experience to the dental setting, complaining of difficulty with breathing or airway maintenance, difficulty with gagging, or inability to tolerate oral injections. **Modeling** is vicarious learning through indirect exposure to traumatic events through parents, siblings, or any other source that affects the patient.

23. Why is understanding the patient's perception of the dentist so important in the control of fear and stress?

According to studies, patients perceive the dentist as both the **controller** of what the patient perceives as dangerous and as the **protector** from that danger. Thus the dentist's behavior and communications assume increased significance. The patient's ability to tolerate stress and to cope with fears depends on the ability to develop and maintain a high level of trust and confidence in the dentist. To achieve this goal, patients must express all the issues that they perceive as threatening, and the dentist must explain what he or she can do to address patient concerns and protect them from the perceived dangers. This is the purpose of the clinical interview. The result of this exchange should be increased trust and rapport and a subsequent decline in fear and anxiety.

24. How are emotions evolved? What constructs are important to understanding dental fears?

Psychological theories suggest that events and situations are evaluated by using interpretations that are personality-dependent (i.e., based on individual history and experience). Emotions evolve from this history. Positive or negative coping abilities mediate the interpretative process (people who believe that they are capable of dealing with a situation experience a different emotion during the initial event than people with less coping ability). The resulting emotional experience may be influenced by vicarious learning experiences (watching others react to an event), direct learning experiences (having one's own experience with the event), or social persuasion (expressions by others of what the event means).

A person's coping ability, or *self-efficacy*, in dealing with an appraisal of an event for its threatening content is highly variable, based on the multiplicity of personal life experiences. Belief that one has the ability to cope with a difficult situation reduces the interpretations that an event will be appraised as threatening, and a lower level of anxiety will result. A history of failure to cope with difficult events or the perception that coping is not a personal accomplishment (e.g., reliance in external aids, drugs) often reduces self-efficacy expectations, and interpretations of the event result in higher anxiety.

25. How can learned fears be eliminated or unlearned?

Because fears of dental treatment are learned, relearning or unlearning is possible. A comfortable experience without the associated fearful and painful elements may eliminate the conditioned fear response and replace it with an adaptive and more comfortable coping response. The secret is to uncover through the interview process which elements resulted in the maladaptation and subsequent response of fear, to eliminate them from the present dental experience by reinterpreting them for the adult patient, and to create a more caring and protected experience. During the interview the exchange of information and the insight gained by the patient decrease levels of fear, increase rapport, and establish trust in the doctor-patient relationship. The clinician needs only to apply expert operative technique to treat the vast majority of fearful patients.

26. What remarks may be given to a patient before beginning a procedure that the patient perceives as threatening?

Opening comments by the dentist to inform the patient about what to expect during a procedure—e.g., pressure, noise, pain—may reduce the fear of the unknown and the sense of helplessness. Control through knowing is increased with such preparatory communications.

27. How may the dentist further address the issue of loss of control?

A simple instruction that allows patients to signal by raising a hand if they wish to stop or speak returns a sense of control.

28. What is denial? How may it affect a patient's behavior and dental treatment-planning decisions?

Denial is a psychologic term for the defense mechanism that people use to block out the experience of information with which they cannot emotionally cope. They may not be able to accept the reality or consequences of the information or experience with which they will have to cope; therefore, they distort that information or completely avoid the issue. Often the underlying experience of the information is a threat to self-esteem or liable to provoke anxiety. These feelings are often unconsciously expressed by unreasonable requests of treatment.

For the dentist, patients who refuse to accept the reality of their dental disease, such as the hopeless condition of a tooth, may lead to a path of treatment that is doomed to fail. The subsequent disappointment of the patient may involve litigation issues.

29. Define dental phobia.

A phobia is an irrational fear of a situation or object. The reaction to the stimulus is often greatly exaggerated in relation to the reality of the threat. The fears are beyond voluntary control, and avoidance is the primary coping mechanism. Phobias may be so intense that severe physiologic reactions interfere with daily functioning. In the dental setting acute syncopal episodes may result.

Almost all phobias are learned. The process of dealing with true dental phobia may require a long period of individual psychotherapy and adjunctive pharmacologic sedation. However, relearning is possible, and establishing a good doctor-patient relationship is paramount.

30. What strategies may be used with the patient who gags on the slightest provocation?

The gag reflex is a basic physiologic protective mechanism that occurs when the posterior oropharynx is stimulated by a foreign object; normal swallowing does not trigger the reflex. When overlying anxiety is present, especially if anxiety is related to the fear of being unable to breathe, the gag reflex may be exaggerated. A conceptual model is the analogy to being "tickled." Most people can stroke themselves on the sole of the foot or under the arm without a reaction, but when the same stimulus is done by someone else, the usual results are laughter and withdrawal. Hence, if patients can eat properly, put a spoon in their mouth, or suck on their own finger, usually they are considered physiologically normal and may be taught to accept dental treatment and even dentures with appropriate behavioral therapy.

In dealing with such patients, desensitization becomes the process of relearning. A review of the history to discover episodes of impaired or threatened breathing is important. Childhood general anesthesia, near drowning, choking, or asphyxiation may have been the initiating event that created increased anxiety about being touched in the oral cavity. Patients may fear the inability to breathe, and the gag becomes part of their protective coping. Thus, reduction of anxiety is the first step; an initial strategy is to give information that allows patients to understand better their own response.

Instruction in nasal breathing may offer confidence in the ability to maintain a constant and uninterrupted air flow, even with oral manipulation. Eye fixation on a singular object may dissociate and distract the patient's attention away from the oral cavity. This technique may be especially helpful for taking radiographs and for brief oral examinations. For severe gaggers, hypnosis and nitrous oxide may be helpful; others may find use of a rubber dam reassuring. For some patients longer-term behavioral therapy may be necessary.

31. What is meant by the term *anxiety*? How is it related to fear?

Anxiety is a subjective state commonly defined as an unpleasant feeling of apprehension or impending danger in the presence of a real or perceived stimulus that the person has learned to associate with a threat to well-being. The feelings may be out of proportion to the real threat, and the response may be grossly exaggerated. Such feelings may be present before the encounter with the feared situation and may linger long after the event. Associated somatic feelings include sweating, tremors, palpations, nausea, difficulty with swallowing, and hyperventilation.

Fear is usually considered an appropriate defensive response to a real or active threat. Unlike anxiety, the response is brief, the danger is external and readily definable, and the unpleasant somatic feelings pass as the danger passes. Fear is the classic "fight-or-flight" response and may serve as an overall protective mechanism by sharpening the senses and the ability to respond to the danger. Whereas the response of fear does not usually rely on unhealthy actions for resolution, the state of anxiety often relies on noncoping and avoidance behaviors to deal with the threat.

32. How is stress related to pain and anxiety? What are the major parameters of the stress response?

When a person is stimulated by pain or anxiety, the result is a series of physiologic responses dominated by the autonomic nervous system, skeletal muscles, and endocrine system. These physiologic responses define stress. In what is termed adaptive responses, the sympathetic responses dominate (increases in pulse rate, blood pressure, respiratory rate, peripheral vasoconstriction, skeletal muscle tone, and blood sugar; decreases in sweating, gut motility, and salivation). In an acute maladaptive response the parasympathetic responses dominate, and a syncopal episode may result (decreases in pulse rate, blood pressure, respiratory rate, muscle tone; increases in salivation, sweating, gut motility, and peripheral vasodilation, with overall confusion and agitation). In chronic maladaptive situations, psychosomatic disorders may evolve. The accompanying figure illustrates the relationships of fear, pain, and stress. It is important to control anxiety and stress during dental treatment. The medically compromised patient necessitates appropriate control to avoid potentially life-threatening situations.

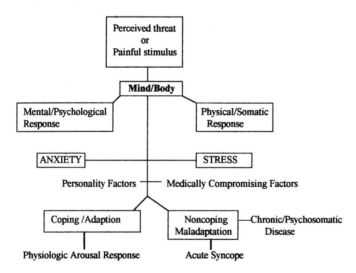

Relationships of pain, anxiety, stress, and reactions. (From Gregg JM: Psychosedation, Part 1. In McCarthy FM (ed): Emergencies in Dental Practice, 3rd ed. Philadelphia, W.B. Saunders, 1979, p 230, with permission.)

33. What is the relationship between pain and anxiety?

Many studies have shown the close relationship between pain and anxiety. The greater the person's anxiety, the more likely it is that he or she will interpret the response to a stimulus as painful. In addition, the pain threshold is lowered with increasing anxiety. People who are debilitated, fatigued, or depressed respond to threats with a higher degree of undifferentiated anxiety and thus are more reactive to pain.

34. List four guidelines for the proper management of pain, anxiety, and stress.

1. Make a careful assessment of the patient's anxiety and stress levels by a thoughtful interview. Uncontrolled anxiety and stress may lead to maladaptive situations that become life-threatening in medically compromised patients. Prevention is the most important strategy.

2. From all information gathered, medical and personal, determine the correct methods for control of pain and anxiety. This assessment is critical to appropriate management. Monitoring the patient's responses to the chosen method is essential.

3. Use medications as adjuncts for positive reinforcement, not as methods of control. Drugs circumvent fear; they do not resolve conflicts. The need for good rapport and communication is always essential.

4. Adapt control techniques to fit the patient's needs. The use of a single modality for all patients may lead to failure; for example, the use of nitrous oxide sedation to moderate severe emotional problems.

35. Construct a model for the therapeutic interview of a self-identified fearful patient.

1. Recognize a patient's anxiety by acknowledgment of what the patient says or observation of the patient's demeanor. Recognition, which is both verbal and nonverbal, may be as simple as saying, "Are you nervous about being here?" This recognition indicates the dentist's concern, acceptance, supportiveness, and intent to help.

2. Facilitate patients' cues as they tell their story. Help them to go from generalizations to specifics, especially to past origins, if possible. Listen for generalizations, distortions, and deletions of information or misinterpretations of events as the patient talks.

3. Allow patients to speak freely. Their anxiety decreases as they tell their story, describing the nature of their fear and the attitude of previous doctors. Trust and rapport between doctor and patient also increase as the patient is allowed to speak to someone who cares and listens.

4. Give feedback to the patient. Interpretations of the information helps patients to learn new strategies for coping with their feelings and to adopt new behaviors by confronting past fears. Thus a new set of feelings and behaviors may replace maladaptive coping mechanisms.

5. Finally the dentist makes a commitment to protect the patient—a commitment that the patient may have perceived as absent in past dental experiences. Strategies include allowing the patient to stop a procedure by raising a hand or simply assuring a patient that you are ready to listen at any time.

36. Discuss behavioral methods that may help patients to cope with dental fears and related anxiety.

1. The first step for the dentist is to become knowledgeable of the patient and his or her presenting needs. Interviewing skills cannot be overemphasized. A trusting relationship is essential. As the clinical interview proceeds, fears are usually reduced to coping levels.

2. Because a patient cannot be anxious and relaxed at the same moment, teaching methods of relaxation may be helpful. Systematic relaxation allows the patient to cope with the dental situation. Guided visualizations may be helpful to achieve relaxation. Paced breathing also may be an aid to keeping patients relaxed. Guiding the rate of inspiration and expiration allows a hyperventilating patient to resume normal breathing, thus decreasing the anxiety level. A sample relaxation script is included below.

Relaxation Script

The following example should be read in a slow, rhythmic, and paced manner while carefully observing the patient's responses. Backing up and repeating parts are beneficial if you find that the patient is not responding at any time. Feel free to change and incorporate your own stylistic suggestions.

Allow yourself to become comfortable . . . and as you listen to the sound of my voice, I shall guide you along a pathway of deepening relaxation. Often we start out at some high level of excitement, and as we slide, down lower, we can become aware of our descent and enjoy the ride. Let us begin with some attention to your breathing. . . taking some regular, slow. . . easy. . . breaths. Let the air flow in . . . and out . . . air in . . . air out . . . until you become very aware of each inspiration . . . and . . . expiration . . . [pause] Very good. Now as you feel your chest rise with each intake and fall with each outflow, notice how different you now feel from a few moments ago, as you comfortably resettle yourself in the chair, adjusting your arms and legs just enough to make you feel more comfortable.

Now with regularly paced, slow, and easy breathing, I would like to ask that you become aware of your arms and hands as they rest [describe where you see them, e.g., "on your lap"]. . . . Move them slightly. [pause] Next become aware of your legs and feel the chair's support under them . . . they may also move slightly. We shall begin our total body relaxation in just this way . . . becoming aware of a part and then allowing it to become at ease . . . resting, floating, lying peacefully. Start at your eyelids, and, if they are not already closed, allow them to become free and rest them downward . . . your eyes may gaze and float upward. Now focusing on your forehead . . . letting the subtle folds become smoother and smoother with each breath. Now let this peacefulness of eyelids and forehead start a gentle warm flow of relaxing energy down over your cheeks and face, around and under your chin, and slowly down your neck. You may find that you have to swallow . . . allow this to happen, naturally. Now continue this flow as a stream ambling over your shoulders and upper chest and over and across to each arm [pause] and when you feel this warmth in your fingertips you may feel them move ever so slightly. [pause for any movement] Very good.

Next allow the same continuous flow to start down to your lower body and over you waist and hips . . . reaching each leg. You may notice that they are heavy, or light, and that they move ever so slightly as you feel the chair supporting them with each breath and each swallow that you take. You are resting easily, breathing comfortably and effortlessly. You may become aware of just how much at ease you are now, in such a short time, from a moment ago, when you entered the room. Very good, be at ease.

3. Hypnosis, a useful tool with myriad benefits, induces an altered state of awareness with heightened suggestibility for changes in behavior and physiologic responses. It is easily taught, and the benefits can be highly beneficial in the dental setting.

4. Informing patients of what they may experience during procedures addresses the specific fears of the unknown and loss of control. Sensory information—that is, what physical sensations may be expected—as well as procedural information is appropriate. Knowledge enhances a patient's coping skills.

5. Modeling, or observing a peer undergo successful dental treatment, may be beneficial. Videotapes are available for a variety of dental scenarios.

6. Methods of distraction may also improve coping responses. Audio or video programs have been reported to be useful for some patients.

37. What are common avoidance behaviors associated with anxious patients?
Commonly, putting off making appointments followed by cancellations and failing to appear are routine events for anxious patients. Indeed, the avoidance of care can be of such magnitude that personal suffering is endured from tooth ailments with emergency consequences. A mutilated dentition often results.

38. Whom do dentists often consider their most "difficult" patient?

Surveys repeatedly show that dentists often view the anxious patient as their most difficult challenge. Almost 80% of dentists report that they themselves become anxious with an anxious patient. The ability to assess carefully a patient's emotional needs helps the clinician to improve his or her ability to deal effectively with anxious patients. Furthermore, because anxious patients require more chair time for procedures, are more reactive to stimuli, and associate more sensations with pain, effective anxiety management yields more effective practice management.

39. What are the major practical considerations in scheduling identified anxious dental patients?

Autonomic arousal increases in proportion to the length of time before a stressful event. A patient left to anticipate the event with negative self-statements and perhaps frightening images for a whole day or at length in the waiting area is less likely to have an easy experience. Thus, it is considered prudent to schedule patients earlier in the day and keep the waiting period after the patient's arrival to a minimum. In addition, the dentist's energy is usually optimal earlier in the day to deal with more demanding situations.

40. What is the opportune time to teach new health information to patients?

Patients are most receptive to learning new health behaviors when there is an immediate *need* for the new skill or behavior. A patient with gingival bleeding at a furcation site wants to know how to resolve the problem and is most receptive to learning how to use a proxybrush.

41. What is a strong motivational tool to use in communicating health improvement issues?

Positive feedback while instructing often yields the greatest acceptance and minimizes patient resistance to compliance. Fear of tooth loss, for example, may not weight as much in communicating the consequences of not brushing as creating a desire for a healthy smile and teeth that serve a lifetime.

42. In introducing new ideas about oral hygiene, what considerations help to maximize compliance?

People learn best when information is presented in a context of their own personal experience. In talking to an avid woodworker, for example, the dentist may speak about "planning down" plaque and debris to create a smooth surface that will stay clean and healthy. Similarly, a gardener may keep plaque weeds suppressed to allow healthy tissues to grow. In each case, context-specific phrasing communicates ideas most effectively.

43. Does self-esteem play a role in adopting new behaviors such as flossing and regular brushing?

Absolutely. Most adults are desirous of learning concepts that enhance or maintain their self-esteem. Enhancing physical appearance is directly related to the acceptance of new health behaviors.

44. List four important elements in maximizing the long-term retention of information given by the dental team to patients.

1. **Repetition** of key ideas enhances patient learning and compliance. A patient may recall only one-third of a conversation after 24 hours and even less after 30 days. By artfully repeating ideas and concepts at the initial presentation, recall is maximized.

2. **Interest and direct relevance** of information to the patient's specific needs yield the greatest learning experience. A patient with a loose tooth is concerned about why the problem occurred and how to prevent tooth loss. This concern may outweigh issues related to the general concepts of periodontal disease and the outcome of full dentures.

3. **Context** of the information presented should been within the personal experience of the patient to maximize acceptance and understanding.

4. **Emotion** relates the patient's feeling about dental issues. Understanding relevant emotional history enhances doctor-patient rapport and the patient's trust and acceptance of the suggests made by the dental team.

45. What do patients describe as qualities of a dentist who makes them feel relaxed and lowers their anxiety?

- Explain procedures before starting.
- Give specific information during procedures.
- Instruct the patient to be calm.
- Verbally support the patient: give reassurance.
- Help the patient to redefine the experience to minimize threat.
- Give the patient some control over procedures and pain.
- Attempt to teach the patient to cope with distress.
- Provide distraction and tension relief.
- Attempt to build trust in the dentist.
- Show personal warmth to the patient.

Corah N: Dental anxiety: Assessment, reduction and increasing patient satisfaction. Dent Clin North Am 32:779–790, 1988.

46. What qualities do patients describe as making them feel satisifed with their dentist and dental experience?

- Assured me that he would prevent pain
- Was friendly
- Worked quickly, but did not rush
- Had a calm manner
- Gave me moral support
- Reassured me that he would alleviate pain
- Asked if I was concerned or nervous
- Made sure that I was numb before starting

Corah N: Dental anxiety: Assessment, reduction and increasing patient satisfaction. Dent Clin North Am 32:779–790, 1988.

BIBLIOGRAPHY

1. The Adult in Learning, P&G Dental Resource Net: <http://www.dentalcare.com/soap/ce3/adltmain.htm>.
2. Corah N: Dental anxiety: Assessment, reduction and increasing patient satisfaction. Dent Clin North Am 32:779–790, 1988.
3. Crasilneck HB, Hall JA: Clinical Hypnosis: Principles and Applications, 2nd ed. Orlando, FL, Grune & Stratton, 1985.
4. Dworkin SF, Ference TP, Giddon DB: Behavioral Science in Dental Practice. St. Louis, Mosby, 1978.
5. Friedman N, Cecchini JJ, Wexler M, et al: A dentist-oriented fear reduction technique: The iatrosedative process. Compend Cont Educ Dent 10:113–118, 1989.
6. Friedman N: Psychosedation. Part 2: Iatrosedation. In McCarthy FM (ed): Emergencies in Dental Practice, 3rd ed. Philadelphia, W.B. Saunders, 1979, pp 236–265.
7. Gelboy MJ: Communication and Behavior Management in Dentistry. London, Williams & Watkins, 1990.
8. Gregg JM: Psychosedation. Part 1: The nature and control of pain, anxiety, and stress. In McCarthy FM (ed): Emergencies in Dental Practice, 3rd ed. Philadelphia, W.B. Saunders, 1979, pp 220–235.
9. Jepsen CH: Behavioral foundations of dental practice. In Williams A (ed): Clark's Clinical Dentistry, vol. 5. Philadelphia, J.B. Lippincott, 1993, pp 1–18.
10. Krochak M, Rubin JG: An overview of the treatment of anxious and phobic dental patients. Compend Cont Educ Dent 14:604–615, 1993.
11. Rubin JG, Kaplan A (eds): Dental Phobia and Anxiety. Dent Clin North Am 32(4), 1988.

2. TREATMENT PLANNING AND ORAL DIAGNOSIS

Stephen T. Sonis, D.M.D., D.M.Sc.

1. What are the objectives of pretreatment evaluation of a patient?
1. Establishment of a diagnosis
2. Determination of underlying medical conditions that may modify the oral condition or the patient's ability to tolerate treatment
3. Discovery of concomitant illnesses
4. Prevention of medical emergencies associated with dental treatment
5. Establishment of rapport with the patient

2. What are the essential elements of a patient history?
1. Chief complaint
2. History of the present illness (HPI)
3. Past medical history
4. Social history
5. Family history
6. Review of systems
7. Dental history

3. Define the chief complaint.
The chief complaint is the reason that the patient seeks care, as described in the patient's own words.

4. What is the history of the present illness?
The HPI is a chronologic description of the patient's symptoms and should include information about duration, location, character, and previous treatment.

5. What elements need to be included in the medical history?
- Current status of the patient's general health
- Hospitalizations
- Medications
- Allergies

6. What areas are routinely investigated in the social history?
- Present and past occupations
- Occupational hazards
- Smoking, alcohol or drug use
- Marital status

7. Why is the family history of interest to the dentist?
The family history often provides information about diseases of genetic origin or diseases that have a familial tendency. Examples include clotting disorders, atherosclerotic heart disease, psychiatric diseases, and diabetes mellitus.

8. How is the medical history most often obtained?
The medical history is obtained with a written questionnaire supplemented by a verbal history. The verbal history is imperative, because patients may leave out or misinterpret questions on the written form. For example, some patients may take daily aspirin and yet not consider it a "true" medication. The verbal history also allows the clinician to pursue positive answers on the written form and, in doing so, to establish rapport with the patient.

9. What techniques are used for physical examination of the patient? How are they used in dentistry?
Inspection, the most commonly used technique, is based on visual evaluation of the patient. Palpation, which involves touching and feeling the patient, is used to determine the consistency

and shape of masses in the mouth or neck. Percussion, which involves differences in sound transmission of structures, has little application to the head and neck. Auscultation, the technique of listening to differences in the transmission of sound, is usually accomplished with a stethoscope. In dentistry it is most typically used to listen to changes in sounds emanating from the temporomandibular joint and in taking a patient's blood pressure.

10. What are the patient's vital signs?
- Blood pressure
- Pulse
- Respiratory rate
- Temperature

11. What are the normal values for the vital signs?
- Blood pressure: 120 mmHg/80 mmHg
- Pulse: 72 beats per minute
- Respiratory rate: 16–20 respirations per minute
- Temperature: 98.6°F or 37°C

12. What is a complete blood count (CBC)?
A CBC consists of a determination of the patient's hemoglobin, hematocrit, white blood cell count, and differential white blood cell count.

13. What are the normal ranges of a CBC?

Hemoglobin:	men, 14–18 g/dl	Differential white blood count
	women, 12–16 g/dl	Neutrophils, 50–70%
Hematocrit:	men, 40–54%	Lymphocytes, 30–40%
	women, 37–47%	Monocytes, 3–7%
White blood count:	4,000–10,000	Eosinophils, 0–5%
	cells/mm^3	Basophils, 0–1%

14. What is the most effective blood test to screen for diabetes mellitus?
The most effective screen for diabetes mellitus is fasting blood sugar.

15. What is the technique of choice for diagnosis of a soft-tissue lesion in the mouth?
With few exceptions, biopsy is the diagnostic technique of choice for virtually all soft-tissue lesions of the mouth.

16. Is there any alternative diagnostic technique to biopsy for the evaluation of suspected malignancies of the mouth?
Exfoliative cytology has been used in the past for the diagnosis of oral lesions. Because of its high false-negative rate, it has never been particularly effective. Recently the technique has been modified to include the use of a brush to obtain a cell sample and then a specific processing and evaluation technique that increases the sensitivity of the assay. The makers of the test emphasize that it is a good, noninvasive screening tool. Biopsy is the still the most popular and reliable way to make a diagnosis.

17. When is immunofluorescence of value in oral diagnosis?
Immunofluorescent techniques are of value in the diagnosis of a number of autoimmune diseases that affect the mouth, including pemphigus vulgaris and mucous membrane pemphigoid.

18. What elements should be included in the dental history?
1. Past dental visits, including frequency, reasons, previous treatment, and complications
2. Oral hygiene practices
3. Oral symptoms other than those associated with the chief complaint, including tooth pain or sensitivity, gingival bleeding or pain, tooth mobility, halitosis, and abscess formation
4. Past dental or maxillofacial trauma
5. Habits related to oral disease, such as bruxing, clenching, and nail biting
6. Dietary history

19. When is it appropriate to use microbiologic culturing in oral diagnosis?

    1. **Bacterial infection.** Because the overwhelming majority of oral infections are sensitive to treatment with penicillin, routine bacteriologic culture of primary dental infections is not generally indicated. However, cultures are indicated in patients who are immunocompromised or myelosuppressed for two reasons: (1) they are at significant risk for sepsis, and (2) the oral flora often change in such patients. Cultures should be obtained for infections that are refractory to the initial course of antibiotics before changing antibiotics.

    2. **Viral infection.** Immunocompromised patients who present with mucosal lesions may well be manifesting herpes simplex infection. A viral culture is warranted. Similarly, other viruses in the herpes family, such as cytomegalovirus, may cause oral lesions in the immunocompromised patient and should be isolated, if possible. Routine culturing for primary or secondary herpes infections is not warranted in healthy patients.

    3. **Fungal infection.** Candidiasis is the most common fungal infection affecting the oral mucosa. Because its appearance is often varied, especially in immunocompromised patients, fungal cultures are often of value. In addition, because candidal infection is a frequent cause of burning mouth, culture is often indicated in immunocompromised patients, even in the absence of visible lesions.

20. How do you obtain access to a clinical laboratory?

    It is easy to obtain laboratory tests for your patients, even if you do not practice in a hospital. Community hospitals provide virtually all laboratory services that your patients may require. Usually the laboratory provides order slips and culture tubes. Simply indicate the test needed, and send the patient to the laboratory. Patients who need a test at night or on a weekend can generally be accommodated through the hospital's emergency department. Commercial laboratories also may be used. They, too, supply order forms. If you practice in a medical building with physicians, find out which laboratory they use. If they use a commercial laboratory, a pick-up service for specimens may well be provided. The most important issue is to ensure the quality of the laboratory. Adherence to the standards of the American College of Clinical Pathologists is a good indicator of laboratory quality.

21. What are the approximate costs of the following laboratory tests: complete blood count, platelet count, PT, fasting glucose, bacterial culture, and fungal culture?

CBC	$18	Fasting glucose	$13
Platelet count	$18	Bacterial culture	$32
PT	$29	Fungal culture	$42

22. What laboratory tests should be used to assess a patient who may be at risk for a deficiency in hemostasis?

    The basic laboratory tests for a possible coagulopathy should include assessments of platelet number and clotting factors of the internal and external pathways. Consequently, the three essential tests are complete blood count that includes platelet number, prothrombin time, and partial thromboplastin time.

23. What positive responses in the medical history should tip you off that a patient may have a problem with hemostasis?

- Family history of a bleeding problem, such as hemophilia
- Taking medications that can cause thrombocytopenia, such as cancer chemotherapy
- History of a disease that may cause thrombocytopenia
- Taking medications known to cause prolonged bleeding, such as aspirin, warfarin, or vitamin E

24. What are the causes of halitosis?

    Halitosis may be caused by local factors in the mouth and by extraoral or systemic factors. Among the local factors are food retention, periodontal infection, caries, acute necrotizing gingivitis, and mucosal infection. Extraoral and systemic causes of halitosis include smoking, alcohol ingestion, pulmonary or bronchial disease, metabolic defects, diabetes mellitus, sinusitis, and tonsillitis.

25. What bacteria are associated with halitosis?
Gram-negative anaerobes.

26. What gases are associated with halitosis?
Volatile sulfur compounds—in particular, hydrogen sulfide, methyl mercaptan, and dimethyl sulfide—are associated with halitosis.

27. What are the most commonly abused drugs in the United States?

Alcohol	Prescription medications
Marijuana	Tricyclic antidepressants
Cocaine	Sedative-hypnotics
Phencyclidine (PCP)	Narcotic analgesics
Heroin	Anxiolytic agents
	Diet aids

28. What are the common causes of lymphadenopathy?
1. Infectious and inflammatory diseases of all types. Common oral conditions causing lymphadenopathy are herpes infections, pericoronitis, aphthous or traumatic ulceration, and acute necrotizing ulcerative gingivitis.
2. Immunologic diseases, such as rheumatoid arthritis, systemic lupus erythematosus, and drug reactions
3. Malignant disease, such as Hodgkin's disease, lymphoma, leukemia, and metastatic disease from solid tumors
4. Hyperthyroidism
5. Lipid storage diseases, such as Gaucher's disease and Niemann-Pick disease
6. Other conditions, including sarcoidosis, amyloidosis, and granulomatosis

29. How can one differentiate between lymphadenopathy associated with an inflammatory process and lymphadenopathy associated with tumor?
1. Onset and duration. Inflammatory nodes tend to have a more acute onset and course than nodes associated with tumor.
2. Identification of an associated infected site. An identifiable site of infection associated with an enlarged lymph node is probably the source of the lymphadenopathy. Effective treatment of the site should result in resolution of the lymphadenopathy.
3. Symptoms. Enlarged lymph nodes associated with an inflammatory process are usually tender to palpation. Nodes associated with tumor are not.
4. Progression. Continuous enlargement over time is associated with tumor.
5. Fixation. Inflammatory nodes are usually freely movable, whereas nodes associated with tumor are hard and fixed.
6. Lack of response to antibiotic therapy. Continued nodal enlargement in the face of appropriate antibiotic therapy should be viewed as suspicious.
7. Distribution. Unilateral nodal enlargement is a common presentation for malignant disease. In contrast, bilateral enlargement often is associated with systemic processes.

30. What is the most appropriate technique for lymph node diagnosis?
The most appropriate technique for lymph node diagnosis is biopsy or needle aspiration. Needle aspiration is preferred, but is technique-sensitive (see question 63).

31. What are the most frequent causes of intraoral swelling?
The most frequent causes of intraoral swelling are infection and tumor.

32. Why does Polly get parrotitis?

Too many crackers.

33. Why do humans get parotitis?

Infection of viral or bacterial origin is the most common cause of parotitis in humans. Viruses causing parotitis are mumps, Coxsackie, and influenza. *Staphylococcus aureus,* the most common bacterial cause of parotitis, results in the production of pus within the gland. Other bacteria, such as actinomyces, streptococci, and gram-negative bacilli, also may cause suppurative parotitis.

34. What are common causes of xerostomia?

- Advanced age
- Certain medications
- Radiation therapy
- Sjögren's syndrome

35. What is the presentation of a patient with a tumor of the parotid gland? How is the diagnosis made?

The typical patient with a parotid gland tumor presents with a firm, fixed mass in the region of the gland. Involvement of the facial nerve is common and results in facial palsy. Fine-needle biopsy is a commonly used technique for diagnosis. However, the small sample obtained by such technique may be limiting. CT and MRI are also often helpful in evaluating suspected tumors.

36. What are the major risk factors for oral cancer?

Tobacco and alcohol use are the major risk factors for the development of oral cancer.

37. What is the most common location of cancers of the tongue?

Lateral or ventral edge of the posterior tongue.

38. Summarize the impact of early detection of mouth cancers on survival.

Although the 5-year survival rate for advanced tongue cancers is only 20%, it is 65% for more localized tumors. For tumors of the floor of the mouth, the differences in survival rates between treatment of early tumors and treatment of advanced cancers is 60%. Patients with early floor mouth tumors have a 5-year survival rate of 78%, but this rate plummets to only 18% for advanced cancers.

39. Cancers of the mouth are typically staged. How?

Tumor staging is system by which cancers are clinically defined based on the parameters of tumor size, involvement of local nodes, and metastases (TNM).

40. What is the possible role of toluidine blue stain in oral diagnosis?

Because toluidine blue is a metachromatic nuclear stain, it has been reported to be preferentially absorbed by dysplastic and cancerous epithelium. Consequently, it has been used as a technique to screen oral lesions. The technique has a reported false-positive rate of 9% and a false-negative rate of 5%.

41. What are the common clinical presentations of oral cancers?

The two most common clinical presentations for oral cancer are a nonhealing ulcer or an area of leukoplakia, often accompanied by erythema.

42. What percent of keratotic white lesions in the mouth are dysplastic or cancerous?

Approximately 10% of such oral lesions are dysplastic or cancerous.

43. What is a simple way to differentiate clinically between necrotic and keratotic white lesions of the oral mucosa?

Necrotic lesions of the mucosa, such as those caused by burns or candidal infections, scrape off when gently rubbed with a moist tongue blade. On the other hand, because keratotic lesions result from epithelial changes, scraping fails to dislodge them.

44. How long should one wait before obtaining a biopsy of an oral ulcer?

Virtually all ulcers caused by trauma or aphthous stomatitis heal within 14 days of presentation. Consequently, any ulcer that is present for 2 weeks or more should be biopsied.

45. What is the differential diagnosis of ulcers of the oral mucosa?

- Traumatic ulcer
- Aphthous stomatitis
- Cancer
- Tuberculosis
- Chancre of syphilis
- Noma
- Necrotizing sialometaplasia
- Deep fungal infection

46. Why is it a good idea to aspirate a pigmented lesion before obtaining a biopsy?

Because pigmented lesions may be vascular in nature, prebiopsy aspiration is prudent to prevent hemorrhage.

47. What are the major causes of pigmented oral and perioral lesions?

Pigmented lesions are due to either endogenous or exogenous sources. Among **endogenous sources** are melanoma, endocrine-related pigmentation (such as occurs in Addison's disease), and perioral pigmentation associated with intestinal polyposis or Peutz-Jegher's syndrome. **Exogenous sources** of pigmentation include heavy metal poisoning (e.g., lead), amalgam tattoos, and changes caused by chemicals or medications. A common example of medication-related changes is black hairy tongue associated with antibiotics, particularly tetracycline, or bismuth-containing compounds, such as Pepto-Bismol.

48. Do any diseases of the oral cavity also present with lesions of the skin?

Numerous diseases can cause simultaneous lesions of the mouth and skin. Among the most common are lichen planus, erythema multiforme, lupus erythematosus, bullous pemphigoid, and pemphigus vulgaris.

49. What is the appearance of the skin lesion associated with erythema multiforme?

The skin lesion of erythema multiforme looks like an archery target with a central erythematous bullseye and a circular peripheral area. Hence, the lesions are called bullseye or target lesions.

50. A 25-year-old woman presents with the chief complaint of spontaneously bleeding gingiva. She also notes malaise. On oral examination you find that her hygiene is excellent. Would you suspect a local or systemic basis for her symptoms? What tests might you order to make a diagnosis?

Spontaneous bleeding, especially in the face of good oral hygiene, is most likely of systemic origin. Gingival bleeding is among the most common presenting signs of acute leukemia, which should be high on the differential diagnosis. A complete blood count and platelet count should provide data to help to establish a preliminary diagnosis. Definitive diagnosis most likely requires a bone marrow biopsy.

51. A 45-year-old, overweight man presents with suppurative periodontitis. As you review his history, he tells you that he is always hungry, drinks water almost every hour, and awakens four times each night to urinate. What systemic disease is most likely a cofactor in his periodontal disease? What test(s) might you order to help you with a diagnosis?

The combination of polyuria, polyphagia, polydipsia, and suppurative periodontal disease should raise a strong suspicion of diabetes mellitus. A fasting blood glucose test is the most efficacious screen.

52. A 60-year-old woman presents with the complaint of numbness of the left side of her mandible. Four years ago she had a mastectomy for treatment of breast cancer. What is the likely diagnosis? What is the first step you take to confirm it?

The mandible is not an infrequent site for metastatic breast cancer. As the metastatic lesion grows, it puts pressure on the inferior alveolar nerve and causes paresthesia. Radiographic evaluation of the jaw is a reasonable first step to make a diagnosis.

53. What endocrine disease may present with pigmented lesions of the oral mucosa?

Pigmented lesions of the oral mucosa may suggest Addison's disease.

54. What drugs cause gingival hyperplasia?
- Phenytoin
- Cyclosporine
- Nifedipine

55. What is the most typical presentation of the oral lesions of tuberculosis? How do you make a diagnosis?

The oral lesions of tuberculosis are thought to result from the presence of organisms brought into contact with the oral mucosa by sputum. A nonhealing ulcer, which is impossible to differentiate clinically from carcinoma, is the most common presentation in the mouth. Ulcers are most consistently present on the lateral borders of the tongue and may have a purulent center. Lymphadenopathy also may be present. Diagnosis is made by histologic examination and demonstration of organisms in the tissue.

56. What are the typical oral manifestations of a patient with pernicious anemia?

The most common target site in the mouth is the tongue, which presents with a smooth, dorsal surface denuded of papillae. Angular cheilitis is a frequent accompanying finding.

57. What is angular cheilitis? What is its cause?

Angular cheilitis or cheilosis is fissuring or cracking at the corners of the mouth. The condition typically occurs because of a localized mixed infection of bacteria and fungi. Cheilitis most commonly results from a change in the local environment caused by excessive saliva due to loss of the vertical dimension between the maxilla and mandible. In addition, a number of systemic conditions, such as deficiency anemias and long-term immunosuppression, predispose to the condition.

58. What is the classic oral manifestation of Crohn's disease?

Mucosal lesions with a cobblestone appearance are associated with Crohn's disease.

59. List the oral changes that may occur in a patient who is receiving radiation therapy for treatment of a tumor on the base of the tongue.
- Xerostomia
- Cervical and incisal edge caries
- Osteoradionecrosis
- Mucositis

60. A patient presents for extraction of a carious tooth. In taking the history, you learn that the patient is receiving chemotherapy for treatment of a breast carcinoma. What information is critical before proceeding with the extraction?

Because cancer chemotherapy nonspecifically affects the bone marrow, the patient is likely to be myelosuppressed after treatment. Therefore, you need to know both the patient's white blood cell count and platelet count before initiating treatment.

61. What oral findings have been associated with the diuretic hydrochlorothiazide?

Lichen planus has been associated with hydrochlorothiazide.

62. Some patients believe that topical application of an aspirin to the mucosa next to a tooth will help odontogenic pain. How may you detect this form of therapy by looking in the patient's mouth?

Because of its acidity, topical application of aspirin to the mucosa frequently causes a chemical burn, which appears as a white, necrotic lesion in the area corresponding to aspirin placement.

63. What are the possible causes of burning mouth syndrome?

1. Dry mouth
2. Nutritional deficiencies
3. Diabetes mellitus
4. Psychogenic factors
5. Medications
6. Acid reflux from the stomach
7. Hormonal imbalances
8. Allergy
9. Chronic infections (especially fungal)
10. Blood dyscrasias
11. Anemia
12. Iatrogenic factors
13. Inflammatory conditions such as lichen planus

64. What is the most important goal in the evaluation of a taste disorder?

The most important goal in evaluating a taste disorder is the elimination of an underlying neurologic, olfactory, or systemic disorder as a cause for the condition.

65. What drugs often prescribed by dentists may affect taste or smell?

1. Metronidazole
2. Benzocaine
3. Ampicillin
4. Tetracycline
5. Sodium lauryl sulfate toothpaste
6. Codeine

66. What systemic conditions may affect smell and/or taste?

1. Bell's palsy
2. Multiple sclerosis
3. Head trauma
4. Cancer
5. Chronic renal failure
6. Cirrhosis
7. Niacin deficiency
8. Adrenal insufficiency
9. Cushing's syndrome
10. Diabetes mellitus
11. Sjögren's syndrome
12. Radiation therapy to the head and neck
13. Viral infections
14. Hypertension

67. What is glossodynia?

Glossodynia, or burning tongue, is relatively common. Although the problem is frequently related to local irritation, it may be a manifestation of an underlying systemic condition.

68. What questions should a clinician consider before ordering a diagnostic test to supplement clinical examination?

1. What is the likelihood that the disease is present, given the history, clinical findings, and known risk factors?
2. How serious is the condition? What are the consequences of a delay in diagnosis?
3. Is an appropriate diagnostic test available? How sensitive and accurate is it?
4. Are the costs, risks, and ease of administering the test worth the effort?

Matthews, et al: The use of diagnostic tests to aid clinical diagnosis. J Can Dent Assoc 61:785, 1995.

69. Distinguish among the accuracy, sensitivity, and specificity of a particular diagnostic test.

The **accuracy** is a measure of the overall agreement between the test and a gold standard. The more accurate the test, the fewer false-negative or false-positive results. In contrast, the **sensitivity** of the test measures its ability to show a positive result when the disease is present. The more sensitive the test, the fewer false negatives. For example, one problem with cytologic evaluation of cancerous keratotic oral lesions is that of 100 patients with cancer, 15 will test as negative (unacceptable false-negative rate). Consequently, cytology for this diagnosis is not highly sensitive. The **specificity** of the test measures the ability to show a negative finding in people who do not have the condition (false positives).

Matthews, et al: The use of diagnostic tests to aid clinical diagnosis. J Can Dent Assoc 61:785, 1995.

70. What is FNA? When is it used?

No, FNA is not an abbreviation for the Finnish Naval Association. It refers to a diagnostic technique called fine-needle aspiration, in which a needle (22-gauge) on a syringe is used to aspirate cells from a suspicious lesion for pathologic analysis. Many otolaryngologists use the technique to aid in the diagnosis of cancers of the head and neck. It seems to be particularly valuable in the diagnosis of submucosal tumors, such as lymphoma, and parapharyngeal masses that are not accessible to routine surgical biopsy. Like many techniques, the efficacy of FNA depends on the skill of the operator and experience of the pathologist reading the slide.

Cramer H, et al: Intraoral and transoral fine needle aspiration. Acta Cytologica 39:683, 1995.

71. Which systemic diseases have been associated with alterations in salivary gland function?

1. Cystic fibrosis
2. HIV infection
3. Diabetes mellitus
4. Affective disorder
5. Metabolic disturbances (malnutrition, dehydration, vitamin deficiency)
6. Renal disease
7. Cirrhosis
8. Thyroid disease
9. Autoimmune disease (Sjögren's syndrome, myasthenia gravis, graft-vs.-host disease)
10. Sarcoidosis
11. Autonomic dysfunction
12. Alzheimer's disease
13. Cancer

72. What is PCR? Why may it become an important technique in oral diagnosis?

Polymerase chain reaction (PCR) is a technique developed by researchers in molecular biology for enzymatic amplification of selected DNA sequences. Because of its exquisite sensitivity PCR appears to have marked clinical potential in the diagnosis of viral diseases of the head and neck.

73. What conditions and diseases may cause blistering (vesiculobullous lesions) in the mouth?

1. Viral disease
2. Lichen planus
3. Pemphigoid
4. Pemphigus vulgaris
5. Erythema multiforme

74. What are the most common sites of intraoral cancer?

The posterior lateral and ventral surfaces of the tongue are the most common sites of intraoral cancer.

75. What is staging for cancer? What are the criteria for staging cancers of the mouth?

Staging is a method of defining the clinical status of a lesion and is closely related to its future clinical behavior. Thus, it is related to prognosis and is of help in providing a basis for treatment planning. The staging system used for oral cancers is called the TNM system and is based on three parameters: T = size of the tumor on a scale from 0 (no evidence of primary tumor) to 3 (tumor > 4 cm in greatest diameter); N = involvement of regional lymph nodes on a scale from 0 (no clinically palpable cervical nodes) to 3 (clinically palpable lymph nodes that are fixed; metastases suspected; and M = presence of distant metastases on a scale from 0 (no distant metastases) to 1 (clinical or radiographic evidence of metastases to nodes other than those in the cervical chain).

BIBLIOGRAPHY

1. Atkinson JC, Fox PC: Sjögren's syndrome: Oral and dental considerations. J Am Dent Assoc 124:74, 1993.
2. Fenlon MR, McCartan BE: Validity of a patient self-completed health questionnaire in a primary dental care practice. Commun Dent Oral Epidemiol 20:130–132, 1992.
3. Harahap M: How to biopsy oral lesions. J Dermatol Surg Oncol 15:1077–1080, 1989.
4. Jones JH, Mason DK: Oral Manifestations of Systemic Disease, 2nd ed. Philadelphia, Baillière Tindall/W.B. Saunders, 1990.
5. Laurin D, Brodeur JM, Leduc N, et al: Nutritional deficiencies and gastrointestinal disorders in the edentulous elderly: A literature review. J Can Dent Assoc 58:738–740, 1992.
6. McCarthy FM: Recognition, assessment and safe management of the medically compromised patient in dentistry. Anesth Prog 37:217–222, 1990.
7. O'Brien CJ, Seng-Jaw S, Herrera GA, et al: Malignant salivary tumors: Analysis of prognostic factors and survival. Head Neck Surg 9:82–92, 1986.
8. Redding SW, Olive JA: Relative value of screening tests of hemostasis prior to dental treatment. Oral Surg Oral Med Oral Pathol 59:34–36, 1985.
9. Replogle WH, Beebe DK: Halitosis. Am Fam Physician 53:1215–1223, 1996.
10. Rose LF, Steinberg BJ: Patient evaluation. Dent Clin North Am 31:53–73, 1987.
11. Shah JP, Lydiatt W: Treatment of cancer of the head and neck. Cancer J Clin 45:352–368, 1995.
12. Sonis ST, Fazio RC, Fang L: Principles and Practice of Oral Medicine, 2nd ed. Philadelphia, W.B. Saunders, 1995.
13. Sonis ST, Woods PD, White BA: Oral complications of cancer therapies. NCI Monogr 9:29–32, 1990.
14. Williams AJ, Wray D, Ferguson A: The clinical entity of orofacial Crohn's disease. Q J Med 79:451–458, 1991.

3. MANAGEMENT OF MEDICALLY COMPROMISED PATIENTS

Joseph W. Costa, Jr., D.M.D., and Dale Potter, D.D.S.

We invariably tell each other, and our students, that the academic tripod consists of patient care, teaching and research. In fact, in the real world where science is performed and medicine is practised, a better understanding of the academic tripod might be: "If it's new, it's not true; if it's true, it's not important; but if it's new and it's true and it's important, then we knew it all along.

Phil Gold, 1995

DISORDERS OF HEMOSTASIS

1. How do you screen a patient for potential bleeding problems?

The best screening procedure for a bleeding disorder is a good medical history. If the review of the medical history indicates a bleeding problem, a more detailed history is needed. The following questions are basic:

1. Is there a family history of bleeding problems?
2. Has bleeding been noted since early childhood, or is the onset relatively recent?
3. How many previous episodes have there been?
4. What are the circumstances of the bleeding?
5. When did the bleeding occur? After minor surgery, such as tonsillectomy or tooth extraction? After falls or participation in contact sports?
6. What medications was the patient taking when the bleeding occurred?
7. What was the duration of the bleeding episode(s)? Did the episode involve prolonged oozing or a massive hemorrhage?
8. Was the bleeding immediate or delayed?

Kupp MA, Chatton MJ: Current Medical Diagnosis and Treatment. East Norwalk CT, Appleton & Lange, 1983, p 324.

2. What laboratory tests should be ordered if a bleeding problem is suspected?

- Platelet count: normal values = 150,000–450,000
- Prothrombin time (PT): normal value = 10–13.5 seconds
- International normalized ratio (INR): normal value = 1–2
- Partial thromboplastin time (PTT): normal value = 25–36 seconds
- Bleeding time: normal value = < 9 minutes (bleeding time is a nonspecific predictor of platelet function)

Normal values may vary from one laboratory to another. It is important to check the normal values for the laboratory that you use. If any of the tests are abnormal, the patient should be referred to a hematologist for evaluation before treatment is performed.

3. What are the clinical indications for use of 1-deamino-8-D-arginine vasopressin (DDAVP) in dental patients?

DDAVP (desmopressin) is a synthetic antidiuretic hormone that controls bleeding in patients with type I von Willebrand's disease, platelet defects secondary to uremia related to renal dialysis, and immunogenic thrombocytopenic purpura (ITP). The dosage is 0.3 mg/kg. DDAVP should not be used in patients under the age of 2 years; caution is necessary in elderly patients and patients receiving intravenous fluids.

23

4. What is hemophilia A?

Hemophilia A is a congenital bleeding disorder characterized by a deficiency of clotting factor VIII.

5. What is hemophilia B?

Hemophilia B is a congenital bleeding disorder characterized by a deficiency of clotting factor IX.

6. How are the hemophilias managed?

In general, hemophilia A and hemophilia B are managed with appropriate concentrates of the deficient factor (in the case of hemophilia A—factor VIII and in the case of hemophilia B—factor IX). Adjunctive treatment with Amicar and tranexamic acid is also appropriate.

7. How does bleeding typically manifest in a patient with thrombocytopenia vs. a patient with hemophilia?

Patients with severe thrombocytopenia typically present with mucosal bleeds. Patients with hemophilia typically present with deep hemorrhage in weight-bearing joints.

8. When do you use epsilon aminocaproic acid or tranexamic acid?

Epsilon aminocaproic acid (Amicar) and tranexamic acid are antifibrinolytic agents that inhibit activation of plasminogen. They are used to prevent clot lysis in patients with hereditary clotting disorders. For epsilon aminocaproic acid, the dose is 75–100 mg/kg every 6 hours; for tranexamic acid, it is 25 mg/kg every 6 hours. Tranexamic acid also comes in a mouth rinse formulation (4.8%), which can be used as a local hemostatic agent. The mouth rinse regimen is 10 ml, 4 times/day. The drug is not currently available for use in the U.S.

9. What is the minimal acceptable platelet count for an oral surgical procedure?

Normal platelet count is 150,000–450,000. In general, the minimal count for an oral surgical procedure is 50,000 platelets. However, emergency procedures may be done with as few as 30,000 platelets if the dentist is working closely with the patient's hematologist and uses excellent techniques of tissue management.

10. For a patient taking warfarin (Coumadin), a dental surgical procedure can be done without undue risk of bleeding if the *PT is below what value?*

Warfarin affects clotting factors II, VII, IX, and X by impairing the conversion of vitamin K to its active form. The normal PT for a healthy patient is 10.0–13.5 seconds. The normal INR is 1–2. Oral procedures with a risk of bleeding should not be attempted if the PT is greater than 1.5 times normal (above 18 seconds). Caution must be taken when the INR is greater than 2. Patients taking warfarin usually have a normal therapeutic INR in the 2–3 range. Simple dental prophylaxis can usually be accomplished with an INR in this range. Simple extractions or other minor surgical procedures can also usually be accomplished in the 2–3 range, using careful surgical technique. When the INR is 3 or above, surgery should be deferred and the patient's physician should be consulted. Consider tapering the dose of warfarin to bring the patient into the 2–3 range.

11. Is the bleeding time a good indicator of peri- and postsurgical bleeding?

The bleeding time is used to test for platelet function. However, studies have shown no correlation between blood loss during cardiac or general surgery and prolonged bleeding time. The best indicator of a bleeding problem in the dental patient is a thorough medical history. The bleeding time should be used in patients with no known platelet disorder to help predict the potential for bleeding.

Lind SE: The bleeding time does not predict surgical bleeding. Blood 77:2547–2552, 1991.

12. Should oral surgical procedures be postponed in patients taking aspirin?

Nonelective oral surgical procedures in the absence of a positive medical history for bleeding should not be postponed because of aspirin therapy, but the surgeon should be aware that bleeding may be exacerbated in a patient with mild platelet defect. However, elective procedures, if at all possible, should be postponed in the patient taking aspirin. Aspirin irreversibly acetylates cyclooxygenase, an enzyme that assists platelet aggregation. The effect is not dose-dependent and lasts for the 7–10-day life span of the platelet.

Tierney LM, McPhee SJ, Papadakis MA, Schroeder SA: Current Medical Diagnosis and Treatment. Norwalk, CT, Appleton & Lange, 1993, p 440.

13. Are patients taking nonsteroidal medications likely to bleed from oral surgical procedures?

Nonsteroidal antiinflammatory medications produce a transient inhibition of platelet aggregation that is reversed when the drug is cleared from the body. Patients with a preexisting platelet defect may have increased bleeding.

14. If a patient presents with spontaneous gingival bleeding, what diagnostic tests should be ordered?

A patient who presents with spontaneous gingival bleeding without a history of trauma, tooth brushing, flossing, or eating should be assessed for a systemic cause. Etiologies for gingival bleeding include inflammation secondary to localized periodontitis, platelet defect, factor deficiency, hematologic malignancy, and metabolic disorder. A thorough medical history should be obtained, and the following laboratory tests should be ordered: (1) PT/INR, (2) PTT, and (3) complete blood count (CBC).

INDICATIONS FOR PROPHYLACTIC ANTIBIOTICS

15. For what cardiac conditions is prophylaxis for endocarditis recommended in patients receiving dental care?

High-risk category
- Prosthetic cardiac valves, including both bioprosthetic and homograft valves
- Previous bacterial endocarditis
- Complex cyanotic congenital heart disease (e.g., single ventricle states, transposition of the great arteries, tetralogy of Fallot)
- Surgically constructed systemic pulmonary shunts or conduits

Moderate-risk category
- Most congenital cardiac malformations other than above and below (see next question)
- Acquired valvular dysfunction (e.g., rheumatic heart disease)
- Hypertrophic cardiomyopathy
- Mitral valve prolapse with valvular regurgitation and/or thickened leaflets

Dajani AS, et al: Prevention of bacterial endocarditis: Recommendations by the American Heart Association. JAMA 277:1794–1801, 1997.

16. What cardiac conditions do *not* require endocarditis prophylaxis?

Negligible-risk category (no higher than the general population)
- Isolated secundum atrial septal defect
- Surgical repair of atrial septal defect, ventricular septal defect, or patent ductus arteriosus (without residua beyond 6 months)
- Previous coronary artery bypass graft surgery
- Mitral valve prolapse without valvular regurgitation
- Physiologic, functional, or innocent heart murmurs
- Previous Kawasaki disease without valvular regurgitation
- Previous rheumatic fever without valvular regurgitation
- Cardiac pacemakers (intravascular and epicardial) and implanted defibrillators

Dajani AS, et al: Prevention of bacterial endocarditis: Recommendations by the American Heart Association. JAMA 277:1794–1801, 1997.

17. What are the antibiotics and dosages recommended by the American Heart Association (AHA) for prevention of endocarditis from dental procedures?

The AHA updates its recommendations every few years to reflect new findings. The dentist has an obligation to be aware of the latest recommendations. The patient's well-being is the dentist's responsibility. Even if a physician recommends an alternative prophylactic regimen, the dentist is liable if the patient develops endocarditis and the latest AHA recommendations were not followed.

Standard regimen

Amoxicillin, 2.0 gm orally 1 hr before procedure

For patients allergic to amoxicillin and penicillin

Clindamycin, 600 mg orally 1 hr before procedure *or*

Cephalexin* or cefadroxil,* 2.0 gm orally 1 hr before procedure *or*

Azithromycin or clarithromycin, 500 mg orally 1 hr before procedure

Patients unable to take oral medications

Ampicillin, intravenous or intramuscular administration of 2 gm 30 min before procedure

For patients allergic to ampicillin, amoxicillin, and penicillin

Clindamycin, intravenous administration of 600 mg 30 min before procedure *or*

Cefazolin,* intravenous or intramuscular administration of 1.0 gm within 30 min before procedure

* Cephalosporins should not be used in patients with immediate-type hypersensitivity reaction (urticaria, angioedema, or anaphylaxis) to penicillins.

Dajani AS, et al: Prevention of bacterial endocarditis: Recommendations by the American Heart Association. JAMA 277:1794–1801, 1997.

18. For what dental procedures is antibiotic premedication recommended in patients identified as being at risk for endocarditis?

- Dental extractions
- Periodontal procedures including surgery, scaling and root planing, probing, and recall maintenance
- Dental implant placement and reimplantation of avulsed teeth
- Endodontic (root canal) instrumentation or surgery only beyond the apex
- Subgingival placement of antibiotic fibers or strips
- Initial placement of orthodontic bands but not brackets
- Intraligamentary local anesthetic injections
- Prophylactic cleaning of teeth or implants if bleeding is anticipated

Dajani AS, et al: Prevention of bacterial endocarditis: Recommendations by the American Heart Association. JAMA 277:1794–1801, 1997.

19. For what dental procedures is antibiotic premedication *not* recommended in patients identified as being at risk for endocarditis?

- Restorative dentistry (including restoration of carious teeth and prosthodontic replacement of teeth) with or without retraction cord (clinical judgment may indicate antibiotic use in selected circumstances that may create significant bleeding)
- Local anesthetic injections (nonintraligamentary)
- Intracanal endodontic treatment (after placement and build-up)
- Placement of rubber dams
- Postoperative suture removal
- Placement of removable prosthodontic or orthodontic appliances
- Making of impressions
- Fluoride treatments
- Intraoral radiographs
- Orthodontic appliance adjustment
- Shedding of primary teeth

Dajani AS, et al: Prevention of bacterial endocarditis: Recommendations by the American Heart Association. JAMA 277:1794–1801, 1997.

20. Should a patient who has had a coronary bypass operation be placed on prophylactic antibiotics before dental treatment?

No evidence indicates that coronary artery bypass graft surgery introduces a risk for endocarditis. Therefore, antibiotic prophylaxis is not needed.

Dajani AS, et al: Prevention of bacterial endocarditis: Recommendations by the American Heart Association. JAMA 277:1794–1801, 1997.

21. What precautions should you take when treating a patient with a central line such as a Hickman or Portacath?

Patients with central venous access are usually receiving intensive antibiotic therapy, chemotherapy, or nutritional support. It is imperative to consult with the patient's physician before performing any dental procedures. If it is determined that the dental procedure is necessary, the patient should receive antibiotic prophylaxis to protect the central venous access line from infection secondary to transient bacteremias. The same antibiotic regimen recommended for the prevention of endocarditis should be prescribed.

22. Should a patient with a prosthetic joint be placed on prophylactic antibiotics before dental treatment?

Case studies support the hematogenous seeding of prosthetic joints. However, it is questionable whether organisms from the oral cavity are a source for late deep infections of prosthetic joints. The decision whether to premedicate should be determined by the dentist's clinical judgment in consultation with the patient's physician or orthopedic surgeon. Patients considered at high risk for developing a late infection of a prosthetic joint should be premedicated. Such patients can be grouped based on predisposing systemic conditions, issues associated with joint prostheses, or presence of acute infection at sites distant to the joint prosthesis.

High-risk Patients with Total Joint Replacements

Predisposing systemic conditions	
Rheumatoid arthritis	Insulin-dependent diabetes mellitus
Systemic lupus erythematosus	Hemophilia
Disease-, drug-, or radiation-induced immunosuppression	Malnourishment
Issues associated with joint prostheses	
First 2 years after joint replacement	Loose prosthesis
History of replacement of prosthesis	History of previous infection of prosthesis
Acute infection located at distant sites: skin, oral cavity, other	

From Fitzgerald RH, et al: Advisory statement: Antibiotic prophylaxis for dental patients with total joint replacements. American Dental Association; American Academy of Orthopaedic Surgeons. J Am Dent Assoc 128: 1004–1007, 1997; and Little JW: Managing dental patients with joint prostheses. J Am Dent Assoc 125:1374–1379, 1994.

23. What are the antibiotics and dosages recommended by the American Dental Association and the American Academy of Orthopaedic Surgeons to prevent late joint infections in patients considered to be at high risk?

Standard regimen

Cephalexin* or cephradine* or amoxicillin, 2 gm orally 1 hr before procedure

For patients allergic to amoxicillin and penicillin

Clindamycin, 600 mg orally 1 hr before procedure

Patients unable to take oral medications

Cefazolin,* intravenous or intramuscular administration of 1.0 gm 1 hr before procedure *or*

Ampicillin, intravenous or intramuscular administration of 2.0 gm 1 hr before procedure

For patients allergic to ampicillin, amoxicillin, and penicillin

Clindamycin, intravenous or intramuscular administration of 600 mg 1 hr before procedure

* Cephalosporins should not be used in patients with immediate-type hypersensitivity reaction (urticaria, angioedema, or anaphylaxis) to penicillins.

Fitzgerald RH, et al: Advisory statement: Antibiotic prophylaxis for dental patients with total joint replacements. American Dental Association; American Academy of Orthopaedic Surgeons. J Am Dent Assoc 128: 1004–1007, 1997.

24. Is it necessary to prescribe prophylactic antibiotics for a patient on renal dialysis?

Patients with arteriovenous (AV) shunts do not require antibiotic prophylaxis because the shunt is derived from native vessels. Patients with grafts or indwelling catheters should receive antibiotic prophylaxis, using the following regimens:

Standard regimen

Amoxicillin, 2.0 gm orally 1 hr before procedure

For patients allergic to amoxicillin and penicillin

Clindamycin, 600 mg orally 1 hr before procedure or

Cephalexin* or cefadroxil,* 2.0 gm orally 1 hr before procedure

Azithromycin or clarithromycin, 500 mg orally 1 hr before procedure

Patients unable to take oral medications

Ampicillin, intravenous or intramuscular administration 2.0 gm within 30 min before procedure

For patients allergic to ampicillin, amoxicillin, and penicillin

Clindamycin, intravenous administration of 600 mg within 30 min before procedure or

Cefazolin,* intravenous or intramuscular administration of 1.0 gm within 30 min before procedure

* Cephalosporins should not be used in patients with immediate-type hypersensitivity reaction (urticaria, angioedema, or anaphylaxis) to penicillins.

TREATMENT OF HIV-POSITIVE PATIENTS

25. What are the considerations in treating patients infected with the HIV virus and treated with azidothymidine (AZT)?

AZT is an antiviral widely used in patients infected with the human immunodeficiency virus (HIV). The drug is toxic to the hematopoietic system and may result in anemia, granulocytopenia, or thrombocytopenia. Patients taking AZT should have a CBC every 2 weeks. Before oral surgical procedures, a CBC should be done to determine whether the patient is neutropenic or thrombocytopenic.

26. What are the common oral manifestations of HIV?

- Oral candidiasis
- Herpes simplex lesions (of lips or intraorally)
- Hairy leukoplakia (EBV-related)
- Aphthous major ulcerations and minor ulcerations
- Petechiae (secondary to thrombocytopenia)
- Lymphoma (B-cell)
- Kaposi's sarcoma
- Acute necrotizing ulcerative gingivitis (ANUG)
- Herpes zoster lesions

Deglin JH, et al: Davis's Drug Guide for Nurses, 2nd ed. Philadelphia, F.A. Davis, 1991.

27. What is the mechanism of action of the HIV-1 protease inhibitors? What precautions must be taken in treating patients that receive protease inhibitors?

The protease inhibitors represent a major advance in the management of HIV disease. Once HIV-1 enters a cell, viral RNA undergoes reverse transcription to produce double-stranded DNA. The viral DNA is integrated into the host genome. It is then transcribed and translated by cellular enzymes to produce large, nonfunctional polypeptide chains, known as polyproteins. Polyproteins are assembled and packaged at the cell surface, and then immature virions are produced and released into the plasma. HIV-1 protease then cleaves the polyproteins into smaller, functional proteins, thereby allowing the virion to mature. In the presence of HIV-1 protease inhibitors, the virion cannot mature and is rapidly cleared from the system. The major protease inhibitors are reviewed below:

HIV-1 Protease Inhibitors and Precautions for the Dental Practitioner

MEDICATION	ADVERSE REACTIONS	INTERACTIONS
Saquinavir (Invirase)	Nausea, diarrhea, abdominal discomfort, and rash, neutropenia, paresthesia, thrombocytopenia	Avoid drugs that alter the cytochrome P450 activity in the liver because they affect the bioavailability of saquinavir. Ketoconazole inhibits cytochrome P450 and may result in increased plasma levels of saquinavir.
Ritonavir (Norvir)	Nausea, vomiting, diarrhea, fatigue, abdominal pain, circumoral paresthesias, taste disturbances, anorexia, elevated triglycerides, creatinine kinase, and transaminases	Use of sedative/hypnotics is contraindicated (e.g., diazepam, midazolam) because of the potential for oversedation. Ritonavir is a powerful inhibitor of cytochrome P450; thus, plasma concentrations of these drugs remain high. Narcotic analgesics, erythromycin, antifungal agents, and corticosteroids must be prescribed with caution for the same reason. NSAIDs may be subject to decreased bioavailability. Ritonavir is formulated in alcohol. Therefore, metronidazole in also contraindicated.
Indinavir (Crixivan)	Nephrolithiasis, abdominal discomfort, asymptomatic hyperbilirubinemia	Generally, indinavir is well-tolerated. No significant contraindications.
Nelfinavir (Viracept)	Diarrhea, loose stools	No significant contraindications, but more testing is necessary.

From Deeks SG, et al: HIV-1 protease inhibitors: A review for clinicians. JAMA 277:145–153, 1997, with permission.

28. A patient with HIV infection requires an oral surgical procedure to remove teeth after severe bone loss due to HIV-related localized periodontitis. What precautions should be taken?

It is estimated that 10–15% of patients with HIV develop immunogenic thrombocytopenic purpura (ITP). The antiplatelet antibodies appear to be found more frequently in advanced stages of the disease. Affected patients should have a CBC before any oral surgical procedure. If the platelets are low (below 150,000), the procedure should be done only after consultation with the patient's physician and with the knowledge that bleeding may be increased. The patient may require platelet transfusions to control postoperative bleeding.

Magnac C, et al: Platelet antibodies in serum of patients with human immunodeficiency virus (HIV) infection. AIDS Res Hum Retroviruses 6:1443–1449,1990.

29. Are there any contraindications to restorative dentistry procedures in patients with HIV infection?

If the patient is not neutropenic or thrombocytopenic, there are no contraindications to preventive and restorative dental care. In fact, patients should receive aggressive dental care to reduce the oral cavity as a source of infection. They should be placed on a 3–6-month recall to maintain optimal oral health and followed closely for opportunistic infections and HIV-related oral conditions.

30. What is a normal CD4 count? At what level is a patient at risk for infections?

A normal CD4 count is greater than 600 cells/mm³. When the CD4 count is less than 400 cells/mm³, the patient is considered to be at risk for acquiring opportunistic infections.

CARDIOVASCULAR DISEASE

31. What is the appropriate response if a patient with a history of cardiac disease develops chest pain during a dental procedure?

1. Discontinue treatment immediately.

2. Take and record vital signs (blood pressure, pulse, respiration), and question the patient about the pain. Chest pain from ischemia may be either substernal or more diffused. Patients of-

ten describe the pain as crushing, pressure, or heavy; it may radiate to the shoulders, arms, neck, or back.

3. If the patient has a history of angina and takes nitroglycerin, give the patient either his or her own nitroglycerin or a tablet from your emergency cart. Continue to monitor the patient's vital signs. If the pain does not stop after 3 minutes, give the patient a second dose. If after 3 doses in a 10-minute period the pain does not subside, contact the medical emergency service and have the patient transported to an emergency department to rule out a myocardial infarction.

4. If the patient does not have a history of heart disease and persistent chest pain for greater than 2 minutes, the medical emergency service should be contacted and the patient transported to a hospital emergency department for evaluation.

5. If the patient is not allergic to aspirin, administer one tablet of aspirin (325 mg) orally. The aspirin acts as an antithrombotic agent.

32. At what blood pressure should elective dental care be postponed?
Elective dental care should be postponed if the systolic blood pressure is > 170 mmHg or the diastolic pressure is > 100 mmHg. Refer to a physician.

33. At what blood pressure should emergency dental care be postponed and the patient treated palliatively until the blood pressure is controlled?
Emergency dental treatment should be postponed if the systolic pressure is > 180 or the diastolic pressure is > 110. Patients must be referred for care immediately to prevent morbidity if they have either (1) asymptomatic severe hypertension with a systolic pressure > 240 mmHg or diastolic pressure > 130 mmHg or (2) symptomatic hypertension, headache, heart failure, angina, or elevated perioperative blood pressure, with a systolic pressure of > 200 mmHg or diastolic pressure of > 120.

Tierney LM, McPhee SJ, Papadakis MA, Schroeder SA: Current Medical Diagnosis and Treatment. Norwalk, CT, Appleton & Lange, 1993, p 366.

34. How long should dental care be postponed after a heart attack?
Dental treatment in a patient who has had a myocardial infarction should be done only after consultation with the patient's physician. Cintron et al. showed that patients treated within 3 weeks of an uncomplicated myocardial infarction experienced no significant hemodynamic changes or complications related to local anesthesia, vigorous dental prophylaxis, or dental extraction. The general guidelines for a patient without angina or heart failure is to wait 6 months for elective dental care.

Cintron G, et al: Cardiovascular effects and safety of dental anesthesia and dental interventions in patients with recent uncomplicated myocardial infarction. Arch Intern Med 146:2203–2204, 1986.

35. How do you differentiate between stable and unstable angina?
Unstable angina is characterized by a change in the pattern of pain. The pain occurs with less exertion or at rest, lasts longer, and is less responsive to medication. Dental care for such patients must be postponed and the patient referred to his or her physician immediately for care. Patients are at increased risk for myocardial infarction. If emergency dental care is necessary before the patient is stable, it should be attempted only with cardiac monitoring and sedation.

Tierney LM, McPhee SJ, Papadakis MA, Schroeder SA: Current Medical Diagnosis and Treatment. Norwalk, CT, Appleton & Lange, 1993, p 298.

36. What precautions should be taken in treating a patient with recent onset of angina?
Patients with recent onset of angina less than 30 days' duration are at increased risk for myocardial infarction and sudden death. The angina may not be severe and may occur only with exercise. However, even though symptoms are mild, dental treatment should be postponed until the patient has had a medical evaluation.

Kilmartin C, Munroe CO: Cardiovascular diseases and the dental patient. J Can Dent Assoc 6:513–518, 1986.

37. Is the use of a vasoconstrictor in local anesthetics contraindicated in patients with cardiac disease?

The use of vasoconstrictors is not necessarily contraindicated in patients with cardiovascular disease. According to conservative recommendations, epinephrine should not exceed 0.04 mg, which equates to 4 carpules of 1/200,000 or 2 carpules of 1/100,000. The use of epinephrine should be minimized in patients with significant cardiac disease, including those diagnosed with an arrhythmia.

Holroyd SV, Wynn RL, Requa-Clark B (eds): Clinical Pharmacology in Dental Practice, 4th ed. St. Louis, Mosby, 1988.

38. Should retraction cord that contains epinephrine be used in a patient with cardiovascular disease?

The concentration of epinephrine in impregnated cord is high, and systemic absorption occurs. Impregnated cord should not be used in patients with cardiac disease, hypertension, or hyperthyroidism. Malamed argues that epinephrine-containing retraction cord should not be used in dental practice.

Kilmartin C, Munroe CO: Cardiovascular diseases and the dental patient. J Can Dent Assoc 6:513–518, 1986.

39. When should vasoconstrictors not be used in either local anesthetic or retraction cord?

Vasoconstrictors should not be used in patients with uncontrolled hypertension or hyperthyroidism. They also should be avoided in patients with significant cardiac disease and/or arrhythmia. Epinephrine should not be used in dental patients under general anesthesia when either halogenated hydrocarbons or cyclopropane are used for anesthesia.

Holroyd SV, Wynn RL, Requa-Clark B (eds): Clinical Pharmacology in Dental Practice, 4th ed. St. Louis, Mosby, 1988, p 58.

40. Is it safe to treat a patient who has had a heart transplant in an outpatient dental office?

Dental treatment should be done only after consultation with the patient's cardiologist. If the patient is stable without rejection, there are no contraindications to dental treatment. Antibiotic prophylaxis is recommended if the patient is severely immunosuppressed. The patient most likely will be taking prednisone and cyclosporine. For restorative and preventive dental procedures and simple extractions, it is not necessary to increase the corticosteroids. Erythromycin and ketoconazole should not be prescribed for a patient on cyclosporine. Erythromycin and ketoconazole inhibit the metabolism of cyclosporine.

41. How long should a dentist wait before performing elective dental treatment on a patient who has undergone cardiac transplant?

3–6 months.

METABOLIC DISORDERS

42. What precautions do you need to take in treating a patient with insulin-dependent diabetes mellitus (IDDM)?

The major concern for the dental practitioner treating the patient with IDDM is hypoglycemia. It is important to question the patient for changes in insulin dosage, diet, and exercise routine before undertaking any outpatient dental treatment. A decrease in dietary intake or an increase in either the normal insulin dosage or exercise may place the patient at risk for hypoglycemia.

Tierney LM, McPhee SJ, Papadakis MA, Schroeder SA: Current Medical Diagnosis and Treatment. Norwalk, CT, Appleton & Lange, 1993, p 928.

43. What are the symptoms of hypoglycemia?

1. Tachycardia
2. Palpitations
3. Sweating
4. Tremulousness
5. Nausea
6. Hunger

The symptoms may progress to coma and convulsions without intervention.

44. What should the dentist be prepared to do for the patient who has a hypoglycemic reaction?

The dental practitioner should have some form of sugar readily available—packets of table sugar, candy, or orange juice. Also available are 3-mg tablets of glucose (Dextrosol). If a patient develops symptoms of hypoglycemia, the dental procedure should be discontinued immediately; if conscious, the patient should be given some form of oral glucose.

If the patient is unconscious, the emergency medical service should be contacted. Then 1 mg of glucagon can be injected intramuscularly, or 50 ml of 50% glucose solution can be given by rapid intravenous infusion. The glucagon injection should restore the patient to a conscious state within 15 minutes; then some form of oral sugar can be given.

Tierney LM, McPhee SJ, Papadakis MA, Schroeder SA: Current Medical Diagnosis and Treatment. Norwalk, CT, Appleton & Lange, 1993, p 932.

45. Is the diabetic patient at greater risk for infection after an oral surgical procedure?

It is important to minimize the risk of infection in diabetic patients. They should have aggressive treatment of dental caries and periodontal disease and then be placed on frequent recall examinations and oral prophylaxis.

After oral surgical procedures, endodontic procedures, and treatment of suppurative periodontitis, diabetic patients should be placed on antibiotics to prevent infection secondary to delayed healing. Antibiotics of choice are amoxicillin, 500 mg 3 times/day, or clindamycin, 300 mg 3 times/day for 7–10 days.

46. When is it necessary to increase the dose of prednisone in patients taking corticosteroids?

Patients taking chronic daily doses of steroids (total dose greater than 15 mg/day of prednisone) should be considered for steroid supplementation, in consultation with their physician. Patients who have taken acute doses of prednisone greater than 15 mg/day within the past two weeks also should be considered for steroid supplementation.

For multiple extractions or extensive mucogingival surgery, the dose of corticosteroids should be doubled on the day of surgery. If the patient is treated in the operating room under general anesthesia, stress level doses of cortisone, 100 mg intravenously or intramuscularly, should be given preoperatively.

47. Should antibiotics be prescribed for oral surgical procedures in patients receiving corticosteroids?

As with the diabetic patient, it is important to minimize the risk of infection in patients taking corticosteroids. Patients on long-term therapy, such as organ transplant recipients, should receive aggressive treatment to eliminate the oral cavity as a source of infection and then be placed on frequent recall examinations and oral prophylaxis.

Patients on corticosteroid therapy should be placed on antibiotic therapy after oral surgical procedures. Antibiotics should be started on the day of the procedure and continued for 5–7 days postoperatively. The antibiotic of choice is amoxicillin, 500 mg 3 times/day. If the patient is allergic to penicillin and taking cyclosporine, clindamycin, 300 mg 3 times/day for 5–7 days, is the antibiotic of choice.

48. What are the clinical symptoms of hypothyroidism? What dental care can be safely provided?

The clinical symptoms of hypothyroidism are weakness, fatigue, intolerance to cold, changes in weight, constipation, headache, menorrhagia, and dryness of the skin. Dental care should be deferred until after a medical consultation in a patient with or without a history of thyroid disease who experiences a combination of the above signs and symptoms. If the patient is myxedematous, he or she should be treated as a medical emergency and referred immediately for medical care. It is important not to prescribe opiates for palliative treatment of the myxedematous patient. The myxedematous patient may be unusually sensitive and die from normal doses of opiates.

Tierney LM, McPhee SJ, Papadakis MA, Schroeder SA: Current Medical Diagnosis and Treatment. Norwalk, CT, Appleton & Lange, 1993, pp 863, 865.

ALLERGIC REACTIONS

49. What would you prescribe for the patient who develops a mild soft-tissue swelling of the lips under the rubber dam?

The patient probably has a contact allergic reaction from the Latex. If the reaction is mild (slight swelling with no extension into the oral cavity) and self-limiting, the patient should be given 50 mg of oral diphenhydramine and observed for at least 2 hours for possible delayed reaction. If the reaction is moderate to severe, the patient should be given 50 mg of diphenhydramine, either intramuscularly or intravenously, and closely monitored. Emergency services should be contacted to transport the patient to the emergency department for treatment and observation. With the advent of the epidemic of HIV infection, Latex gloves and condoms are now widely used. Allergic patients should be instructed to inform health care providers of their Latex allergy and referred to an allergist.

50. What should you do if a patient for whom you prescribed the prophylactic antibiotic amoxicillin approximately 1 hour previously reports urticaria, erythema, and pruritus (itching)?

If the reaction is delayed (longer than 1 hour) and limited to the skin, the patient should be given 50 mg of diphenhydramine, intramuscularly or intravenously, then observed for 1–2 hours before being released. If no further reaction occurs, the patient should be given a prescription for 25–50 mg of diphenhydramine to be taken every 6 hours until symptoms are gone.

If the reaction is immediate (less than 1 hour) and limited to the skin, 50 mg of diphenhydramine should be given immediately either intravenously or intramuscularly. The patient should be monitored and emergency services contacted to transport the patient to the emergency department. If other symptoms of allergic reaction occur, such as conjunctivitis, rhinitis, bronchial constriction, or angioedema, 0.3 cc of aqueous 1/1000 epinephrine should be given by subcutaneous or intramuscular injection. The patient should be monitored until emergency services arrive. If the patient becomes hypotensive, an intravenous line should be started with either Ringer's lactate or 5% dextrose/water.

Malamed SF, Robbins KS: Medical Emergencies in the Dental Office, 5th ed., Yearbook Medical Publishers, 2000.

51. What are the signs and symptoms of anaphylaxis? How should it be managed in the dental office?

Anaphylaxis is characterized by bronchospasm, hypotension or shock, and urticaria or angioedema. It is a medical emergency in which death may result from respiratory obstruction, circulatory failure, or both. With the first indication of anaphylaxis, 0.2–0.5 cc of 1/1000 aqueous epinephrine should be injected subcutaneously or intramuscularly, and emergency services should be contacted. The injection of epinephrine may be repeated every 20–30 minutes, if necessary, for as many as 3 doses. Oxygen at a rate of 4 L/min must be delivered with a face mask. The patient must be continuously monitored, and an intravenous line containing either Ringer's lactate or normal saline should be infused at 100 cc/hour. If the patient becomes hypotensive, the intravenous infusion should be increased. If airway obstruction occurs from edema of the larynx or hypopharynx, a cricothyrotomy must be done. If the airway obstruction is due to bronchospasm, an albuterol or terbutaline nebulizer should be administered or intravenous aminophylline, 6 mg/kg, infused over 20–30 minutes.

Tierney LM, McPhee SJ, Papadakis MA, Schroeder SA: Current Medical Diagnosis and Treatment. Norwalk, CT, Appleton & Lange, 1993, p 634.

HEMATOLOGY/ONCOLOGY

52. What are the normal values for a CBC?

White blood cell count		Hemoglobin (Hgb)	
18 years and older	4,000–10,000/ml	18 years and older	
12–17 years	4,500–13,000/ml	Male	13.5–18.0 gm/dl
6 months to 11 years	4,500–13,500/ml	Female	11.5–16.4 gm/dl
Red blood cell count		12–17 years	
18 years and older		Male and female	12.0–16.0 gm/dl
Male	4.5–6.4 M/ml	6 months to 11 years	
Female	3.9–6.0 M/ml	Male and female	10.5–14.0 gm/dl
12–17 years		**Platelet count (PLT)**	
Male and female	4.1–5.3 M/ml	8 days and older	150,000–450,000/ml
6 months to 11 years			
Male and female	3.7–5.3 M/ml	Up to 7 days	150,000–350,000/ml

Hematocrit (Hct)	
18 years and older	
Male	40–54%
Female	36–48%
12–17 years	
Male and female	36–39%
6 months to 11 years	
Male and female	34–45%

53. What precautions should be taken in providing dental care to a patient with sickle-cell anemia?

1. Patients with sickle-cell disease should not receive dental treatment during a crisis, except for the relief of dental pain and treatment of acute dental infections. Dental infections should be treated aggressively; if facial cellulitis develops, the patient should be admitted to the hospital for treatment.

2. The patient's physician should be consulted about the patient's cardiovascular status. Myocardial damage secondary to infarctions and iron deposits is common.

3. Patients with sickle-cell anemia are at increased risk for bacterial infections and should receive prophylactic antibiotics before any dental procedure that may cause a transient bacteremia. The prophylactic antibiotic regimen used for the prevention of endocarditis should be followed. After a surgical procedure, antibiotics (amoxicillin, 500 mg 3 times/day, or clindamycin, 300 mg 3 times/day) should be continued for 7–10 days postoperatively.

Sams DR, et al: Managing the dental patient with sickle cell anemia: A review of the literature. Pediatr Dent 12(5):317–320, 1990.

Smith HB, et al: Dental management of patients with sickle cell disorders. J Am Dent Assoc 114:85, 1987.

54. What hematologic disorders are characterized by a "hair-on-end" appearance of bone on radiographic surveys?

Thalassemia major and sickle cell anemia.

55. Can local anesthetic with a vasoconstrictor be used in a patient with sickle-cell disease?

Because of the possibility of impairing local circulation, the use of vasoconstrictors in patients with sickle-cell disease is controversial. It is recommended that the planned dental procedure dictate the choice of local anesthetic. If the planned procedure is a routine, short procedure that can be performed without discomfort by using an anesthetic without a vasoconstrictor, the vasoconstrictor should not be used. However, if the procedure requires long, profound anesthesia, 2% lidocaine with 1/100,000 epinephrine is the anesthetic of choice.

Smith HB, et al: Dental management of patients with sickle cell disorders. J Am Dent Assoc 114:85, 1987.

56. Can nitrous oxide be used to help manage anxiety in patients with sickle-cell anemia?

Nitrous oxide can be safely used in patients with sickle-cell anemia as long as the concentration of oxygen is greater than 50%, the flow rate is high, and the patient is able to ventilate adequately.

Smith HB, et al: Dental management of patients with sickle cell disorders. J Am Dent Assoc 114:85, 1987.

57. Can a dental infection cause a crisis in a patient with sickle-cell anemia?

Preventive dental care—routine scaling and root planing, topical fluorides, sealants and treatment of dental caries—is important in patients with sickle-cell anemia. The literature reports some cases of a sickle-cell crisis precipitated by periodontal infections.

Sams DR, et al: Managing the dental patient with sickle cell anemia: A review of the literature. Pediatr Dent 12(5):317–320, 1990.

58. What are the oral symptoms of acute leukemia?

Over 65% of patients with acute leukemia have oral symptoms. The symptoms result from myelosuppression due to the overwhelming numbers of malignant cells in the bone marrow and/or large numbers of circulating immature cells (blasts).

1. Symptoms from thrombocytopenia: gingival oozing, petechiae, hematoma, and ecchymosis

2. Symptoms from neutropenia: recurrent or unrelenting bacterial infections, lymphadenopathy, oral ulcerations, pharyngitis, and gingival infection

3. Symptoms from circulating immature cells (blasts): gingival hyperplasia from blast infiltration

Patients with the above signs or symptoms should be evaluated to rule out a hematologic malignancy. The dentist should consider carefully whether the symptoms can be explained by local factors or are disproportionate to the local factors. If a hematologic malignancy is suspected, a CBC with a differential white cell count should be ordered.

Sonis ST, et al: Principles and Practice of Oral Medicine, 2nd ed. Philadelphia, W.B. Saunders, 1995, pp 262–275.

59. Which leukemia is typically referred to as the "leukemia of childhood"?

Acute lymphocylic leukemia almost always occurs in children. The condition can be successfully treated, with a 50–70% 5-year survival.

60. Is it safe to extract a tooth in a patient who is receiving chemotherapy?

The major organ system affected by cytotoxic chemotherapy is the hematopoietic system. When a patient receives chemotherapy, the white cell count and platelets may be expected to decrease in about 7–10 days. If the patient's absolute neutrophil count (calculated by multiplying the white cell count by the number of neutrophils in the differential count and dividing by 100) drops below 500 neutrophils, the patient is considered neutropenic and at risk for infection. If the platelet count drops below 50,000, the patient is at risk for bleeding.

Dental procedures should be scheduled, if possible, 2 weeks before planned chemotherapy or after the counts begin to recover, usually 14 days for white cells and 21 days for platelets. Dental treatment should be attempted only after consultation and in coordination with the patient's physician and after the patient has had a CBC.

61. What precautions should be taken in treating a patient who has received bone marrow transplantation for a hematologic malignancy?

Dental care should be done only in consultation with the patient's physician. As a rule, elective dental treatment should be postponed for 6 months after transplant. However, emergency dental treatment can be done. If dental care must be done before the recommended postponement, a CBC should be checked and if the results are acceptable (platelets > 50,000 and neutrophils > 500), the patient should be premedicated with the same regimen used for the prevention of endocarditis.

62. What should be done if a patient has enlarged lymph nodes?

Lymphadenopathy may be secondary to a sore throat or upper respiratory infection or the initial presentation of a malignancy. A thorough history and clinical examination help to determine the etiology of the lymphadenopathy.

Patients with lymphadenopathy and an identifiable inflammatory process should be reexamined in 2 weeks to determine whether the lymphadenopathy has responded to treatment. If no inflammatory process can be identified or if the lymphadenopathy does not resolve after treatment, the patient should be referred to a physician for further evaluation and possible biopsy.

	Inflammatory Process	*Granulomatous Disease/ Neoplasia*
Onset	Acute	Progressive enlargement
Pain on palpation	Tender	Neoplasia: asymptomatic Granulomatous: painful
Symmetry	Bilateral for systemic infections Unilateral for localized infections	Usually unilateral
Consistency	Firm, movable	Firm, nonmovable

From Sonis ST, et al: Principles and Practice of Oral Medicine, 2nd ed. Philadelphia, W.B. Saunders, 1995, pp 269–271, with permission.

KIDNEY DISEASE

63. What precautions should be taken before beginning treatment of a patient on dialysis?

Patients typically receive dialysis 3 times/week, usually on a Monday, Wednesday, Friday schedule or a Tuesday, Thursday, Saturday schedule. Dental treatment for a patient on dialysis should be done on the day between dialysis appointments to avoid bleeding difficulties (patients receive the anticoagulant, heparin, on dialysis days). Patients with grafts or indwelling catheters should be premedicated to prevent infection of the graft or catheter. Patients with an arteriovenous (AV) shunt do not need to be premedicated.

64. What adjustments in the dosage of oral antibiotics should you make for a patient on renal dialysis who has a dental infection?

Penicillin	500 mg orally every 6 hr; dose after hemodialysis
Amoxicillin	500 mg orally every 24 hr; dose after hemodialysis
Ampicillin	250 mg to 1 g orally every 12–24 hr; dose after hemodialysis
Erythromycin	250 mg orally every 6 hr; not necessary to dose after hemodialysis
Clindamycin	300 mg every 6 hr; not necessary to dose after hemodialysis

Bennett WM, et al: Drug Prescribing in Renal Failure, 2nd ed. Philadelphia, American College of Physicians, 1991.

65. Which regional lymph nodes are most commonly involved in the presentation of *early* Hodgkin's disease?

Hodgkin's disease typically presents with cervical, subclavicular, axillary or mediastinal lymph node involvement and less commonly with inguinal and abdominal lymph node involvement.

66. What pain medications can be safely prescribed for patients on dialysis?

- **Codeine** is safe to use in dialysis but may produce more profound sedation. The dose should be titrated beginning with one-half the normal dose for patients on dialysis and one-half to three-fourths the normal dose for patients with severely decreased renal function.
- **Acetaminophen** is nephrotoxic in overdoses. However, it may be prescribed in patients on

dialysis at a dose of 650 mg every 8 hours. For patients with decreased renal function, the regimen should be 650 mg every 6 hours.
- **Aspirin** should be avoided in patients with severe renal failure and in patients on renal dialysis because of the possibility of potentiating hemorrhagic diathesis.
- **Propoxyphene** (Darvon) should not be prescribed for a patient on renal dialysis. The active metabolite norpropoxyphene accumulates in patients with end-stage renal disease.
- **Meperidine** (Demerol) should not be prescribed in patients on renal dialysis. The active metabolite, normeperidine, accumulates and may cause seizures.

Bennett WM, et al: Drug Prescribing in Renal Failure, 2nd ed. Philadelphia, American College of Physicians, 1991.

67. What changes do you expect to see in the dental radiographs of a patient on renal dialysis?

The most common changes are decreased bone density with a ground-glass appearance, increased bone density in the mandibular molar area compatible with osteosclerosis, loss of lamina aura, subperiosteal cortical bone resorption in the maxillary sinus and the mandibular canal, and brown tumor.

Spolnik KJ: Dental radiographic manifestations of end-stage renal disease. Dent Radiogr Photogr 54(2): 21–31, 1981.

68. What is uremic stomatitis?

Uremic stomatitis is an ulcerative condition of the oral mucosa which develops in patients that have chronic renal failure. It is thought to be caused by ammonia metabolites.

69. What is a common oral complication of renal transplant patients that are on chronic doses of cyclosporin A?

Gingival hyperplasia

70. What other medications are known to cause gingival hyperplasia?

Phenytoin (Dilantin) and nifedipine (Procardia) are known to cause gingival hyperplasia.

71. What precautions should be taken in treating a patient after renal transplantation?

After renal transplant patients receive immunosuppressive drugs and have an increased susceptibility to infection. Dental infections should be treated aggressively. Prophylactic antibiotics should be considered whenever the risk of bacteremia is present. Erythromycin should not be prescribed for any patient taking cyclosporine.

72. What antibiotic, used often in dentistry, should be avoided in a patient taking cyclosporine?

Cyclosporine is used to prevent organ rejection in renal, cardiac, and hepatic transplantation and to prevent graft-vs.-host disease in patients with bone marrow transplants. Erythromycin should not be prescribed for patients taking cyclosporine. Erythromycin increases the levels of cyclosporine by decreasing its metabolism.

PULMONARY DISEASE

73. What precautions should be taken in treating a patient with chronic obstructive pulmonary disease (COPD)?

Patients with COPD and a history of hemoptysis should be prescribed drugs with antiplatelet activity (aspirin and nonsteroidals) with caution. Hemoptysis has been reported after the use of aspirin in patients with COPD.

Tierney LM, McPhee SJ, Papadakis MA, Schroeder SA: Current Medical Diagnosis and Treatment. Norwalk, CT, Appleton & Lange, 1993, p 197.

74. What antibiotic should not be prescribed for patients with COPD who take theophylline?

Erythromycin should not be prescribed for patients taking theophylline. Erythromycin decreases the metabolism of theophylline and may cause toxicity.

Deglin JH, et al: Davis's Drug Guide for Nurses, 2nd ed. Philadelphia, F.A. Davis, 1991.

75. What intervention is appropriate for a dental patient who has an asthma attack in the office?

The medical history should provide an indication of the severity of the asthma and the medications that the patient takes for an asthma attack. The symptoms of an acute asthma attack are shortness of breath, wheezing, dyspnea, anxiety, and, with severe attacks, cyanosis. As with all medical emergencies, the first two steps are (1) to discontinue treatment and (2) to remain calm and not increase the patient's anxiety. Patients should be allowed to position themselves for optimal comfort and then placed on oxygen, 2–4 L/min. If patients have their own nebulizer, they should be allowed to use it. If the patient does not have a nebulizer, he or she should be given either a metaproterenol or albuterol nebulizer from the emergency cart or case and take 2 inhalations.

If the symptoms do not subside or increase in severity, emergency services should be contacted; the patient must be closely monitored and given either 0.3–0.5 ml of a 1:1000 solution of epinephrine subcutaneously or intravenous aminophylline, 5.6 mg/kg in 150 ml of either D-5 1/2 normal saline or normal saline infused over 30 minutes. (To calculate kg weight, divide the patient's weight in pounds by 2.2.) The dose of epinephrine may be repeated every 30 minutes for as many as 3 doses. Epinephrine should not be used in patients with severe hypertension, severe tachycardia, or cardiac arrhythmias. Aminophylline should not be used in patients who have had theophylline in the past 24 hours.

76. Can nitrous oxide be used safely to sedate a patient with COPD?

Sedation with nitrous oxide should be avoided in patients with COPD. The high flow of oxygen may depress the respiratory drive. Low-flow oxygen via a nasal cannula may be safely used without risk of respiratory depression.

Little JW, Falace DA: Dental Management of the Medically Compromised Patient, 5th ed. St. Louis, Mosby, 1996.

LIVER DISEASE

77. What laboratory blood tests should be ordered for a patient with alcoholic hepatitis?

Alcoholic hepatitis is the most common cause of cirrhosis, which is one of the most common causes of death in the United States. There are a number of concerns in treating the patient with alcoholic hepatitis:

1. Increased risk of peri- and postoperative bleeding, secondary to a decrease in vitamin K-dependent coagulation factors
2. Qualitative and quantitative effects of alcohol on platelets
3. Anemia secondary to dietary deficiencies and/or hemorrhage

Before attempting a surgical procedure, the minimal laboratory tests are PT/INR, PTT, CBC, and bleeding time.

78. What precautions should be taken with patients on anticonvulsant medications?

It is important to obtain a detailed history of the seizure disorder to determine whether the patient is at risk for seizures during dental treatment. Important information includes the type and frequency of seizures, the date of the last seizure, prescribed medications, the last blood test to determine therapeutic ranges, and activities that tend to provoke seizures. For patients taking valproic acid or carbamazepine, periodic tests for liver function should be performed. Blood counts for patients taking carbamazepine and ethosuximide should be done by the patient's physician. Both liver function and blood counts should be checked before any oral surgical procedure is planned.

Deglin JH, et al: Davis's Drug Guide for Nurses, 2nd ed. Philadelphia, F.A. Davis, 1991.

Little JW, Falace DA: Dental Management of the Medically Compromised Patient, 6th ed. St. Louis, Mosby, 2002.

Tierney LM, McPhee SJ, Papadakis MA, Schroeder SA: Current Medical Diagnosis and Treatment. Norwalk, CT, Appleton & Lange, 1993.

Seizure Medications and Precautions for the Dental Practitioner

MEDICATION	ADVERSE REACTIONS	INTERACTIONS
Valproic acid (Depakote) Heparin	Prolonged bleeding time, leukopenia, thrombocytopenia	Increased risk of bleeding with aspirin and NSAIDs or warfarin. Additive depression of CNS with other depressants, including narcotic analgesics and sedative/hypnotics.
Carbamazepine (Tegretol)	Aplastic anemia, agranulocytosis, thrombocytopenia, leukopenia, leukocytosis	Erythromycin increases levels of carbamazepine and may cause toxicity.
Phenytoin (Dilantin)	Aplastic anemia, agranulocytosis, leukopenia, thrombocytopenia	Additive depression of CNS with other depressants, including narcotics and sedative/hypnotics.
Phenobarbital		Additive depression of CNS with other depressants, including narcotics and sedative/hypnotics. May increase risk of hepatic toxicity of acetaminophen.
Primidone	Blood dyscrasias, orthostatic hypotension	Additive depression of CNS with other depressants, including narcotics and sedative/hypnotics.
Ethosuximide	Aplastic anemia, granulocytosis, leukopenia	Additive depression of CNS with other depressants.
Clonazepam	Anemia, thrombocytosis, leukopenia	Additive depression of CNS with other depressants.

79. What emergency procedures should be taken for a patient having a seizure?

It is important to determine whether the patient has a history of seizure disorder. Any patient who has a seizure in the dental office without a history of seizures must be treated as a medical emergency. The emergency medical service should be contacted as the dentist proceeds with management. There are two stages of a seizure: the ictal phase and the postictal phase. The management of each is described below.

Ictal phase

1. Place the patient in a supine position away from hard or sharp objects to prevent injury; a carpeted floor is ideal. If the patient is in the dental chair, it is important to protect the patient by moving equipment as far as possible out of the way.

2. Airway must be maintained and vital signs monitored during the tonic stage. If suctioning equipment is available, it should be ready with a plastic tip for suctioning secretions to maintain the airway. The patient may experience periods of apnea and develop cyanosis. The head should be extended to establish a patent airway, and oxygen should be administered. Vital signs, pulse, respiration and blood pressure must be monitored throughout the seizure.

3. If the ictal phase of the seizure lasts more than 5 minutes, emergency services should be called. Tonic-clonic status epilepticus is a medical emergency. If the dentist is trained to do so, an intravenous line should be initiated, and a dose of 25–50 ml of 50% dextrose should be given immediately in case the cause of the seizure is hypoglycemia. If there is no response, the patient should be given 10 mg of diazepam intravenously over a 2-minute period. The patient's vital signs must be monitored, because the diazepam may cause respiratory depression. The dose of diazepam may be repeated after 10 minutes, if necessary.

Postictal phase

1. Once the seizure activity has stopped and the patient enters the postictal phase, it is important to continue to monitor the vital signs and, if necessary, to provide basic life support. If respiratory depression is significant, emergency services should be called, the airway maintained, and respiration supported. Blood pressure may be initially depressed but should recover gradually.

2. If the patient recovers from the postictal phase without basic life support or other complications, the patient's physician should be contacted, and the patient, if stable, should be discharged from the dental office, accompanied by a responsible adult.

Malamed SF, Robbins KS: Medical Emergencies in the Dental Office, 5th ed. St. Louis, Yearbook Medical Publishes, 2000.

80. What dental considerations must be considered in treating patients with seizure disorders?

Patients taking phenytoin are at risk for gingival hyperplasia. Tissue irritation from orthodontic bands, defective restorations, fractured teeth, plaque, and calculus accelerate the hyperplasia.

The dental practitioner should consider the patient's seizure status. A rubber dam with dental floss tied to the clamp should be used for all restorative dental procedures to enable the rapid removal of materials and instruments from the patient's oral cavity. Fixed prosthetics, when indicated, should be fabricated rather than removable prosthetics. If removable prosthetics are indicated, they should be fabricated with metal for all major connectors. Acrylic partial dentures should be avoided because of the risk of breaking and aspiration during seizure activities. Unilateral partial dentures are contraindicated. Temporary crowns and bridges should be laboratory-cured for strength.

81. Is general anesthesia contraindicated in patients with a seizure disorder?

No. However, general anesthesia lowers the seizure threshold, and precautions must be taken to ensure that serum levels of the antiseizure drug are within therapeutic range.

82. What are the common causes of unconsciousness in dental patients?

The most common cause of loss of consciousness in the dental office is syncope. The signs and symptoms are diaphoresis, pallor, and loss of consciousness. Place the patient in the supine position with the feet elevated, monitor vital signs, and give oxygen, 3–4 L/minute, via nasal cannula.

RADIATION THERAPY

83. What are the risk factors for the development of osteoradionecrosis?

Bone exposed to high radiation therapy is hypovascular, hypocellular, and hypoxic tissue. Osteoradionecrosis develops because the radiated tissue is unable to repair itself. The risk for osteoradionecrosis increases as the dose of radiation increases from 5,000 rads to over 8,000 rads. Tissues receiving less than 5,000 rads are at low risk for necrosis. In addition, the risk increases with poor oral health. Oral surgical procedures after radiation therapy place the patient at high risk for developing osteoradionecrosis. Soft-tissue trauma from dentures and oral infections from periodontal disease and dental caries also put the patient at risk.

84. How should the dentist prepare the patient for radiation therapy of the head and neck?

The dentist should consult with the radiotherapist to determine what oral structures will be in the field as well as the maximal radiation dose. If teeth are in the field and the dose is greater than 5,000 rads, periodontally involved teeth and teeth with periapical lucencies should be extracted at least 2 weeks before radiation therapy begins. The dentist should prepare the patient for postradiation xerostomia, provide custom fluoride trays, and prescribe 0.4% stannous fluoride gel to be used for 3–5 minutes twice daily. The patient must he placed on a 2–3-month recall schedule. On recall, the teeth must be carefully examined for root caries, and instruction in oral hygiene should be reviewed.

BIBLIOGRAPHY

1. Bennett WM, et al: Drug Prescribing in Renal Failure, 2nd ed. Philadelphia, American College of Physicians, 1991.
2. Cintron G, et al: Cardiovascular effects and safety of dental anesthesia and dental interventions in patients with recent uncomplicated myocardial infarction. Arch Intern Med 146:2203–2204, 1986.
3. Dajani AS, et al: Prevention of bacterial endocarditis recommendations by the American Heart Association. JAMA 277:1794–1801, 1997.
4. Deeks SG, et al: HIV-1 protease inhibitors: A review for clinicians. JAMA 277:145–153, 1997.
5. Deglin JH, et al: Davis's Drug Guide for Nurses, 2nd ed. Philadelphia, F.A. Davis, 1991.
6. Dialysis therapy. N Engl J Med 338:1428–1437, 1998.
7. Fitzgerald RH, et al: Advisory statement: Antibiotic prophylaxis for dental patients with total joint replacements. American Dental Association; American Academy of Orthopaedic Surgeons. J Am Dent Assoc 128:1004–1007, 1997.
8. Holroyd SV, Wynn RL, Requa-Clark B (eds): Clinical Pharmacology in Dental Practice, 4th ed. St. Louis, Mosby, 1988.
9. Ifudu O: Care of patients undergoing hemodialysis. N Engl J Med 339:1054–1062, 1998.
10. Kilmartin C, Munroe CO: Cardiovascular diseases and the dental patient. J Can Dent Assoc 6:513–518, 1986.
11. Krasner AS: Glucocorticoid-induced adrenal insufficiency. JAMA 282:671, 1999.
12. Kupp MA, Chatton MJ: Current Medical Diagnosis and Treatment. Norwalk, CT, Appleton & Lange, 1983.
13. Lind SE: The bleeding time does not predict surgical bleeding. Blood 77:2547–2552, 1991.
14. Little JW: Managing dental patients with joint prostheses. J Am Dent Assoc 125:1374–1379, 1994.
15. Little JW, Falace DA: Dental Management of the Medically Compromised Patient, 6th ed. St. Louis, Mosby, 2002.
16. Magnac C, et al: Platelet antibodies in serum of patients with human immunodeficiency virus (HIV) infection. AIDS Res Hum Retroviruses 6:1443–1449, 1990.
17. Malamed SF, Robbins KS: Medical Emergencies in the Dental Office, 5th ed. St. Louis, Yearbook Medical Pub, 2000.
18. Sams DR, et al: Managing the dental patient with sickle cell anemia: A review of the literature. Pediatr Dent 12:317–320, 1990.
19. Smith HB, et al: Dental management of patients with sickle cell disorders. J Am Dent Assoc 114:85, 1987.
20. Sonis ST, et al: Principles and Practice of Oral Medicine, 2nd ed. Philadelphia, W.B. Saunders, 1995.
21. Spolnik KJ: Dental radiographic manifestations of end-stage renal disease. Dent Radiogr Photogr 54(2): 21–31, 1981.
22. Tierney LM, McPhee SJ, Papadakis MA, Schroeder SA: Current Medical Diagnosis and Treatment. Norwalk, CT, Appleton & Lange, 1993.
23. Troulis M, et al: Dental extractions in patients on oral anticoagulants: A survey of practices in North America. J Oral Maxillofac Surg 56:914, 1998.

4. ORAL PATHOLOGY

Sook-Bin Woo, D.M.D., M.M.Sc.

DEVELOPMENTAL CONDITIONS

Tooth-related Problems

1. True or false: Dental fluorosis increases pitting and porosity of the enamel and therefore increases the risk of dental caries.

It is true that fluorosis causes increased pitting and porosity because fluoride increases retention of amelogenin, which results in hypomineralization of the enamel. This causes an unesthetic chalky white or even brown discoloration of the enamel, which may be pitted and fissured. However, because this enamel is more caries-resistant, the risk of dental caries is lower.

2. Name the three main forms of amelogenesis imperfecta.

Hypoplastic form: inadequate deposition of enamel matrix. Whatever is deposited calcifies normally. The teeth have thin enamel that may be pitted.

Hypomaturation form: adequate deposition of enamel, but the enamel crystal does not mature normally. The result is soft pigmented enamel that chips easily.

Hypocalcified form: inadequate mineralization. The result is enamel that gets lost a few years after eruption.

3. Describe the two main types of dentin dysplasia.

Radicular type. The roots are poorly-formed, short and distorted with poorly formed pulp chambers. Periapical lucencies develop early and teeth exfoliate prematurely.

Coronal type. The crowns contain large pulp chambers that extend into the root. Pulp stones often develop.

4. Describe the different types of dentinogenesis imperfecta.

Dentinogenesis imperfecta (DI) causes the teeth to be opalescent and affects both the primary and permanent dentition. The teeth are bluish-brown and translucent. Enamel is lost early, and the exposed dentine undergoes rapid attrition.

Type I	DI with osteogenesis imperfecta
Type II	DI without osteogenesis imperfecta
Type III	Brandywine type, which also occurs in the absence of osteogenesis imperfecta but is clustered within a racial isolate in Maryland. This is likely a variant of type II disease. In addition to classic findings of DI, radiographs may exhibit multiple periapical radiolucencies, and large pulp chambers may lead to multiple pulp exposures.

5. What is the difference between fusion and concrescence? Twinning and gemination?

Fusion is a more complete process than concrescence and may involve either (1) fusion of the entire length of two teeth (enamel, dentin, and cementum) to form one large tooth, with one less tooth in the arch, or (2) fusion of the root only (dentin and cementum) with the maintenance of two clinical crowns. Concrescence involves fusion of cementum only.

Twinning is more complete than gemination and results in the formation of two separate teeth from one tooth bud (one extra tooth in the arch). In gemination, separation is attempted, but the two teeth share the same root canal.

6. What is a Turner's tooth?

A Turner's tooth is a solitary, usually permanent tooth with signs of enamel hypoplasia or hypocalcification. This phenomenon is caused by trauma or infection in the overlying deciduous tooth that damages the ameloblasts of the underlying tooth bud and thus leads to localized enamel hypoplasia or hypocalcification.

7. What are "bull teeth"?

Bull teeth, also known as taurodonts, have long anatomic crowns, large pulp chambers, and short roots, resembling teeth found in bulls. They are most dramatic in permanent molars but may affect teeth in either dentition. They occur more frequently in certain syndromes, such as Klinefelter syndrome.

8. What is the difference between dens evaginatus and dens invaginatus?

Dens evaginatus occurs primarily in persons of mongoloid descent and affects the premolars. **Evagination** of the layers of the tooth germ results in the formation of a tubercle that arises from the occlusal surface and consists of enamel, dentin, and pulp tissue. This tubercle tends to break when it occludes with the opposing dentition and may result in pulp exposure and subsequent pulp necrosis. Dens invaginatus occurs mainly in maxillary lateral incisors and ranges in severity from an accentuated lingual pit to a "dens in dente." This phenomenon is caused by **invagination** of the layers of the tooth germ. Food becomes trapped in the pit, and caries begin early.

9. What are the causes of generalized intrinsic discoloration of teeth?

Amelogenesis imperfecta	Fluorosis	Congenital porphyria
Dentinogenesis imperfecta	Rh incompatibility	Biliary atresia
Tetracycline staining		

10. Why do teeth discolor from ingestion of tetracycline during odontogenesis?

Tetracycline binds with the calcium component of bones and teeth and is deposited at sites of active mineralization, causing a yellow-brown endogenous pigmentation of the hard tissues. Because teeth do not turn over like some bone tissues, this stain becomes a permanent "label" that fluoresces under ultraviolet light.

11. Which teeth are most commonly missing congenitally?

Third molars, maxillary lateral incisors, and second premolars.

12. What conditions are associated with multiple supernumerary teeth?

Gardner's syndrome and cleidocranial dysplasia are two important ones.

13. What are the most common sites for supernumerary teeth?

Midline of the maxilla (mesiodens), posterior maxilla (fourth molar or paramolar), and mandibular bicuspid areas.

Intrabony Lesions

14. A 40-year-old African-American woman presents with multiple radiolucencies and radiopacities. What is the diagnosis?

The African-American population is prone to developing benign fibroosseous lesions of various kinds. They range from localized lesions, such as periapical cemental dysplasia involving one tooth (usually mandibular anterior), to florid cementoosseous dysplasia, involving all four quadrants. The second condition also has been referred to as familial gigantiform cementoma, multiple enostoses, and sclerotic cemental masses.

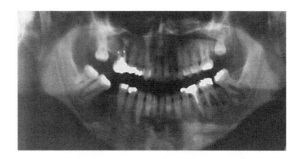

Florid cementoosseous dysplasia affecting at least three quadrants.

15. Are fibrous dysplasias of bone premalignant lesions?

Fibrous dysplasia, a developmental malformation of bone, is of unknown etiology and is not premalignant. The monostotic form often affects the maxilla unilaterally. The polyostotic form is associated with various other abnormalities, such as skin pigmentations and endocrine dysfunction (Albright and Jaffe-Lichtenstein syndromes). Cherubism, which used to be termed familial fibrous dysplasia, is probably not a form of fibrous dysplasia. In the past, fibrous dysplasia was treated with radiation, which sometimes caused the development of osteosarcoma.

16. True or false: The globulomaxillary cyst is a fissural cyst.

False. Historically, the globulomaxillary cyst was classified as a nonodontogenic or fissural cyst thought to result from enclavement of epithelial rests along the line of fusion between the lateral maxillary and nasomedial processes. Current thinking puts it in the category of odontogenic cysts, probably of developmental origin and possibly related to the development of the lateral incisor or canine. The two embryonic processes mentioned above do not fuse. The fold between them fills in and becomes erased by mesodermal invasion so that there is no opportunity for trapping of epithelial rests. This cyst occurs between the roots of the maxillary lateral incisor and cuspid, both of which are vital.

17. True or false: The median palatal cyst is a true fissural cyst.

True. The epithelium of this intrabony cyst arises from proliferation of entrapped epithelium when the right and left palatal shelves fuse in the midline. This should be distinguished from a nasopalatine duct cyst, which arises from remnants of the duct in the area of the nasopalatine foramen. The soft tissue counterpart, which also occurs in the midline of the palate and is known as the palatal cyst of the newborn (Epstein's pearl), is congenital and exteriorizes on its own.

18. A neonate presents with a few white nodules on the mandibular alveolar ridge. What are they?

They are most likely dental lamina cysts of the newborn (Bohn's nodules). The epithelium of these cysts arises from remnants of dental lamina on the alveolar ridge after odontogenesis. Dental lamina cysts of the newborn tend to involute and do not require treatment.

19. A boy presents to the dental clinic with multiple jaw cysts and a history of jaw cysts in other family members. What syndrome does he most likely have?

The boy most likely has the bifid rib-basal cell nevus syndrome, which is inherited as an autosomal dominant trait. The cysts are odontogenic keratocysts, which have a higher incidence of recurrence than other odontogenic cysts. Other findings include palmar pitting, palmar and plantar keratosis, calcification of the falx cerebri, hypertelorism, ovarian tumors, and neurologic manifestations such as mental retardation and medulloblastomas.

20. Are all jaw cysts that produce keratin considered odontogenic keratocysts?

No. The odontogenic keratocyst is a specific histologic entity. The epithelial lining exhibits corrugated **parakeratosis**, uniform thinness (unless altered by inflammation), and palisading of the basal cell nuclei. The recurrence rate is high, and the condition is associated with the basal cell carcinoma-bifid rib (Gorlin-Goltz) syndrome. Odontogenic cysts that produce **orthokeratin** do not show the basal cell nuclei changes, do not have the same tendency to recur, and are not associated with the syndrome. However, some pathologists use the term "orthokeratinized variant" after odontogenic keratocyst to denote the difference, which often causes confusion. The preferred term is orthokeratinizing odontogenic cyst. The clinical differences are important.

21. What neoplasms may arise in a dentigerous cyst?

Ameloblastoma, mucoepidermoid carcinoma, and squamous cell carcinoma may arise in a dentigerous cyst. Odontogenic tumors that may arise in a dentigerous relationship, although not within a dentigerous cyst, include adenomatoid odontogenic tumor and calcifying epithelial odontogenic tumor (Pindborg tumor).

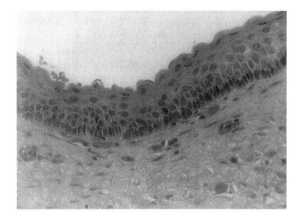

Classic parakeratinized odontogenic keratocyst.

22. What is the difference between a lateral radicular cyst and a lateral periodontal cyst?

A lateral radicular cyst is an **inflammatory** cyst in which the epithelium is derived from rests of Malassez (like a periapical or apical radicular cyst). It is in a lateral rather than an apical location because the inflammatory stimulus is emanating from a lateral canal. The associated tooth is always nonvital. The lateral periodontal cyst is a **developmental** cyst in which the epithelium probably is derived from rests of dental lamina. It is usually located between the mandibular premolars, which are vital.

23. What is the incidence of cleft lip and/or cleft palate?

Cleft lip and cleft palate should be considered as two entities: (1) cleft palate alone and (2) cleft lip with or without cleft palate. The former is more common in females and the latter in males. The incidence of cleft palate alone is 1 in 2,000–3,000 births, whereas the incidence of cleft lip with or without cleft palate is 1 in 700–1,000 births. Of all cases, 25% are cleft palate alone and 75% are cleft lip with or without cleft palate.

Soft Tissue Conditions

24. Name the organism that colonizes lesions of median rhomboid glossitis.

Candida sp. colonizes these atrophic areas on the midline dorsum of tongue, although it is unclear why this area is particularly susceptible. However, even with elimination of candidal organisms, the area of papillary atrophy persists. It was originally thought that median rhomboid glossitis was a developmental malformation, possibly caused by failure of the tuberculum impar to retract completely. However, the fact that this condition is almost never seen in childhood goes against this theory.

25. Is benign migratory glossitis ("geographic tongue") associated with any systemic conditions?

Most cases of benign migratory glossitis occur in the absence of a systemic condition, although some cases have been associated with fissured tongue. However, patients with psoriasis, especially generalized pustular psoriasis, have a higher incidence of benign migratory glossitis. There may be an association with atopy and some HLA types.

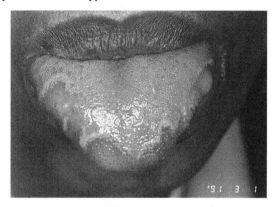

Benign migratory glossitis.

26. What predisposes to the formation of a hairy tongue?

Hyposalivation, broad-spectrum antibiotics, systemic steroids, debilitation, and oxygenating mouth rinses predispose to the formation of a hairy tongue. The "hairs" are filiform papillae with multiple layers of keratin that fail to shed adequately. The papillae are putatively colonized by chromogenic bacteria, so that the tongue may appear black, brown, or even green. It does not represent a fungal infection.

INFECTIONS

Fungal Infection

27. Discuss the two clinical forms of candidiasis.

Acute forms: pseudomembranous candidiasis (the typical type with curdy white patches, also known as thrush) and atrophic or erythematous candidiasis, often seen in HIV infection, or at corners of mouth (angular cheilitis).

Chronic forms: hyperplastic candidiasis (leukoplakia-like patches that do not wipe off easily), atrophic candidiasis (denture sore mouth), mucocutaneous candidiasis (associated with skin candidiasis and an underlying systemic condition such as an endocrinopathy).

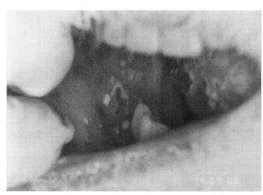

Acute pseudomembranous candidiasis.

28. What factors predispose to candidal infection?

Predisposing factors include (1) poor immune function, which may be due to age (very young and very old), malignancies, immunomodulating drugs, endocrine dysfunction, or HIV infection; (2) malnutrition; (3) antibiotics that upset the normal balance of flora; (4) dental prostheses, especially dentures; and (5) alteration in saliva flow and constituents.

29. A culture performed on an oral ulcer grows *Candida* sp. Does this mean that the patient has candidiasis?

No. Approximately one-quarter to one-third of the adult population harbors *Candida* sp. in the mouth. These persons grow the organisms on culture in the complete absence of a candidal infection.

30. How do you make a diagnosis of candidiasis?

1. **Good clinical judgment.** Pseudomembranous plaques of candidiasis usually wipe off with difficulty, leaving a raw, bleeding surface.

2. **Potassium hydroxide (KOH) preparation.** The plaque is scraped, and the scrapings are put onto a glass microscopic slide. A few drops of KOH are added, the slide is warmed over an alcohol flame for a few seconds, and a coverslip is placed over the slide. The hyphae, if present, can be seen with a microscope.

3. **Biopsy** to show hyphae penetrating the tissues (too invasive for routine use).

4. **Cultures.** Although cultures are not the ideal way to diagnose candidiasis, the quantity of candidal organisms that grow on culture correlates somewhat with clinical candidiasis. Cultures are particularly important for recalcitrant candidiasis to identify drug-resistant species.

31. What are common antifungal agents for treating oral candidiasis?

- Polyenes: nystatin (topical), amphotericin (topical, systemic)
- Imidazoles: chlortrimazole, ketoconazole
- Triazoles: fluconazole

32. True or false: Actinomycosis represents a fungal infection.

False. Actinomycetes is a gram-positive bacteria. Do not be fooled by the suffix *mycosis*.

33. What are sulphur granules?

These yellowish granules (hence the name) are seen within the pus of lesions of actinomycosis. They represent aggregates of *Actinomyces israelii*, which are invariably surrounded by neutrophils.

34. Name two opportunistic fungal diseases that often present in the orofacial region.

Aspergillosis and zygomycosis tend to infect immunocompromised hosts; the latter causes rhinocerebral infections in patients with diabetes mellitus.

35. Name two deep fungal infections that are endemic in North America.

Histoplasmosis (caused by *Histoplasma capsulatum*) is endemic in the Ohio–Mississippi basin, and coccidioidomycosis (caused by *Coccidioides immitis*) is endemic in the San Joaquin Valley in California.

Viral Infection

36. Name the five most common viruses of the Herpesviridae family that often present in the orofacial area.

Herpes simplex virus (HSV 1 and 2)   Varicella zoster virus (VZV)
Cytomegalovirus (CMV)   Epstein-Barr virus (EBV)
Human herpes virus 8 (causes Kaposi's sarcoma)

37. True or false: Antibodies against HSV-1 protect against further outbreaks of the disease.

False. The herpes viruses are unique in that they exhibit latency. Once one has been infected by HSV 1, the virus remains latent within the trigeminal ganglion for life. When conditions are favorable (for the virus, not the patient), HSV travels along nerve fibers and causes a mucocutaneous lesion at a peripheral site, such as a cold sore on the lip. A positive antibody titer (IgG) indicates that the patient has been previously exposed, and at the time of reactivation the titer may rise.

38. How do you differentiate between recurrent aphthous ulcers and recurrent herpetic ulcers?

Clinically, recurrent aphthous ulcers (minor) occur only on the nonkeratinized mucosae of the labial mucosa, buccal mucosa, sulci, ventral tongue, soft palate, and faucial pillars. Recurrent herpetic ulcers occur on the vermilion border of the lips (cold sores or fever blisters) and on the keratinized mucosae of the palate and attached gingiva. A culture confirms the presence of virus. In immunocompromised hosts, however, recurrent herpetic lesions may occur on both the keratinized and nonkeratinized mucosae and may mimic aphthous ulcers.

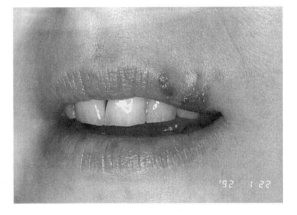

Recurrent herpes labialis (cold sores or fever blisters).

39. An elderly patient with long-standing rheumatoid arthritis presents with a history of upper respiratory tract infection, ulcers of the right hard palate, right facial weakness, and vertigo. What does he have?

Herpes zoster infection, which typically is unilateral. The patient also has Ramsay-Hunt syndrome, which is caused by infection of cranial nerves VII and VIII with herpes zoster, leading to facial paralysis, tinnitus, deafness, and vertigo.

40. What lesions associated with the Epstein-Barr virus may present in the orofacial region?

Infectious mononucleosis	Nasopharyngeal carcinoma
Burkitt's lymphoma (African type)	Hairy leukoplakia

41. How does infectious mononucleosis present in the mouth?

Infectious mononucleosis usually presents as multiple, painful, punctate ulcers of the posterior hard palate and soft palate in young adults or adolescents. It is often associated with regional lymphadenopathy and constitutional signs of a viral illness.

42. What oral lesions have been associated with infection by human papillomavirus (HPV)?

- Focal epithelial hyperplasia (Heck's disease)
- Oral condylomas
- Verruca vulgaris
- Squamous papilloma
- Some squamous cell and verrucous carcinomas
- Some verrucous leukoplakias

The benign conditions are usually associated with HPV 6 and 11; the malignant ones with HPV 16 and 18. Heck's disease is associated with HPV-13 and HPV-32.

43. What oral conditions does Coxsackievirus cause?

Herpangina and hand-foot-mouth disease are caused by the type A Coxsackievirus and generally affect children, who then develop oral ulcers associated with an upper respiratory tract viral prodrome.

44. What are Koplik spots?

Koplik spots are early manifestations of measles or rubeola (hence they also are called herald spots). They are 1–2-mm, yellow-white, necrotic ulcers with surrounding erythema that occur on the buccal mucosa, usually a few days before the body rash of measles is seen. Koplik spots are not seen in German measles.

Other Infections

45. What are the organisms responsible for noma?

Noma, which is a gangrenous stomatitis resulting in severe destruction of the orofacial tissues, is usually encountered in areas where malnutrition is rampant. The bacteria are similar to those associated with acute necrotizing ulcerative gingivitis, namely, spirochetes and fusiform bacteria. It is sometimes seen in patients with AIDS.

46. What are the oral findings in syphilis?

Primary: oral chancre
Secondary: mucous patches, condyloma lata
Tertiary: gumma, glossitis
Congenital: enamel hypoplasia, mulberry molars, notched incisors

47. What is a granuloma?

Strictly speaking, a granuloma is a collection of epithelioid histiocytes that often is associated with multinucleated giant cells like the Langhans-type giant cells seen in granulomas of tuberculosis. Many infectious agents, including fungi (such as *Histoplasma* spp.) and those causing tertiary syphilis and cat-scratch disease, can produce granulomatous reactions. Foreign body reactions are often granulomatous. Some granulomatous diseases, such as orofacial granulomatosa, Crohn's disease, and sarcoidosis, are of unclear etiology.

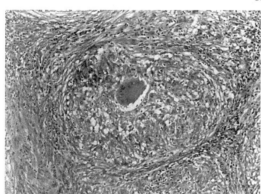

Tuberculous granuloma with Langhans giant cell.

48. What are Langhans cells?

Langhans cells are multinucleated giant cells seen in granulomas, usually those caused by *Mycobacterium tuberculosis*. Their nuclei have a characteristic horseshoe distribution. Do not confuse them with Langerhans cells, which are antigen-processing cells.

REACTIVE, HYPERSENSITIVITY, AND AUTOIMMUNE CONDITIONS

Intrabony and Dental Tissues

49. True or false: The periapical granuloma is composed of a collection of histiocytes, that is, a true granuloma.

False. The periapical granuloma is a tumorlike (-oma) proliferation of granulation tissue found around the apex of a nonvital tooth. It is associated with chronic inflammation from pulp devitalization. The inflammation can stimulate proliferation of the epithelial rests of Malassez to form a cyst, either apical radicular or periapical.

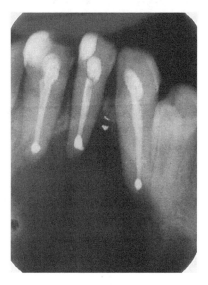

Apical radicular cyst.

50. What is condensing osteitis?

Condensing osteitis, a relatively common condition, manifests as an area of radiopacity in the bone, usually adjacent to a tooth that has a large restoration or endodontic therapy, although occasionally it may lie adjacent to what appears to be a sound tooth. It is asymptomatic. Histologically, condensing osteitis consists of dense bone with little or no inflammation. It probably arises as a bony reaction to a low-grade inflammatory stimulus from the adjacent tooth. It also has been referred to as idiopathic osteosclerosis and bone scar, but these two terms should be used for similar lesions unassociated with teeth.

51. What are the etiologic differences among the wearing down of teeth caused by attrition, abrasion, erosion, and abfraction?

Attrition: tooth-to-tooth contact

Abrasion: a foreign object-to-tooth contact, e.g., toothbrush bristles, bobby pins, nails

Erosion: a chemical agent-to-tooth contact, e.g., lemon juice, gastric juices

Abfraction: occlusal stress leading to excessive tensile forces, which cause damage to enamel at cervical areas of teeth

Soft Tissue Conditions

52. Aphthous ulcers may be associated with certain systemic conditions. Name them.

Iron, folate or vitamin B12 deficiency	Hypersensitivity to food or medications
Inflammatory bowel disease	HIV infection
Behçet's disease	Conditions predisposing to neutropenia

53. True or false: An aphthous ulcer is the same as a traumatic ulcer.

False but with reservations. A traumatic ulcer is the most common form of oral ulcer and, as its name suggests, occurs at the site of trauma such as the buccal mucosa, lateral tongue, lower labial mucosa, or sulci. It follows a history of trauma such as mastication or toothbrush injury. An aphthous ulcer may occur at the same sites, but often with no history of trauma. However, patients prone to developing aphthae tend to do so after episodes of minor trauma.

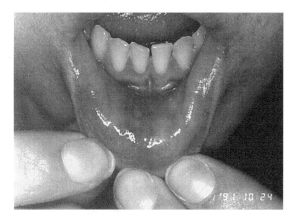

Recurrent aphthous ulcer (minor) of lower labial mucosa.

54. A child returns one day after a visit to the dentist at which several amalgam restorations were placed. He now has ulcers of the lateral tongue and buccal mucosa on the same side as the amalgams. What is your diagnosis?

Factitial injury. Children may inadvertently chew their tongues and buccal mucosae while tissues are numb from local anesthesia, because the tissues feel strange to the child. Children and parents should be advised to be on the look-out for such behavior.

55. Is the mucocele a true cyst?

It depends. The term *mucocele* refers loosely to a cystlike lesion that contains mucus and usually occurs on the lower lip or floor of the mouth. However, it may occur wherever mucus glands are present. In most cases, it is not a true cyst because it is not lined by epithelium. It is caused by escape of mucus into the connective tissue when an excretory salivary duct is traumatized. Therefore, the mucocele is lined by fibrous and granulation tissue. In a small number of cases, it is caused by distention of the excretory duct due to a distal obstruction. In such a case, the mucocele is a true cyst, because the lining is the epithelium of the duct.

56. What is the etiology of necrotizing sialometaplasia?

This painless ulcer usually develops on the hard palate but may occur wherever salivary glands are present. It represents vascular compromise and subsequent infarction of the salivary gland tissue, with reactive squamous metaplasia of the salivary duct epithelium that may mimic squamous cell carcinoma. The lesion resolves on its own.

57. Name the major denture-related findings in the oral cavity.

- Chronic atrophic candidiasis, especially of the palate (denture sore mouth)
- Papillary hyperplasia of the palatal mucosa
- Fibrous hyperplasia of the sulcus where the denture flange impinges (epulis fissuratum)
- Traumatic ulcers from overextension of flanges
- Angular cheilitis from overclosure
- Denture-base hypersensitivity reactions

58. A patient is suspected of having an allergy to denture materials. What do you recommend?
The patient should be patch-tested by an allergist or dermatologist to a panel of denture-base materials, which include both metals and products of acrylic polymerization. Usually, the lesions resolve with topical steroids.

59. What is a gum boil (parulis)?
A gum boil is an erythematous nodule usually located on the attached gingiva. It may have a yellowish center that drains pus and may be asymptomatic. The nodule consists of granulation tissue and a sinus tract that usually can be traced to the root of the underlying tooth with a thin gutta percha point. It indicates an infection of either pulpal or periodontal origin.

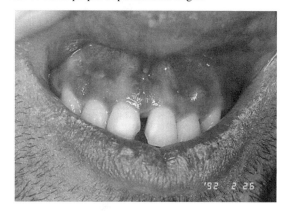

Two parulides. The one on the left is about to drain.

60. What is plasma cell gingivitis?
Plasma cell gingivitis, reported in the 1970s, presented as an intensely erythematous gingivitis and was likely due to an allergic reaction to a component of chewing gum or other allergen. It still occurs sporadically.

61. Some patients have a reaction to tartar-control toothpaste. What is the offending ingredient?
The offending ingredient is cinnamaldehyde. Susceptible patients develop burning of the mucosa and sometimes bright red gingivitis, akin to plasma cell gingivitis, after using the product. They often also have a reaction to chewing gum that contains cinnamon.

62. What is the differential diagnosis for desquamative gingivitis? What special handling procedures are necessary if you obtain a biopsy?

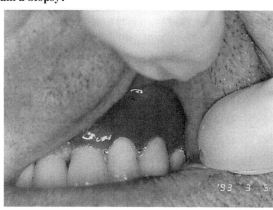

Desquamative gingivitis.

Desquamative gingivitis, which usually affects middle-aged women, is characterized by painful, red, eroded, and denuded areas of the gingiva. Definitive diagnosis requires direct immunofluorescence studies of the gingiva with various commerically available antibodies directed against autoantibodies. To preserve the integrity of immune reactants, the biopsy specimen should be split: one-half should be submitted in formalin for routine histopathology and the other half in Michel's solution or fresh on ice.

The immunofluorescence patterns show that 40% of lesions are cicatricial pemphigoid, 40% are lichenoid reactions or lichen planus, 10% have nonspecific immunoreactivity, and 10% are bullous pemphigoid, pemphigus vulgaris or other autoimmune conditions, such as lupus erythematosus, linear IgA disease, and epidermolysis bullosa acquisita.

63. What is the Grinspan syndrome?

As reported by Grinspan, this syndrome consists of hypertension, diabetes mellitus, and lichen planus. Current thinking suggests that the lichen planus is caused by medications that the patients take for hypertension (especially hydrochlorothiazides) and diabetes mellitus.

64. What drugs can give a lichen planus-like (lichenoid) mucosal reaction?

- Drugs for treating hypertension, such as hydrochlorothiazide, ACE inhibitors, and beta blockers
- Hypoglycemic agents, such as chlorpropamide and tolazamide
- Antiarthritic agents, such as penicillamine
- Antigout agents, such as allopurinol
- Nonsteroidal antiinflammatory drugs.

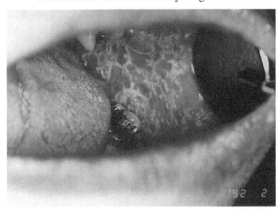

Lichenoid stomatitis associated with hydrochlorothiazide.

65. Name the drugs that can be used to treat symptomatic lichen planus.

Most of the drugs involved are immunomodulating agents. The most commonly used are corticosteroids, applied topically, injected intralesionally, or taken systemically. Hydroxychloroquine, azathioprine, cyclosporine A, and retinoics have been used with some success.

66. True or false: Dental restorations may cause lichen planus-like reactions.

True. Amalgam and composite restorations have been shown to cause a lichenoid reaction in some people in the mucosa in contact with the restoration. Replacement of the restoration leads to resolution.

67. What are the typical skin lesions of erythema mulitforme called?

Target, iris, or "bull's eye" lesions. Erythema multiforme is an acute mucocutaneous inflammatory process that may recur periodically in chronic form. It may be idiopathic but also may occur after ingestion of drugs or after a herpes simplex virus infection.

68. Name the most common factors responsible for recurrent erythema multiforme.

Herpes simplex virus reactivation and hypersensitivity to certain foods, such as benzoates. Do not expect to be able to culture herpes simplex virus from the lesions of recurrent erythema multiforme, which is a hypersensitivity reaction to some component of the virus. Usually the viral infection precedes the lesions of erythema multiforme.

69. What is Stevens-Johnson syndrome?

Stevens-Johnson syndrome is a severe form of erythema multiforme with extensive involvement of the mucous membranes of the oral cavity, eyes, genitalia, and occasionally the upper gastrointestinal and respiratory tracts. Desquamation and ulceration of the lips, with crusting, is usually dramatic. Typical target lesions may be seen on the skin.

70. What is the difference between pemphigus and pemphigoid?

Both are autoimmune, vesiculobullous diseases. In pemphigus (usually vulgaris), autoantibodies attack desmosomal plaques of the epithelial cells, leading to acantholysis and formation of an intraepithelial bulla. In pemphigoid (usually mucous membrane), autoantibodies attack the junction between the epithelium and connective tissue, leading to the formation of a subepithelial bulla.

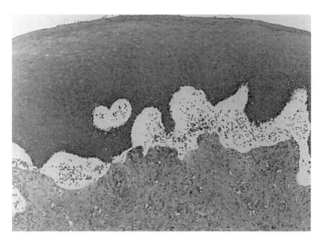

Subepithelial bulla formation in mucous membrane pemphigoid.

71. What two forms of pemphigoid involve the oral cavity?

Mucous membrane pemphigoid and bullous pemphigoid. These autoimmune vesiculobullous diseases have antigens located in the lamina lucida of the basement membrane. Mucous membrane pemphigoid presents primarily with oral mucosal and ocular lesions and occasionally with skin lesions, whereas bullous pemphigoid presents primarily with skin lesions and occasionally with mucosal lesions. IgG and/or C3 localize at the basement membrane zone.

72. Differentiate between a Tzanck test and a Tzanck cell.

The **Tzanck test** entails direct examination of cells that may indicate a herpes simplex virus infection. The test is done by scraping the lesion (which may be a vesicle, ulcer, or crust) and smearing the debris on a slide. The slide is then stained and examined under a microscope for virally infected cells, which show multinucleation and "ground-glass" nuclei. **Tzanck cells** are acantholytic cells seen within the bulla of pemphigus vulgaris.

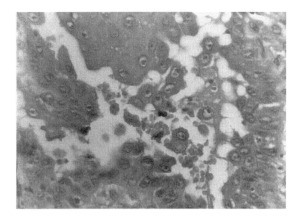

Tzanck (acantholytic) cells of pemphigus vulgaris.

73. What is the difference between systemic lupus erythematosus (SLE) and discoid lupus erythematosus (DLE)?

SLE is the prototypical multisystem autoimmune disease characterized by circulating antinuclear antibodies; the principal sites of injury are skin, joints, and kidneys. The oral mucosa is often involved, and the lesions may appear lichenoid, with white striae, and atrophic or erythematous. DLE is the limited form of the disease; most manifestations are localized to the skin and mucous membranes with no systemic involvement. DLE does not usually progress to SLE, although certain phases of SLE are clinically indistinguishable from DLE. The oral findings are similar in both.

74. Define midline lethal granuloma/midline destructive disease.

This term describes a destructive, ulcerative process, usually located in the midline of the hard palate, that may lead to palatal perforation. Although the clinical picture is dramatic and ominous, the histologic picture may be somewhat nonspecific, showing only inflammation and occasionally vasculitis. Conditions that may cause this clinical entity include fungal infections, syphilitic gummas, Wegener's granulomatosis, chronic cocaine use, and malignant neoplasms such as sinonasal lymphomas.

CHEMOTHERAPY AND HIV DISEASE

75. What are the common oral manifestations in patients who have undergone chemotherapy?

Chemotherapy can produce direct stomatotoxicity by acting on mitotically active cells in the basal cell layer of the epithelium. The mucosa becomes atrophic and, when traumatized, ulcer-

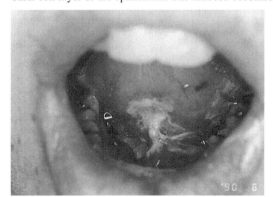

Chemotherapy-associated oral ulcerative mucositis.

ates. The chemotherapeutic agents also act on other rapidly dividing cells in the body, such as hematopoietic tissues. The results are neutropenia, anemia, and thrombocytopenia. Neutropenia may have an indirect stomatotoxic effect by allowing oral bacteria to colonize the ulcers. Usually, these ulcers develop in the period of profound neutropenia and resolve when neutrophils reappear in the blood circulation. In addition, patients are at increased risk for developing oral candidiasis, oral herpetic lesions, and deep fungal infections. Thrombocytopenia may cause oral petechiae, ecchymoses, and hematomas, especially at sites of trauma.

76. A patient who underwent cancer chemotherapy now has recurrent intraoral herpetic lesions but no history of cold sores or fever blisters. Is this likely?

Yes. Many people have been exposed to herpes simplex virus without their knowledge and are completely asymptomatic. The virus becomes latent within sensory ganglia and reactivates to give rise to recurrent or recrudescent herpetic lesions. The prevalence of people who have been exposed to HSV increases with age.

77. What are the complications of leukemia in the oral cavity, aside from those associated with chemotherapy?

Leukemic infiltration of the bone marrow leads to reduced production of functional components of the marrow. Granulocytopenia results in more frequent and more aggressive odontogenic infections; thrombocytopenia results in petechiae, ecchymoses, and hematomas in the oral cavity, which is subject to trauma from functional activities. The patient may have a more than adequate white cell count, but many of the white cells are malignant and do not necessarily function like normal white cells. In addition, some leukemias, especially acute monocytic leukemia, have a propensity to infiltrate the gingiva, causing localized or diffuse gingival enlargement.

78. A patient underwent a matched allogenic bone marrow transplantation for the treatment of leukemia. Three months later he has erosive and lichenoid lesions in his mouth. What is your diagnosis?

The likely diagnosis is chronic oral graft-vs.-host disease. The allogenic bone marrow transplant or graft contains immunocompetent cells that recognize the host cells as foreign and attack them. The oral lesions of chronic graft-vs.-host disease resemble the lesions of lichen planus.

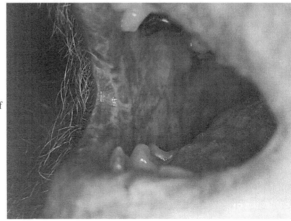

Chronic oral graft-vs.-host disease of buccal mucosa.

79. What are the effects of radiation on the oral cavity?

Short-term: oral erythema and ulcers, candidiasis, dysgeusia, parotitis, acute sialadenitis, hyposalivation

Long-term: hyposalivation, dental caries, osteoradionecrosis, epithelial atrophy and fibrosis

80. What factors predispose to osteoradionecrosis?

This necrotic process affects bone that has been in the radiation field. Predisposing factors include high total dose of radiation (especially if > 6,500 cGy), presence of odontogenic infection (such as periapical pathosis and periodontal disease), trauma (such as extractions), and site (the mandible is less vascular and more susceptible than the maxilla).

81. What is the basic cause of osteoradionecrosis?

The breakdown of hypocellular, hypovascular, and hypoxic tissue readily results in a chronic, nonhealing wound containing sequestra that can be secondarily infected.

82. What are the common oral manifestations of HIV infection?

Soft tissue: candidiasis, recurrent herpetic infections, deep fungal infections, aphthous ulcers, hairy leukoplakia, viral warts, acute necrotizing stomatitis

Periodontium: nonspecific gingivitis, acute necrotizing ulcerative gingivitis, severe and rapidly destructive periodontal disease, often with unusual pathogens

Tumors: Kaposi's sarcoma, B-cell lymphoma, squamous cell carcinoma

83. A patient who tested positive for HIV antibodies presents with a CD4 count of 150 but has never had an opportunistic infection or been symptomatic. Does he have AIDS?

Yes. By the CDC definition (February 1993), patients with CD4 counts below 200 are considered to have AIDS.

84. True or false: Like other leukoplakias, hairy leukoplakia has a tendency to progress to malignancy.

False. Hairy leukoplakia is associated with EBV infection and usually a superimposed hyperplastic candidiasis. However, patients infected with HIV are more susceptible to oral cancer in general.

85. Are HIV-associated aphthous ulcers similar to recurrent major aphthae?

Yes. They tend to be greater than 1 cm, persist for long periods (weeks to months), and are difficult to treat. They may be associated with neutropenia.

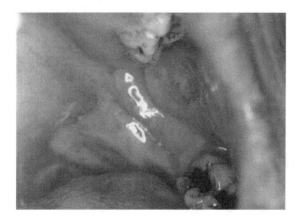

HIV-associated aphthous ulcers of the soft palate and oropharynx.

86. Should HIV-associated aphthous ulcers be routinely cultured?

Yes. Often the culture is positive for HSV or even CMV, and the patient needs to be treated appropriately.

87. True or false: Kaposi's sarcoma (KS) is seen equally in the different population risk groups.

False. Over 90% of the epidemic cases of KS are diagnosed in homosexual or bisexual men. KS is an AIDS-defining lesion that is seen much less frequently in the other risk groups for HIV infection. It is associated with Kaposi's sarcoma-associated human herpesvirus 8.

88. What management issues other than infection control and diagnosis of oral lesions should you keep in mind when treating patients with AIDS?

Hematologic dysfunction is common. HIV infection is associated with autoimmune thrombocytopenic purpura, granulocytopenia and anemia. In addition, antiretroviral agents such as zidovudine are myelosuppressive, as are drugs used as prophylaxis against *Pneumocystis carinii* pneumonia, such as trimethoprim-sulfamethoxazole. The patient's blood picture should be known before treatment, especially surgical procedures, begins.

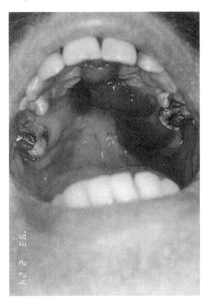

HIV-related Kaposi's sarcoma of the palate.

89. How do you treat intraoral Kaposi's sarcoma?

Surgical excision, intralesional injections of vinca alkaloids, radiation, and possibly interferon.

BENIGN NEOPLASMS AND TUMORS

Odontogenic Tumors

90. Name the benign odontogenic tumors that are purely epithelial.

- Ameloblastoma
- Calcifying epithelial odontogenic tumor (Pindborg tumor)
- Adenomatoid odontogenic tumor
- Solid variant of the calcifying odontogenic cyst
- Squamous odontogenic tumor
- Clear-cell odontogenic carcinoma

91. Which odontogenic tumor is associated with amyloid production? With ghost cells?

Calcifying epithelial odontogenic tumor (Pindborg tumor) is associated with amyloid production; calcifying odontogenic cyst (Gorlin cyst) is associated with ghost cells.

92. Which two lesions, one in the long bones and one in the cranium, resemble the ameloblastoma?

In the long bones, adamantinoma; in the cranium, craniopharyngioma.

93. True or false: All forms of ameloblastoma behave aggressively and tend to recur.

False. One form of ameloblastoma, which occurs in adolescents and young adults, behaves less aggressively and has a lower tendency to recur. It is is called unicystic ameloblastoma.

94. True or false: Because ameloblastoma is so aggressive, it can be considered a malignancy.

False. Ameloblastoma is a locally destructive lesion that has no tendency to metastasize. However, it has two malignant counterparts: ameloblastic carcinoma and malignant ameloblastoma.

95. To which teeth are cementoblastomas usually attached?

The mandibular permanent molars.

96. Name two odontogenic tumors that produce primarily mesenchymal tissues.

Odontogenic fibroma and odontogenic myxoma.

97. An adolescent presents with a mandibular radiolucency with areas that histologically resemble ameloblastoma as well as dental papilla. What is your diagnosis?

The diagnosis is ameloblastic fibroma, one of the rare odontogenic tumors that has both a neoplastic epithelial and mesenchymal component.

Fibroosseous Tumors

98. True or false: Ossifying fibromas arise from bone-producing cells, and cementifying fibromas are odontogenic in origin.

In real life and real pathology, the line of demarcation between the two is not so clear. They are clinically indistinguishable. Histologically, although pure ossifying and pure cementifying fibromas exist, it is much more common to see a mixture of bone/osteoid and cementum in any given lesion, with either predominating or in equal proportions. Many pathologists use the term cemento-ossifying fibroma as a unifying concept. The cell of origin is likely to be a mesenchymal cell in the periodontal ligament that is capable of producing either bone or cementum, therefore duplicating the two anchoring sites for Sharpey's fibers. From that point of view, both are odontogenic in origin.

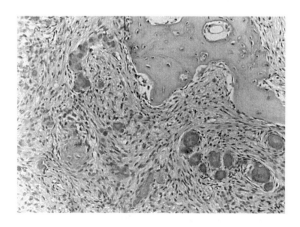

Central cementoossifying fibroma with round globules of cementum and trabeculae of osteoid.

99. Is it possible to distinguish histologically between fibrous dysplasia and central ossifying fibroma?

No. The clinical and radiographic findings are the most important for differentiating between the two. Fibrous dysplasia tends to occur in the maxilla of young people and presents as a poorly defined radiolucent or radiopaque area that is nonencapsulated. The radiographic appearance has been described as "ground glass." The central ossifying fibroma is a well-demarcated radiolucency, often with a distinct border, and may contain areas of radiopacity within the lesion. It is more common in the mandible.

Soft Tissue Tumors

100. True or false: Fibroma of the oral cavity is a true neoplasm.

False. As its name suggests, fibroma of the oral cavity is a tumor ("-oma") composed of fibrous tissue. It tends to occur as a result of trauma and therefore usually presents on the buccal mucosa, lower labial mucosa, and lateral tongue. It is nonencapsulated and grows as long as the inciting factor, such as trauma, is present. By Willis's definition of neoplasm ("new growth"), the growth, once established, continues in an excessive manner even after cessation of the stimuli that first evoked the change. Therefore it is not a true neoplasm. Some pathologists prefer the term *fibrous hyperplasia* or fibroepithelial polyp rather than fibroma because it more accurately reflects its nature. The pathogenesis is similar to that of fibrous hyperplasias caused by poorly fitting dentures.

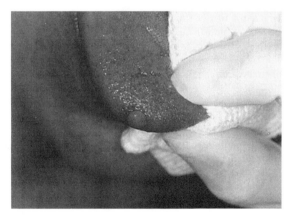

Fibroma of tongue.

101. What are verocay bodies?

Verocay bodies consist of amorphous-looking, eosinophilic material that forms between parallel groups of nuclei in the schwannoma. They actually represent duplicated basement membrane produced by Schwann cells and are an important component of Antoni A tissue.

102. What is the cell of origin of the granular cell tumor? How is it different from the cell of origin of the congenital epulis of the newborn?

The cell of origin of the granular cell tumor is probably a neural cell, such as the Schwann cell. This tumor used to be called the granular cell myoblastoma because it was believed that the cell of origin was a myocyte. The cell appears granular because it contains many lysosomes. By light microscopy, these cells resemble cells of the congenital epulis of the newborn. Whereas the granular cell tumor stains for S-100 protein, a marker for neural tissues, among others, the congenital epulis does not.

103. A patient presents with multiple neuromas of the lips and tongue. What do you suspect?

The patient probably has multiple endocrine neoplasia type III, which is inherited as an autosomal dominant condition. Patients also have pheochromocytomas, café-au-lait macules, neurofibromas of the skin, and medullary carcinoma of the thyroid. Recognition of the oral findings may lead to early diagnosis of the thyroid carcinoma.

104. What are venous lakes?

Venous lakes or varices are purplish-blue nodules or papules, often present on the lips of older people, that represent dilated venules.

105. What is the most common benign salivary gland tumor?

Pleomorphic adenoma.

106. Why is pleomorphic adenoma sometimes called the benign "mixed tumor"?

Pleomorphic adenoma is called a "mixed tumor" because histologically it may have a mixture of both epithelial and connective tissue components. The tumor arises from an epithelial reserve cell. The connective tissue components may be prominent because one of the cells responsible for the tumor is the myoepithelial cell, which, as its name suggests, has properties of both epithelial and connective tissue. This cell is responsible for the areas of cartilage and bone formation as well as for the myxoid nature of many "mixed tumors." In addition, there are areas of epithelial cell proliferation in the form of ducts, islands, and sheets of cells.

107. What is the brown tumor?

The brown tumor is histologically a central giant-cell granuloma associated with hyperparathyroidism. It appears brown when excised because it is a highly vascular lesion. Because it is indistinguishable from banal central giant-cell granuloma, all patients diagnosed with central giant-cell granuloma should have their serum calcium levels checked.

MALIGNANT NEOPLASMS

108. What percentage of the population has leukoplakia? What percentage of leukoplakias have dysplasia or carcinoma when first biopsied compared with erythroplakias?

Leukoplakia occurs in 3–4% of the population, and 15–20% of leukoplakias have dysplasia or carcinoma at the time of biopsy, whereas 90% of erythroplakias show such changes at the time of biopsy.

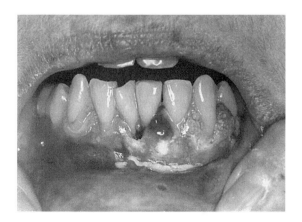

Squamous cell carcinoma presenting as leukoplakia with erythematous and verrucous areas.

109. What is proliferative verrucous leukoplakia?
It is a clinically aggressive and progressive form of leukoplakia with a higher rate of malignant transformation than banal leukoplakia.

110. What is the prevalence of oral cancer in the United States? Which country in the world has the highest prevalence of oral cancer?
Oral cancer accounts for 3% of all cancers in the United States if one includes oropharyngeal lesions. India has the highest prevalence of oral cancer, which is the most common cancer in that country and is related to the use of areca nut and tobacco products.

111. What are the risk factors for oral cancer?
- Tobacco products
- Alcohol (especially in conjunction with smoking)
- Areca nut products (especially in East Indians and some Southeast Asian cultures)
- Sunlight (especially for cancer of the lip in men)
- Plummer-Vinson syndrome
- History of submucous fibrosis
- Immunosuppression
- History of oral cancer or other cancer
- Preexisting oral mucosal dysplasia
- Age

112. What do snuff-associated lesions look like?
At the site where the snuff is placed (usually the sulcus), the mucosa is whitened with a translucent hue, and linear white ridges run parallel to the sulcus.

113. What is the difference in prognosis between a squamous cell carcinoma and a verrucous carcinoma?
Approximately one-half of squamous cell carcinomas have metastasized at the time of diagnosis. The larger they are, the more likely that metastases will develop. Verrucous carcinomas do not tend to metastasize despite the rather large size of some lesions; they are locally aggressive lesions. Whereas many squamous cell carcinomas are radiosensitive, verrucous carcinomas have been reported to become aggressive and histologically anaplastic when treated with radiation.

114. What is a "rodent ulcer"?
A rodent ulcer refers to a basal cell carcinoma that, despite its low tendency to metastasize, erodes through adjacent tissues like the gnawing of a rodent and through persistence may cause destruction of the facial complex.

115. What are the three most common intraoral malignant salivary gland tumors?
Mucoepidermoid carcinoma, polymorphous low-grade adenocarcinoma, and adenoid cystic carcinoma.

116. Which two salivary gland tumors often show perineural invasion (neurotropism)?
Adenoid cystic carcinoma and polymorphous low-grade adenocarcinoma. However, any malignancy (particularly carcinomas) can show perineural invasion.

117. True or false: Myoepithelial sialadenitis (formerly known as benign lymphoepithelial lesion) of Sjögren's syndrome is an innocuous autoimmune sialadenitis.
False. The "benign" lymphoepithelial lesion is not so benign. Many experts believe that these lesions are premalignant. Affected patients have a higher incidence of lymphoma than the general population.

118. A patient with Sjögren's syndrome is referred for a labial salivary gland biopsy to identify a myoepithelial sialadenitis. Does this sound right?

No. The myoepithelial sialadenitis of Sjögren's syndrome is found in the major glands, mainly the parotid, especially if parotid enlargement is present. A labial salivary gland biopsy will show an autoimmune sialadenitis characterized by lymphocytic infiltrates that form foci. The more foci, the more likely the diagnosis of an autoimmune sialadenitis; foci are less specific than myoepithelial sialadenitis.

119. Do lymphomas of the oral cavity occur outside Waldeyer's ring?

Yes. Oral lymphomas are most common in Waldeyer's ring, but they may occur in the palate (a condition formerly described as lymphoproliferative disease of the palate), buccal mucosa, tongue, floor of the mouth, and retromolar areas. Not infrequently they are also primary lesions in the jaw bones.

120. What does a monoclonal plasma cell proliferation mean?

Plasma cells produce immunoglobulin that contains heavy and light chains. Each plasma cell and its progeny produce either kappa or lambda light chains. A group of plasma cells that produces only kappa or lambda light chains but not both is most likely due to a proliferation of a single malignant clone of plasma cells, such as a plasmacytoma or multiple myeloma. The presence of both light chains in a plasma cell proliferation is more in keeping with a polyclonal proliferation, which characterizes inflammatory lesions.

121. Name the different epidemiologic forms of Kaposi's sarcoma.

1. Classic or European form: usually Eastern European men (often Jewish); multiple red papules on the lower extremities, with rare visceral involvement and a more indolent course.

2. Endemic or African form: young men or children in equatorial Africa; frequent visceral involvement that may be fulminant.

3. Epidemic form: HIV-associated; may be widely disseminated to mucocutaneous and visceral sites; variable course.

4. Renal transplant-associated form: patients who have undergone renal transplantation with immunosuppressive therapy; lesions usually regress when immunosuppressive therapy is discontinued.

122. A patient has a suspected metastatic tumor to the mandible. What are the likely primary tumors?

- Lung
- Breast
- Prostate
- Kidney
- Gastrointestinal tract
- Skin
- Thyroid

123. True or false: Osteosarcoma of the jaws occurs in younger patients more often than osteosarcoma of the long bones.

False. Patients with osteosarcoma of the jaws are 1–2 decades older than patients with osteosarcoma of the long bones.

124. What conditions predispose to osteosarcoma?

Many cases of osteosarcoma in young adults occur de novo. However, there are well-documented cases of osteosarcoma in association with Paget's disease, chronic osteomyelitis, a history of retinoblastoma, and prior radiation to the bone for fibrous dysplasia.

NONVASCULAR PIGMENTED LESIONS

125. What drugs can cause mucosal melanosis?

- Oral contraceptives
- Antimalarial agents (e.g., hydroxychloroquin)
- Minocycline
- Zidovudine (possible)
- Methyldopa

126. Why does heavy metal poisoning primarily cause staining of the gingiva?

Heavy metals such as lead, bismuth, and silver may cause a grayish-black line to appear on the gingival margins, especially in patients with poor oral hygiene. Plaque bacteria can produce hydrogen sulfide, which combines with the heavy metals to form heavy metal sulfides that are usually black.

127. What can cause mucosal melanosis?

Benign: physiologic pigmentation, postinflammatory hyperpigmentation (especially in dark-skinned people), oral melanotic macule, smoking, mucosal nevus, melanoacanthosis

Malignant: melanoma

Systemic conditions: Peutz-Jegher's syndrome, Albright's syndrome, Addison's disease, neurofibromatosis, drug ingestion

128. What are the different forms of oral melanocytic nevi?

Intramucosal nevus: tends to be elevated, papular or nodular

Junctional nevus: tends to be macular

Compound nevus: tends to be papular or nodular

Blue nevus: tends to be macular

129. What is the most common site for oral melanoma?

Hard palate.

130. What is the difference between a melanocyte and a melanophage?

A melanocyte is a neuroectodermally derived dendritic cell that contains the intracellular apparatus to manufacture melanin. A melanophage is a macrophage that has phagocytosed melanin pigment and therefore can look like a melanocyte because it contains melanin. However, it lacks the enzymes to produce melanin.

METABOLIC LESIONS ASSOCIATED WITH SYSTEMIC DISEASE

131. What are the three presentations of Langerhans cell disease (histiocytosis X)?

Chronic localized disease: eosinophilic granuloma; usually in adults.

Chronic disseminated disease: limited to a few organ systems in adults. Hand-Schuller-Christian disease is a well-recognized form, characterized by exophthalmos; diabetes insipidus and bony lesions; sometimes with skin and visceral involvement.

Acute disseminated disease: Letterer-Siwe disease in children; widespread involvement of multiple organ systems, especially skin; usually runs a rapidly progressive, often fatal course; considered a malignancy for the most part.

132. What are Birbeck granules?

Birbeck granules are racket-shaped cytoplasmic inclusions seen in Langerhans cells of histiocytosis X.

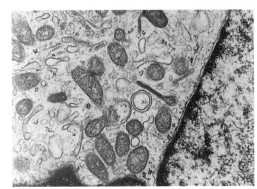

Racket-shaped Birbeck granule of Langerhans cell histiocytosis.

133. What are two common oral changes associated with pregnancy?
Gingivitis and pyogenic granuloma (epulis gravidarum).

134. An elderly man complains that his jaw seems to be getting too big for his dentures and that his hat does not fit him anymore. What do you suspect?
Paget's disease (osteitis deformans), a metabolic bone disease in which initial bone resorption is followed by haphazard bone repair, with resulting marked sclerosis. This condition may lead to narrowing of skull base foramina and neurologic deficits. The maxilla is often affected; a "cotton-wool" appearance has been described on radiographs.

135. What oral lesions are associated with gastrointestinal disease?
The most common gastrointestinal disease associated with oral signs is inflammatory bowel disease, especially Crohn's disease. Patients may manifest with cobblestoning of the mucosa and papulous growths, which represent granulomatous inflammation similar to what is seen in the gastrointestinal tract. Occasionally, patients also develop a pyostomatitis vegetans. In addition, they may have aphthouslike ulcers as well as symptoms of glossitis associated with vitamin B12 deficiency if part of the ileum has been resected for the disease. Patients with gluten-sensitive enteropathies also may present with aphthouslike ulcers.

136. What is primary and secondary Sjögren's syndrome?
Primary Sjögren's syndrome, which used to be called the sicca syndrome, consists of dry eyes (keratoconjunctivitis sicca) and dry mouth (hyposalivation) in the absence of other systemic conditions. Secondary Sjögren's syndrome consists of primary Sjögren's syndrome plus a connective-tissue disorder such as rheumatoid arthritis, systemic lupus erythematosus, or progressive systemic sclerosis. Most patients with Sjögren's syndrome have circulating autoantibodies.

137. What is the dental significance of the Sturge-Weber syndrome?
This syndrome is characterized by vascular malformations of the leptomeninges, facial skin innervated by the fifth nerve (nevus flammeus), and the corresponding ipsilateral areas in the oral mucosa and bone. Bleeding is therefore an important consideration in dental treatment. Patients also may exhibit mental retardation and seizure disorders. Treatment may include phenytoin.

DIFFERENTIAL DIAGNOSES AND GENERAL CONSIDERATIONS

Intrabony Lesions

138. What are pseudocysts of the jaw bones? Give examples.
These conditions appear cystlike on radiograph but are not true cysts. Examples include:
- Traumatic (simple) bone cyst: scallops between roots of teeth; empty at surgery
- Aneurysmal bone cyst: giant cells lining blood-filled spaces
- Static bone cyst (Stafne bone cavity): salivary gland depression beneath inferior alveolar canal
- Hematopoietic marrow defect: hematopoietic marrow

139. What is the differential diagnosis for a multiloculated radiolucency?
- Dentigerous cyst
- Odontogenic keratocyst
- Ameloblastoma
- Vascular malformations, such as hemangiomas
- Odontogenic myxoma
- Intraosseous salivary gland tumors
- Lesions that contain giant cells, such as aneurysmal bone cyst, central giant cell granuloma, and cherubism

Soft Tissue Lesions

140. What is the differential diagnosis for an upper lip nodule?

Salivary gland lesion: sialolith, benign salivary gland tumor (especially pleomorphic adenoma and canalicular adenoma), malignant salivary gland tumor

Vascular lesion: hemangioma, lymphangioma, other vascular anomaly

Neural lesion: neurofibroma, schwannoma, neuroma

Skin appendage tumors

141. What may cause diffuse swelling of the lips?

- Vascular malformations, such as lymphangiomas and hemangiomas
- Angioedema
- Hypersensitivity reactions
- Cheilitis glandularis
- Orofacial granulomatosis (e.g., Melkersson-Rosenthal syndrome)
- Crohn's disease

142. What is the differential diagnosis for a solitary gingival nodule?

The most common diagnoses are fibroma or fibrous hyperplasia, pyogenic granuloma (especially in a pregnant patient), peripheral giant cell granuloma, and peripheral ossifying fibroma (essentially a fibrous hyperplasia with metaplastic bone formation). Other less common conditions include benign and malignant tumors, especially of odontogenic origin, gingival cysts and (in elderly patients) metastatic tumors.

143. What may cause generalized overgrowth of gingival tissues?

Common causes include plaque accumulation; drugs such as phenytoin, cyclosporine A, sodium valproate, diltiazem, and nifedipine (the last two are calcium channel blockers); hormonal factors (puberty and pregnancy); Wegener's granulomatosis, orofacial granulomatosis; fibromatosis gingivae; and leukemic infiltrate.

144. A labial salivary gland biopsy is useful for diagnosis of certain systemic conditions. What are they?

- Sjögren's syndrome
- Autoimmune sialadenitis associated with connective-tissue disease
- Amyloidosis
- Sarcoidosis

145. What may cause chronic hyposalivation?

Common causes include ingestion of anticholinergic drugs, autoimmune sialadenitis (such as Sjögren's syndrome and graft-vs.-host disease), aging (although many experts believe this to be drug-related), radiation to the gland, primary neurologic dysfunction, and nutritional deficiencies (e.g., vitamin A, vitamin B, and iron).

146. Name possible causes of bilateral parotid swelling.

Mumps	Malnutrition	Lymphoepithelial
Sjögren's syndrome	Alcoholism	cysts in HIV
Radiation-induced acute parotitis	Bulimia	infection
Diabetes mellitus	Warthin's tumor	

147. What may cause depapillation of the tongue?

Vitamin B, iron and/or folate deficiency	Median rhomboid glossitis (focally)
Benign migratory glossitis (focally)	Syphilis
Plummer-Vinson syndrome	Lichen planus

148. What may cause diffuse enlargement of the tongue?

Congenital macroglossia	Angioedema
Lymphangioma	Acromegaly
Hemangioma	Trisomy 21
Neurofibromatosis	Amyloidosis
Hyperpituitarism	Hypothyroidism

149. What is the differential diagnosis of midline swellings of the floor of the mouth?

Ranula (mucocele)	Dermoid cyst
Epidermoid cyst	Oral lymphoepithelial cyst

150. What may cause diffuse white plaques in the buccal mucosa?

Cannon's white sponge nevus	Pachyonychia congenita
Leukedema	Dyskeratosis congenita
Hereditary benign intraepithelial dyskeratosis	Extensive leukoplakia (especially proliferative verrucous leukoplakia)
Candidiasis	Chronic bite injury

151. Name the conditions that may give rise to papillary lesions of the oral cavity.

Possible underlying conditions include papilloma, verruca vulgaris, condyloma, papillary hyperplasia of the palatal mucosa (denture injury), Heck's disease, oral florid papillomatosis, verrucous carcinoma, papillary squamous cell carcinoma, pyostomatitis vegetans (associated with inflammatory bowel disease), and verruciform xanthoma.

152. What lesions may occur in the oral cavity of neonates?

Lesions in the oral cavity of neonates include neuroectodermal tumor of infancy, congenital epulis of the newborn, gingival cyst of the newborn, palatal cyst of the newborn (Bohn's nodules and Epstein's pearls), lymphangiomas of the alveolar ridge, and natal teeth.

153. What may cause "burning mouth" syndrome?

This sensation usually results from mucosa that is atrophic or inflamed, which, in turn, may be caused by candidiasis (especially atrophic candidiasis of the tongue or of the palate caused by dentures), hyposalivation, allergies (especially to denture materials), and specific inflammatory mucosal lesions, such as lichen planus and migratory glossitis. However, this syndrome may also occur in the absence of any organic mucosal disease. In such cases, there is a strong association with anxiety and depression, and it represents a form of neuropathic pain.

154. What may cause oral paresthesia?

Oral paresthesia may be caused by manipulation or inflammation of a nerve or tissues around a nerve, direct damage to a nerve or tissues around a nerve, tumor impinging on or invading a nerve, primary neural tumor, and central nervous system tumor.

155. Why do lesions appear white in the oral cavity?

Lesions appear white because the epithelium has been changed, usually thickened, causing the underlying blood vessels to be deeper, as in hyperkeratosis, epithelial hyperplasia (acanthosis), and swelling of the epithelial cells (leukedema). Lesions may appear white if exudate or necrosis is present in the epithelium (candidiasis, ulcers) or if there are fewer vessels in the connective tissue (scar). Finally, a change in the intrinsic nature of the epithelial cell, such as epithelial dysplasia, may cause the mucosa to appear white (leukoplakia).

156. Why do lesions appear red in the oral cavity?

Lesions appear red because the epithelium is thinned and the underlying vessels are now closer to the surface, as in epithelial atrophy, desquamative conditions, healing ulcers, and loss of the keratin layer. Redness also may be caused by an increase in the number or dilatation of blood vessels in the connective tissue, as in inflammation. Finally, a change in the intrinsic nature of the epithelial cell, such as epithelial dysplasia, may cause the mucosa to look red (erythroplakia).

157. Distinguish macules, papules, and plaque.

A macule is a localized lesion that is not raised and is better seen than felt. It is often used to describe localized pigmented lesions, such as amalgam tattoos and melanotic macules. Both papules and plaque are broad-based, raised lesions; the papule is < 5 mm, and the plaque is larger.

158. What is the difference between a bulla and vesicle?

The bulla is usually >5 mm in size; the vesicle is <5 mm.

159. Differentiate between a hamartoma and a choristoma.

A **hamartoma** is a tumorlike growth consisting of an overgrowth of tissues that histologically appears mature and is native to the area (e.g., hemangioma, odontoma). A **choristoma** is a tumorlike growth consisting of an overgrowth of tissues that histologically appears mature but is not native to the area (e.g., cartilaginous choristoma or bony choristoma of the tongue). A hamartoma of the skin and mucosa is sometimes called a nevus (e.g., vascular, epidermal, or melanocytic nevus).

160. What are oncocytes?

Oncocytes are eosinophilic, swollen cells found in many salivary gland tumors, such as on-cocytomas and Warthin's tumor, and in oncocytic metaplasia of salivary ducts. They are swollen because they contain many mitochondria.

161. What are Russell bodies?

Russell bodies are round, eosinophilic bodies found in reactive lesions and represent glob-ules of immunoglobulin within plasma cells.

BIBLIOGRAPHY

Developmental Conditions
 1. Christ TF: The globulomaxillary cyst: An embryologic misconception. Oral Surg 30:515, 1970.
 2. Cohen DA, et al: The lateral penodontal cyst. J Periodontol 55:230, 1984.
 3. Waldron CA: Fibro-osseous lesions of the jaws. J Oral Maxillofac Surg 43:249, 1985.
 4. Wright JM: The odontogenic keratocyst: Orthokeratinized variant. Oral Surg 51:609, 1981.
Infections
 5. Dismukes WE: Azole antifungal drugs: Old and new. Ann Intern Med 109:177, 1988.
 6. Lehner T: Oral candidosis. Dent Pract Dent Res 17:209, 1967.
 7. Scully C, et al: Papillomaviruses: The current status in relation to oral disease. Oral Surg Oral Med Oral Pathol 65:526, 1988.
 8. Weathers DR, Griffin JW: Intraoral ulcerations of recurrent herpes simplex and recurrent aphthae: Two distinct clinical entities. J Am Dent Assoc 81:81, 1970.
Reactive, Hypersensitivity, and Autoimmune Conditions
 9. Bean SF, Quezada RK: Recurrent oral erythema multiforme. Clinical experience with 11 patients. JAMA 249:2810, 1983.
10. Kerr DA, McClatchey KD, Regezi JA: Idiopathic gingivostomatitis. Oral Surg Oral Med Oral Pathol 32: 402, 1971.
11. Nisengard RJ, Rogers RS III: The treatment of desquamative gingival lesions. J Periodontol 58: 167, 1987.
12. Rennie JS: Recurrent aphthous stomatitis. Br Dent J 159:361, 1985.
13. Schiodt M, Halberg P, Hentzer B: A clinical study of 32 patients with oral discoid lupus erythematosus. Int J Oral Surg 7:85, 1978.
14. Silverman S, Lozada-nur F: A prospective follow-up study of 570 patients with oral lichen planus: Per-sistence, remission, and malignant association. Oral Surg Oral Med Oral Pathol 60:30, 1985.
Chemotherapy and HIV Disease
15. Greenberg MS, et al: Oral herpes simplex infections in patients with leukemia. J Am Dent Assoc 1145: 483, 1987.

16. Libman H, Witzburg RA (eds): HIV Infection: A Clinical Manual. Boston, Little, Brown, 1993.
17. Marks RE, Johnson RP: Studies in the radiobiology of osteoradionecrosis and their clinical significance. Oral Surg Oral Med Oral Pathol 64:379, 1987.
18. Peterson DE, Elias KG, Sonis ST (eds): Head and Neck Management of the Cancer Patient. Boston, Martinus Nijhoff, 1986, p 351.
19. Schubert MM, et al: Oral manifestations of chronic graft-v.-host disease. Ann Intern Med 144:1591, 1984.

Benign Neoplasms and Tumors
20. Ellis GL, Auclair PL, Gnepp DR: Surgical Pathology of the Salivary Glands. Philadelphia, W.B. Saunders, 1991.
21. Eversole LR, Leider AS, Nelson K: Ossifying fibroma: A clinicopathologic study of 64 cases. Oral Surg Oral Med Oral Pathol 60:505-511, 1985.
22. Hansen LS, Eversole LR, Green TL, Powell NB: Clear cell odontogenic tumor—A new histologic variant with aggressive potential. Head Neck Surg 8:115, 1985.
23. Robinson L, Martinez MG: Unicystic ameloblastoma: A prognostically distinct entity. Cancer 40:2278, 1977.

Malignant Neoplasms
24. Batsakis JG: The pathology of head and neck tumors: The lymphoepithelial lesion and Sjögren's syndrome. Head Neck Surg 5:150, 1982.
25. Batsakis JG, et al: The pathology of head and neck tumors: Verrucous carcinoma. Head Neck Surg 5:29, 1982.
26. Freedman PD, Lumerman H: Lobular carcinoma of intraoral minor salivary glands. Oral Surg Oral Med Oral Pathol 56:157, 1983.
27. Hansen L, Olson J, Silverman S: Proliferative verrucous leukoplakia. Oral Surg Oral Med Oral Pathol 60:285, 1985.
28. Waldron CA, Shafer WG: Leukoplakia revisited. Cancer 36:1386, 1975.

Nonvascular Pigmented Lesions
29. Argenyi ZB, et al: Minocycline-related cutaneous hyperpigmentation as demonstrated by light microscopy, electron microscopy, and x-ray energy spectroscopy. J Cutan Pathol 14:176, 1987.
30. Buchner A, Hansen L: Pigmented nevi of the oral mucosa. Oral Surg Oral Med Oral Pathol 63:566, 1987.

Metabolic Lesions Associated with Systemic Disease
31. Beitman RG, Frost SS, Roth JLA: Oral manifestations of gastrointestinal disease. Digest Dis Sci 26:741, 1981.
32. Little JW, Falace DA: Dental Management of the Medically Compromised Patient, 6th ed. St. Louis, Mosby, 2002.
33. Writing Group of the Histiocytosis Society: Histiocytosis syndromes in children. Lancet i:208, 1987.

Differential Diagnoses and General Considerations
34. Neville BW, Damm DD, Allen CM, Bouquot JE: Oral and maxillofacial pathology, 2nd ed. Philadelphia, W.B. Saunders, 2002.
35. Regezi JA, Sciubba JJ: Oral Pathology: Clinical-Pathologic Correlations, 3rd ed. Philadelphia, W.B. Saunders, 1999.
36. Shafer WG, Hine MK, Levy BM: A Textbook of Oral Pathology, 4th ed. Philadelphia, W.B. Saunders, 1983.

5. ORAL RADIOLOGY

Bernard Friedland, B.Ch.D., M.Sc., J.D.

RADIATION PHYSICS AND BIOLOGY

1. How are x-rays produced?

X-rays are produced by "boiling off" electrons from a filament (the cathode) and accelerating the electrons to the target at the anode. The accelerated x-rays are decelerated by the target material, resulting in bremsstrahlung. Characteristic x-rays are produced when the incoming electrons knock out an inner K- or L-shell electron in the target and an electron from the L or M shell falls in to fill the void.

2. At the energies typically used in dental radiography, what interactions do the x-rays undergo with tissues?

X-rays undergo three interactions with tissue: elastic scatter, Compton scatter (also known as inelastic or incoherent scatter), and photoelectric absorption. Pair production occurs at much higher energy values (1.02 megaelectron volts [MeV]) than are used in dentistry.

3. Which of the interactions is primarily responsible for patient dose?

In the photoelectric process the incoming x-ray transfers all of its energy to the tissue. Photoelectric absorption, therefore, contributes the most to patient dose.

4. Why are filters used?

Filters are used to remove the low-energy x-rays, which are primarily responsible for photoelectric interactions and patient dose. Removing these x-rays increases the average energy of the beam and reduces the likelihood of photoelectric interactions, thereby reducing patient dose.

5. Why are intensifying screens used in extraoral radiography? How do they work?

Intensifying screens are used to reduce patient dose. They do so by converting x-rays to light. Since one x-ray gives rise to many light photons, the number of x-rays required to produce the same density on the film is markedly reduced.

6. What radiosensitive organs are in the field of typical dental x-ray examinations?

The thyroid is an extremely radiosensitive organ, along with lymphoid tissue and bone marrow in the exposed areas.

7. What evidence suggests a risk of carcinogenesis from exposures to low levels of ionizing radiation such as those in dentistry?

No single study proves the association between carcinogenesis and exposure to x-rays at the low levels used in dentistry. Many studies that follow patients exposed to higher levels, however, provide evidence of a link. Populations that have been studied include atomic bomb survivors in Nagasaki and Hisoshima, radium watch-dial painters, patients exposed to multiple fluoroscopies for tuberculosis, and others.

8. What units are used to describe radiation exposure and dose? What do they measure?

1. The roentgen (R) is the basic unit of radiation exposure for x- and gamma radiation. It is defined in terms of the number of ionizations produced in air.

2. The rad (roentgen absorbed dose) is a measure of the amount of energy absorbed by an organ or tissue. Different organs or tissues absorb a different amount of energy when exposed to the same amount of radiation or roentgens.

3. The rem (roentgen equivalent man or mammal) is a measure of the degree of damage caused to different organs or tissues. Different organs or tissues show differing amounts of damage even when they have absorbed the same amounts of rads.

The International System of Units (SIs) are the coulomb/kilogram, the Gray, and the Sievert for the roentgen, rad, and rem, respectively.

9. Explain the basic principles of conventional or plain-film tomography.

Conventional tomography is a technique that shows images of structures in one plane, while blurring images of structures in other planes. The technique achieves its objective by having the x-ray tube and film move in opposite directions. The structures most clearly depicted lie in the same plane that serves as the fulcrum of movement for the particular exposure. Thus, in the sketch below, the images of structures in plane B, which serves as the fulcrum of movement for the x-ray tube and film, will be visualized, whereas the images of structures on either side of plane B will be blurred out. In essence, tomography is a radiograph of a selected layer, achieving its aim by a controlled blurring of structures (Fig. 1).

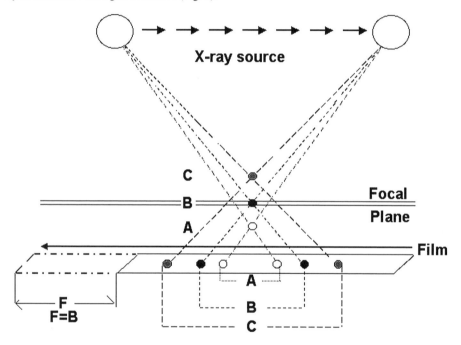

Figure 1. Conventional or plain-film tomography.

10. What is the difference between density and contrast?

Density refers to the overall degree of blackening of a film. Contrast refers to the differences in densities between adjacent areas of the film.

11. Which technique factors control film density?

The longer a film is exposed, the darker it will be; hence, time of exposure controls density. The milliampere (mA) determines how hot the filament gets and how many electrons are boiled off. The greater the filament current, the hotter the filament and the more electrons are boiled off to reach the anode and to produce x-rays; hence mA also controls density. As a result of the kilo-volt peak (kVp), which is the potential voltage difference between the cathode (filament) and anode, electrons that are boiled off are accelerated to the anode. The greater the potential difference between the cathode and anode, the greater the acceleration of the electrons toward the anode. Electrons that hit the anode at greater speed result in x-rays with higher energies. X-rays with higher energies are more likely to reach the film and blacken it. Thus, kVp also controls film density. The distance from the source to the film also has a great effect on film density (see question 17).

12. Which technique factors control film contrast? How do they affect contrast?

Contrast is controlled by the kVp only. The higher the kVp, the lower the contrast, and vice versa. Time, mA, and distance affect only density and not contrast.

13. What is subtraction radiography? Discuss its primary advantage and technical difficulty.

Subtraction radiography is a technique used to make radiographic changes that occur over time easier to see. It requires two radiographs exposed at different times and "subtracted" from one another, leaving only the changes between the two intact. Subtraction radiograph does not add information; it merely clarifies it. The different gray-scale levels in one of the radiographs are subtracted from the gray-scale levels in the same positions in the other radiograph. Where no changes have occurred, structures cancel each other out. Areas with changes stand out (Fig. 2).

The primary advantage of subtraction radiography is its extreme sensitivity. Small changes that would otherwise be virtually impossible to see are rendered clearly visible.

To get an accurate subtracted radiograph, the first and second radiographs must be exposed with virtually identical geometry—a goal difficult to achieve in dental practice without the aid of customized stents. Work is under way on programs that eliminate this limitation. Researchers have presented a technique that can be used to align radiographs taken with either a standardized technique or free hand. Digital radiography has also transformed subtraction radiography, making it much easier to apply clinically.

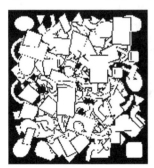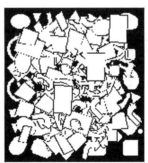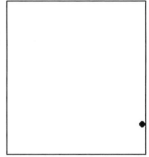

Figure 2. This schematic illustration shows radiographs A and B exposed at different times and with the same geometry in a patient. Viewing only figures A and B, it is virtually impossible to see any difference between them. Subtracting one film from the other readily shows the one difference between them.

14. What is tomosynthesis or tuned-aperture computed tomography (TACT)?

Tomosynthesis, also known as TACT, is a relative new modality that uses conventional two-dimensional projections to reconstruct images. TACT requires the acquisition of multiple conventional images of an object from different projection angles. One can apply the modality to static views, such as periapical films, or tomographic views. From the initial projections, TACT can construct three-dimensional displays much like CT. It can produce images suitable for digital subtraction without the need to mechanically secure the projection geometry. From a finite number of radiographic projections TACT can generate an infinite number of slices for viewing. The technology is not yet available for routine clinical use but looks promising.

15. How is the latent image on an x-ray film converted into a visible image?

When a film is developed, the exposed silver halide crystals are converted to metallic silver, which blackens film and thus makes the image visible.

16. How do you trouble-shoot a dental radiograph that is too dark or too light?

Changes in radiographic quality most commonly result from errors in processing and less commonly, but not rarely, from errors in technique factors. Check the exposure factors (kVp, mAs) to ensure that they were appropriate for the patient. Check the chemicals to ensure that they are at the correct temperature, that they have been stirred, and that they are fresh. If all of these factors are satisfactory, evaluation of the x-ray unit or film may be necessary. A problem with either is rare.

17. What is the inverse square law?

The intensity or exposure rate of radiation at a given distance from the source is inversely proportional to the square of the distance. If we double the distance from the source, for example, the intensity of the radiation is reduced fourfold.

18. How do we control scatter radiation?

In intraoral radiography, we do not control scattered x-rays that result from the interaction of x-rays with the patient. We do try, however, to minimize the scatter by use of a lead-lined long cone. In extraoral radiography, such as cephalometric radiography, scattered radiation is controlled by the use of a grid that is situated between the patient and the x-ray film.

19. What is meant by film speed? How is film speed expressed?

Film speed refers to the amount of radiation required to produce a particular density. Thus, the faster a film, the less radiation is needed to produce the same density than for a slower film. The speed of a film is expressed as the reciprocal value of the number of roentgens required to produce a density of one. Thus, if 5 roentgens are required to produce a density of one, the film speed is 0.20. If 8 roentgens are required to produce a density of one, the film speed is 0.125.

20. What is meant by the terms *sensitivity, specificity*, and *predictive value* when applied to the efficacy of radiographic examinations?

Sensitivity refers to the ability of a test, in this case a radiograph, to detect disease in patients who have disease. Thus, sensitivity is a measure of the frequency of positive (true-positive rate) and negative (false-negative rate) test results in patients with disease. Specificity refers to the ability of a test to screen out patients who do not in fact have the disease. Thus, specificity is a measure of the frequency of negative (true-negative rate) and positive (false-positive) test results in patients without disease. The predictive value of a radiograph is the probability that a patient with a positive test result actually has the disease (positive predictive value) or the probability that a patient with a negative test result actually does not have the disease (negative predictive value).

21. What is the basic technology behind magnetic resonance imaging (MRI)?

Atoms in the body act like bar magnets. In the MRI procedure, the area to be examined is subjected to an external magnetic field. The atoms line up with the magnetic field so that their long axes point in the same direction, just as one finds when bar magnets are subjected to a magnetic field. Once the atoms are so aligned, they are also subjected to a radio wave. The atoms absorb some of the radio wave's energy and lean over. When the radio wave is turned off, the atoms "relax" and emit the energy that they absorbed. This energy can be picked up by appropriate receivers and converted into a picture.

22. What is the trend with respect to use of a lead apron and thyroid collar to protect a patient from radiation?

Although as yet there is no consensus on the issue, there is an increasing tendency **not** to use lead aprons and thyroid collars in dental radiology. The feeling is that with modern machines, well-collimated beams, and fast films, the use of a lead apron offers no additional protection because virtually all of the patient dose is a result of internal scatter radiation. An exception, even among those who have discontinued use of the lead apron and thyroid collar, is occlusal films in younger patients. In occlusal radiography, the sensitive thyroid gland of younger patients is frequently in the path of the primary beam.

RADIOGRAPHIC TECHNIQUES

23. From the standpoint of the detector, what kinds of intraoral digital radiographic systems are available today? How do they differ from one another? What are the advantages of each system?

There are basically three kinds: the charge-coupled device (CCD), complementary metal oxide semiconductor (CMOS), and storage phosphor (PSP).

The most basic clinical differences among the systems lie in the physical nature of the detector and the manner in which images are transferred to the computer monitor. CCD and CMOS detectors are rigid, whereas PSP detectors are flexible. In the rigid-detector systems, the detector is connected directly (hard-wired) to a computer, whereas with PSP systems the latent image must first be "processed" by putting the detector into a laser-scanning device. The latter is connected to be computer.

Advantages of storage phosphor

- Detectors are thin and flexible, more comfortable for the patient, and easier for the operator to use.
- Cheaper, especially when multiple operatories are involved.

Advantages of rigid-detector systems

- The image appears on the monitor instantaneously.
- Infection control is easier and quicker. The detector is merely enclosed in a protective latex sleeve. With a storage phosphor system, in which a full-mouth series is done using multiple detectors just as with film, each detector must be wrapped before use and then unwrapped after use before placement in the scanner

24. What are the advantages of the long-cone technique?

The long-cone technique has two primary benefits. The long cone reduces patient dose by reducing the field size. It also increases the target-film distance, thereby reducing magnification.

25. Why is it important to obtain right-angle views of any radiographic abnormality?

Radiographs are two-dimensional representations of three-dimensional objects. To obtain a three-dimensional view with film, one needs to obtain views at right angles to each other. For example, a periapical film suggesting a cyst of the mandible should be supplemented with an occlusal view and a posteroanterior (PA) view of the mandible.

26. If you intend to remove a tooth surgically — for example, an impacted second bicuspid — how can you determine whether the impacted tooth lies buccal or lingual to the erupted teeth?

A periapical view shows only the mesiodistal location of a tooth relative to other teeth. To determine its buccolingual relation, you need a view at right angles to the periapical view. An occlusal view is generally the easiest view to take and is the only intraoral view that you can take at 90° to the periapical view. In areas where it may not be possible to get an occlusal view, such as the third molar region, a PA mandibular film may be the best solution. This, of course, is an extraoral view. You could also determine the impacted tooth's buccolingual relation by exposing a second periapical view with the tube positioned either more mesially or distally compared with the first periapical exposure. By applying the buccal object rule, you can then determine the impacted tooth's buccolingual relation to the erupted teeth.

27. What are the indications for an occlusal film?
- To determine the buccolingual position of an impacted tooth
- To demonstrate the buccal and lingual cortices, particularly in the mandible
- To visualize the intermaxillary suture
- To demonstrate arch form
- To replace periapical films in young children

An occlusal film also may be used when one wishes to visualize on one film a lesion that is too large to fit on a single periapical film.

28. What operator error results in a foreshortened image?
Foreshortening results when the vertical angulation of the tube is too great; that is, the tube is angled too steeply. Elongation, by contrast, results from a vertical angle that is too shallow. A good way to remember cause and effect is to think of the sun and your shadow. Your shadow is shortest at noon when the sun is highest in the sky (a steep vertical angle) and longest in the late afternoon when the sun is low in the sky (a shallow vertical angle).

29. Is it preferable to err on the side of foreshortening or elongation? Why?
If one is going to err, it is best to foreshorten. Think again of the sun and shadows. The short shadows produced by the high-noon sun have crisp, well-delineated margins, whereas the long shadows produced by the low late-afternoon sun disappear into the distance with ill-defined margins. It is better to have a foreshortened image that is crisp rather than an elongated image that is difficult to read. This is particularly true when one is examining the apical area.

30. Which radiographic view is considered the primary view for evaluating the alveolar bone for periodontal disease? What are the radiographic manifestations of periodontal disease?
The bitewing view is the primary view for evaluating radiographic changes consistent with periodontal disease, which include loss of crestal cortication, changes in the contour of the interdental bone, horizontal and angular bone loss, and furcation involvement. The bitewing film is superior to a periapical film because distortion, including elongation or foreshortening, is slight. The reason is that the vertical angle is small (approximately 5°), and the central ray is directed at right angles to the film.

31. Is there a generally accepted protocol for the frequency of radiographic evaluation in adult dental patients?
Yes. The United States Food and Drug Administration, in cooperation with the American Dental Association and other major organizations, has developed and disseminated protocols for exposing dental patients to x-ray examinations. These protocols require a history and clinical examination before prescribing an individualized radiographic examination.

32. How should radiographic protocols be altered for pregnant dental patients?
With the use of standard radiation protection, there should be no additional risk to the fetus from x-ray exposures commonly used in dentistry. However, because of the concerns many women have during pregnancy, it is advisable to limit x-ray exposures to the necessary minimum.

33. What type of information that can be gleaned from radiographs is it desirable to have before undertaking implant surgery? What types of imaging are available to gather the necessary information?
The anatomic structures of primary concern in implant surgery include the sinuses, nasal fossae, and incisive foramen and canal in the maxillae; the mandibular canals; and mental foramina in the mandible. Other structures that are of importance, but which are often overlooked, include depressions in the buccal cortical plate, commonly seen in the incisor and canine regions in the maxillae, and the submandibular and sublingual gland fossae and genial tubercles in the mandible. Additional information that is necessary to the successful placement and restoration of an implant includes the height and buccolingual width of the alveolar bone, the angulation of the bone, and the presence of other potentially complicating factors, such as remaining roots or pathology.

The presence or absence of root pathology is probably best ruled out through the use of conventional dental radiography, such as intraoral (best) and panoramic films. Conventional dental radiographs do not permit accurate measurement, nor do they show the buccolingual bone width or the angulation of the bone. To get this information, one needs more advanced imaging. Plain-film (conventional) tomography (Fig. 3) and CT can provide this information. MRI is not a good modality for examining the bone.

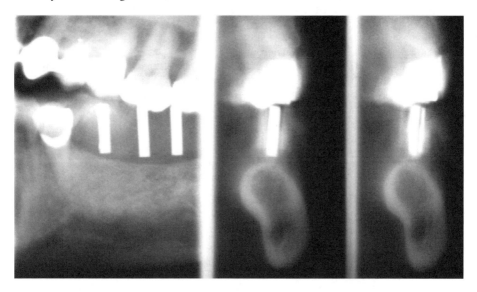

Figure 3. Plain-film (conventional) tomography for implant surgery.

34. What are the differences between standard intraoral radiography (bitewings and periapicals) and panoramic radiography?

1. Bitewing and periapical techniques use direct-exposure film while the panoramic technique uses intensifying screens.

2. The panoramic view uses a tube movement that results in loss of detail and resolution.

35. What imaging techniques are available to evaluate the soft tissue components of the temporomandibular joints (TMJs)?

Three imaging procedures are available for evaluation of the soft tissue components of the TMJs: arthrography, computed tomography (CT), and MRI. MRI studies are becoming more widely used because they image soft tissue well, do not employ ionizing radiation, and are non-invasive. Arthrography is the most invasive and involves the introduction of contrast into one or both joint spaces.

36. Name the paranasal sinuses and the radiographic views commonly used to evaluate the sinuses.

The paranasal sinuses are the frontal sinuses, the maxillary sinuses, the sphenoid sinuses, and the ethmoid sinuses. The views used to evaluate them are the Waters view (maxillary sinus), the Caldwell view (maxillary and frontal sinus), the lateral view (maxillary and frontal sinus), and the submentovertex view (sphenoid and ethmoid sinus). A panoramic film may be used as an adjunct to these views. The panoramic film shows the maxillary sinus.

The view of choice depends on precisely what is under examination. For example, the submentovertex view permits excellent visualization of the lateral wall of the maxillary sinus, whereas the Waters view depicts the medial, lateral, and inferior borders of the maxillary sinus.

37. What plain film views may be used to visualize the TMJ?

The transpharyngeal or Parma view provides an image mainly of the lateral aspect of the condyle. The lateral transcranial view also provides an image mainly of the lateral aspect of the condyle. Its main purpose is to depict the condyle-glenoid fossa relationship. The Zimmer or trans- or periorbital view provides a mediolateral image of the condyle as well as the condylar neck. A reverse Towne view is useful for visualizing the condylar neck. Keep in mind that tomography provides better visualization of the TMJ than plain film views. The above views, however, are relatively easy to take.

38. What are the indications for a panoramic film?

There is no specific indication for the panoramic film. Virtually any structure that is portrayed on a panoramic film can be displayed by another view, which often provides greater detail. For example, the panoramic film is often used to visualize impacted third molars. A lateral oblique view of the jaws provides the same information with greater detail. A Waters view provides greater information about the maxillary and other sinuses than a panoramic film.

39. Which intraoral view is best for visualizing the greater palatine foramina?

The greater palatine foramina cannot be visualized on any intraoral film. On some maxillary occlusal films, a foramen can be seen in the area of the second or third molars. This foramen is the nasolacrimal canal and not the greater palatine foramen.

40. What are the names of the major salivary glands? How are they studied radiographically?

The three major salivary glands are the parotid, submandibular, and sublingual glands. Because the salivary glands consist of soft tissue, they cannot be seen on radiographs unless special steps are taken to make them visible. In a technique called sialography, a radiopaque dye or contrast is injected through the duct openings into the gland. Iodine is the agent normally used to provide contrast. If patients are allergic to iodine, a different contrast agent must be used. Calcifications of the duct may be seen on intraoral films, especially calcifications of Wharton's duct, the submandibular gland duct. The stones or sialoliths may be seen on either periapical or more commonly on occlusal films. MRI is increasingly replacing sialography as the modality of choice for studying the salivary glands.

41. What are the major advantages of digital radiography over conventional film-based systems?

- With a charge-coupled device (CCD) and complementary metal oxide semiconductor (CMOS) detectors, images are visible instantaneously.
- The need for a film processor and/or darkroom is eliminated.
- Archiving of images is easier, and so is retrieval. Depending on the digital radiography software and the office management software, it may be possible to integrate the two, thus enabling one to recall images and all other patient data from a single window.
- Digital images can be manipulated (density and contrast can be changed; images can be magnified).
- Built-in digital rulers enable one to perform measurements on the image.
- Patient dose is reduced. Importantly, however, it is unclear whether the reduction in dose has any biologic benefits (e.g. reduced number of cancers, cataracts). There is much controversy in the radiation biology and radiation physics literature over this issue.

42. What are the typical magnifications of radiographs commonly used in dentistry?

The magnification of periapical and bitewing films is about 4%; of cephalometric films, about 10%; and of panoramic films, 20–25%.

43. What are the indications for the use of MRI vs. CT?

There is no simple answer to this question. In general, MRI is better for imaging lesions based in soft tissues—for example, a tumor in the tongue. CT, on the other hand, provides better images of bone; thus, for an intraosseous tumor, CT is the technique of choice. Not uncommonly one may want to use both MRI and CT. For example, when a patient has a tumor in the floor of the mouth, one may use MRI to determine its extent in the soft tissue and CT to determine whether there is any bone involvement. For TMJ imaging, MRI is better at imaging the soft tissue of the disk, but CT is better for almost all other investiagions of the TMJ.

BASIC RADIOLOGIC INTERPRETIVE CONCEPTS

44. What are the radiographic features of any lesion or area of interest on the film that always should be defined and recorded?
1. Location of the lesion as exactly as possible
2. Size
3. Shape
4. Appearance of borders
5. Density, with particular attention to whether it is radiolucent, radiopaque, or mixed
6. Effects of the lesion on adjacent structures

45. Once you have described the features of a lesion (see previous question), you need to arrive at a differential diagnosis. Describe a method or algorithm for doing so.
Although there is no one correct way, everyone's first question should be whether the area in question is normal or abnormal. If it's normal, you should be able to identify the structure. If you decide that the area in question is abnormal, one way to proceed is presented in Figure 4.
One reason for following at least the initial steps outlined in the above scheme is that patients typically want to know (1) whether something is normal and (2) if it is not, whether the abnormality is benign or malignant. After that, there is more leeway. Some clinicians, for example, may prefer to decide on the odontogenic vs non-odontogenic nature of a lesion before deciding whether it is a cyst or tumor.

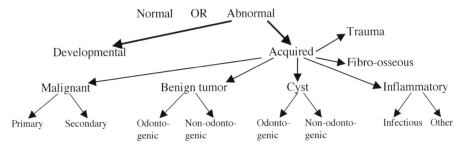

Figure 4. Algorithm for arriving at a differential diagnosis.

46. What is by far the most likely interpretation of a bilaterally symmetric radiographic appearance in the jaws?
A bilateral symmetric appearance, with extremely few exceptions, is indicative of normality. Among the few exceptions to this rule are cherubism and infantile cortical hyperostosis (Caffey's disease).

47. The location of a lesion may be a clue to its origin. What single anatomic structure in the mandible is most useful in differentiating between a lesion of possible odontogenic vs. nonodontogenic origin?
The mandibular or inferior alveolar canal is extremely useful in distinguishing between a lesion of odontogenic vs. nonodontogenic origin. Because one does not expect to find odontogenic tissues below the canal, it is most unlikely that lesions situated below the canal are odontogenic in origin.

Indeed, the lesion of odontogenic origin rarely, if ever, begins below the canal. Of course, any lesion, including one of odontogenic origin, may begin above the canal and extend below it.

48. What is the most likely tissue of origin for a tumor in the mandibular canal?

Because a nerve and a blood vessel run in the canal, the tissue of origin is most likely to be either neural or vascular, resulting in tumors such as neurolemmoma, neurofibroma, traumatic neuroma, or hemangioma.

49. What broad categories of possible disease entities need to be considered in developing a differential diagnosis of any abnormality noted during a radiographic examination?

- Trauma
- Metabolic, nutritional, and endocrinologic diseases
- Congenital anomalies and abnormalities of growth and development
- Iatrogenic lesions
- Neoplastic diseases (benign and malignant)
- Inflammation and infection

50. What general radiographic features or principles permit the diagnosis of an underlying systemic cause for a particular condition or appearance?

When a systemic cause underlies a problem, both the mandible and maxilla are affected. Furthermore, the jaws are typically affected bilaterally, often symmetrically. If the condition affects the teeth, one would expect them to be affected in a bilaterally symmetrical fashion, too.

51. What technique can be used to determine the track of a fistula that exits on the soft tissue adjacent to the teeth?

Insert a gutta percha point into the fistula, and allow it to track as far as it can. Obtain a periapical view with the gutta percha point in place.

52. What are the usual radiographic signs of inflammatory disease involving the paranasal sinuses?

- Mucous membrane thickening
- Air-fluid levels
- Opacification of a sinus cavity
- Presence of a soft-tissue mass
- Changes in the cortical margins of a sinus

53. What common radiographic signs help to distinguish among a cyst, benign neoplasm, or malignant neoplasm?

Cysts tend to be radiolucent and round or oval in shape and to have intact cortical margins. Benign neoplasms are more variable than cysts in density, shape, and definition of margins. Malignant neoplasms of the jaws tend to be aggressive, with ragged margins and poor definition of shape and borders. Malignant lesions often grow quickly, leaving roots of teeth in position and giving the appearance of roots floating in space. Both cysts and benign neoplasms are more likely than malignant neoplasms to resorb tooth roots.

54. When should bitewing views first be obtained for the typical child?

The first bitewing views should be obtained after the establishment of contacts on the posterior teeth.

55. How do primary teeth differ from permanent teeth radiographically? How does the difference affect the radiographic evidence of caries in primary teeth?

Primary teeth are smaller and have relatively larger pulp chambers with pulp horns in closer proximity to the external surface of the crown. The enamel layer is thinner in dimension. Primary teeth are slightly less opaque on film because of a higher inorganic content. As a result, caries in primary teeth tends to progress more rapidly from initial surface demineralization to involvement of the dentin. Thus careful interpretation is especially important in evaluating the primary dentition.

56. What is the correlation between the histologic and radiographic progress of dental caries?
There must be 30–60% loss in mineralization before caries is radiographically evident with standard D- and E-speed intraoral films. Therefore, the histologic or clinical progress of a carious lesion is advanced, sometimes significantly, compared with its radiographic progress.

57. What is the rule of 3's for radiographic assessment of the development of permanent teeth?
It takes approximately 3 years for a permanent tooth bud to calcify after matrix formation is complete, approximately 3 more years for the tooth to erupt after calcification is complete, and about 3 more years after initial eruption for root formation to be complete.

58. What is the difference in the progress of pit and fissure caries and proximal or smooth-surface caries on a radiograph?
In smooth surface caries in enamel the base of the triangle is at the surface, whereas the apex is at the amelodentinal junction. Once smooth surface caries penetrates, it spreads rapidly along the amelodentinal junction so that the base of the triangle is now at the amelodentinal junction and the apex is directed toward the dentin. Pit and fissure caries are not usually visible radiographically until the caries has reached the dentin. Pit or fissure caries then have a triangular appearance with the base of the triangle at the amelodentinal junction and the apex directed toward the deeper surface of the tooth. (See Figure 5.)

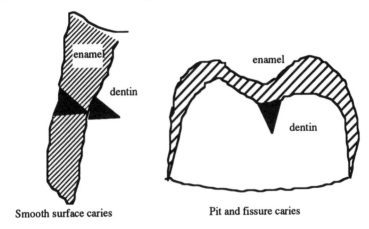

Smooth surface caries   Pit and fissure caries

Figure 5. *Left,* smooth surface caries. *Right,* pit and fissure caries.

59. In pathology of the maxilla, what feature is most useful in determining whether the pathology arose inside or outside the sinus?
The floor of the sinus is the most useful feature. If the pathology arose inside the sinus, the floor is intact and in its normal position or perhaps depressed inferiorly. If the pathology arose outside the sinus, the floor of the sinus is intact and in its normal position or moved or pushed superiorly. If the sinus floor has been destroyed, it may not be possible to determine whether the pathology arose from without or within the sinus.

60. Foramina may be superimposed over the apices of teeth, mimicking the presence of periapical disease. What radiographic features are most useful in distinguishing between normal structures and apical pathology?
If the lucency is due to the superimposition of a foramen, the periodontal ligament space and the lamina aura around the tooth are intact. The exposure of a second radiograph, with the tube in a different position from the first exposure, also is frequently useful. If the lucency moves rela-

tive to the apex of the tooth, the lucency is not associated with the tooth and is not due to peri-apical pathology. This exercise, however, does not rule out the possibility that the lesion is abnormal; it means merely that the lesion is not related to the tooth.

61. What is the differential diagnosis of a radiopacity in the soft tissues in and around the jaws?

It is easiest to answer this question if one first classifies the radiopacities into varies groups: tooth, bone, foreign body, and calcification (although bone is a form of calcification or mineralization, it is distinctive enough to warrant a separate category). Although in a given case it may be difficult to distinguish even among these categories, the classification is nevertheless useful. In most cases one can easily rule out a tooth in soft tissue, although in cases of trauma fragments of a tooth or even a whole tooth may be found in the lips or tongue. Bone in soft tissue is rare, but choristomas and ossifying hematomas are examples. Foreign bodies tend to be metallic but need not be. Gutta percha, endodontic cements, some composites, and contrast media are opaque but not metal. A host of entities fall under calcification. Fortunately, only a few are common: sialoliths, lymph node calcification (e.g., in granulomatous diseases such as tuberculosis), and tonsilloliths. Less common examples include phleboliths, calcified acne lesions, and parasitic larva (e.g., cysticercosis). Antroliths and rhinoliths are calcifications ("stones") that occur within a sinus or the nasal cavity, respectively. When an opacity is seen in a cavity, such as the sinus, fluids and soft tissue should be added as two separate groups.

62. Is it possible for a patient to be in acute pain as a result of a periapical abscess, yet to have a completely normal periapical film?

This finding is not unusual because 30–60% of mineralization must be lost before bone destruction is radiographically evident. In an acute situation, there frequently has not been sufficient time for this amount of bone destruction to occur. Thus, the radiograph lags behind the clinical picture. The same may be true in the healing phase. A patient may be improving clinically yet still show radiographic signs of pathology.

63. Is a widened periodontal ligament space at the apex of a tooth always indicative of pathology?

No. When a radiolucency such as the mental foramen or mandibular canal is superimposed over the periodontal ligament space, the ligament space appears to be widened. Such a widening is purely artifactual. The periodontal ligament space also may appear wider at the neck of a tooth. If the lamina aura is normal in this area, the widened periodontal ligament space is probably a variant of normal.

64. Can a patient refuse an x-ray examination that is considered necessary, given signs and symptoms, and sign a release of responsibility in the chart?

A patient may legally refuse to undergo a radiographic examination. Such patients probably waive their right to seek damages later if an adverse event occurs that may have been detected by the radiograph. The patient's decision to refuse a radiographic examination is a matter of informed consent. The dentist may not be protected from suit if the record reflects merely that the patient was told of the need for an x-ray and declined to undergo the examination. The record should show clearly that the patient was told why the examination was necessary, what information the dentist needed, and how the lack of that information may lead to improper diagnosis and/or treatment.

65. What are the radiographic manifestations in the jaws of patients infected with the human immunodeficiency virus (HIV)?

There are no unique oral or maxillofacial radiographic manifestations of HIV infection, although infected patients are at a significantly higher risk for aggressive periodontal disease.

66. What is the efficacy of dental radiographs?

Studies of standard dental radiography (bitewing, periapical, and panoramic views) show considerable variance in the ability to detect common dental diseases such as caries, periodontal disease, and apical periodontitis. Radiographs should not be considered to be perfect, but they are most valuable when combined with a thorough history and clinical examination.

RADIOGRAPHIC INTERPRETATION

67. What is the earliest radiographic sign of periapical disease of pulpal origin?

The earliest radiographic sign is widening of the periodontal ligament space around the apex of the tooth.

68. What is the next radiographic sign of periapical disease of pulpal origin?

The next radiographic sign is loss of the lamina aura around the apex of the tooth.

69. Describe the radiographic differences that allow one to distinguish among periapical abscess, granuloma, radicular (periapical) cyst, and an apical surgical scar.

One cannot distinguish among periapical abscess, granuloma, or radicular (periapical) cyst on radiographic grounds alone. All of these lesions are radiolucent with well-defined borders. Whereas an abscess may be expected to be less well corticated than a radicular cyst, this feature is not marked or constant enough to be of real utility. An apical surgical scar may be radiographically distinguishable from the other three lesions if there is radiographic evidence of surgery, such as a retrograde amalgam. Of course, a history should elicit the fact of surgery.

70. How does the radiographic appearance of pulpal pathology that has extended to involve the bone differ in primary posterior teeth from the picture commonly seen in permanent posterior teeth?

In permanent teeth, widening of the periodontal ligament space is seen around the apex of the tooth. In primary teeth, by contrast, the infection presents as widening of the periodontal ligament space or an area of lucency in the furcation area.

71. Does any radiographic sign permit the diagnosis of a nonvital tooth?

It is frequently stated that tooth vitality cannot be determined by radiographs alone, but this is not so. The presence of a root canal filling in a tooth provides virtually conclusive proof of its nonvitality, as does the presence of a retrograde filling, usually amalgam.

72. At times it may be difficult to distinguish between hypercementosis and condensing or sclerosing osteitis around the apex of a tooth. What radiographic feature permits a definitive diagnosis when one is confronted with this dilemma?

If hypercementosis is present, the periodontal ligament space is visible around the added cementum; that is, the cementum is contained within and is surrounded by the periodontal ligament space. Condensing osteitis, by contrast, is situated outside the periodontal ligament space.

73. What is the differential diagnosis for delayed tooth eruption?

This condition can be broken down into delayed eruption of one or a few teeth vs. many or all teeth.

One or a few teeth
- Normal variation
- Hyperplastic follicle
- Cyst (dentigerous, eruption)
- Tumor (some typically occur in association with the follicle space, such as adenomatoid odontogenic tumor, ameloblaslc fibroma)

- Occlusion (e.g., tipped teeth sandwiching another tooth)
- Supernumeraries
- Fibrous dysplasta
- Fibromatosis

Many or all teeth

- Normal variation
- Fibrous dysplasta
- Fibromatosis
- Iatrogenic (e.g., phenytoin hyperplasia)
- Cherubism
- Cleidocranial dysostosis (supernumeraries)
- Gardner's syndrome (supernumeraries)

- Osteopetrosis
- Turner syndrome (XO)
- Hypothyroidism (cretinism)
- Pycnodysostosis
- Romberg's disease
- Hurler's syndrome

74. What is the earliest radiographic sign of periodontal disease?

The earliest radiographic sign of periodontal disease is loss of density of the crestal cortex, which is best seen in the posterior regions. In the anterior part of the mouth, the alveolar crests lose their pointed appearance and become blunted. In the posterior areas, the alveolar crests usually meet the lamina aura at right angles. In the presence of periodontal disease, these angles become rounded.

75. What is the earliest radiographic sign of furcation involvement due to periodontal disease?

In periodontal disease, one may see the loss of a cortical plate, either the buccal or lingual plate, on an intraoral film. The plate may be lost so that the crest now occupies a position apical to the furcation. This appearance, however, does not permit a diagnosis of furcation involvement. Widening of the periodontal ligament space in the furcation area is the earliest radiographic sign of furcation involvement.

76. What is the radiographic differential diagnosis of a radiolucency on the root of a periodontally healthy tooth?

Internal resorption, external resorption, and superimposition are the most common causes. Note that the question refers to a periodontally healthy tooth. If bone loss has resulted in exposure of the root, caries and abrasion, among other potential possibilities, enter the picture.

77. How can you distinguish among the above radiolucencies on the root of a tooth?

In internal resorption, the canal is widened, whereas it is unaffected in external resorption. If the resorption began below the bone level, it has to be internal resorption because, without adjacent bone, there are no osteoclasts in the area to cause external resorption. Of course, if either internal or external resorption involves both the canal and other tooth structure, it is not possible to distinguish between the two conditions. A superimposed radiolucency moves relative to the root if another view is obtained with the tube in a different position. The most common such lucencies are normal anatomy, such as foramina, sinus, mandibular canal, and accessory or nutrient foramina or canals. Artifacts such as cervical burnout also may produce a lucency on the root at the junction of the enamel and cementum.

78. What is the radiographic differential diagnosis of a radiolucency on the crown of a tooth?

Caries, internal resorption, restorations, abrasions, erosions, and enamel hypoplasia are among the more common possibilities. Caries typically have irregular margins; they may also have typical shapes, such as the triangular appearance of interproximal caries. Internal resorption has smooth, well-defined margins. The same is true of radiolucent restorations, which frequently can be recognized by their shape and sometimes by the presence of an opaque base, such as calcium hydroxide, lining the floor of the preparation. Abrasions, particularly at the cervical margins, often have a V-shaped appearance. Other abrasions, such as those caused by a clasp on a denture, typically have well-defined borders and straight lines, unlike most naturally occurring phenomena. Erosions also have well-defined borders, and their shape is typically round or oval. Hypoplasia usually is not a single lucency on a tooth but rather many small lucencies.

79. What is the differential diagnosis of a root that appears short on the radiograph?

A root that appears short may indicate an incompletely formed tooth, which may be either vital and still developing or nonvital; a short but otherwise normal root (the root may be congenitally short or underdeveloped because of an acquired condition such as radiation); root resorption; foreshortening; surgery, such as apicoectomy; or iatrogenic causes, such as orthodontic treatment. In certain conditions, such as dentinogenesis imperfecta, the teeth also have short roots.

80. How can one distinguish among the various possibilities for a radiographically short-appearing root?

In a normal root, the canal is not radiographically visible to the apex and appears to end just before the apex. In the case of a foreshortened normal root, the canal is not open at the apex. Foreshortening can be distinguished from a normal short root by the fact that other structures in the radiograph point to the steep angulation of the tube. Alternatively, a second film can be exposed to ensure that the correct vertical angle is used. If the root still looks short, it cannot be due to foreshortening. In teeth with an open apex, the shape of the canal is important. In a still-developing tooth, the ends of the canal diverge ("blunderbuss"), whereas in resorption the walls of the canal converge. Surgical intervention is usually easily spotted by the presence of a retrograde amalgam. The involvement of multiple teeth with short roots points to a condition such as dentinogenesis imperfecta. A history of orthodontic treatment confirms an iatrogenic cause.

81. What is the differential diagnosis for teeth with pulps that are reduced in size?

In dentinogenesis imperfecta all of the teeth are involved. In dentinal dysplasia all or or only some of the teeth may be involved. Less commonly, reduced chambers may be seen in amelogenesis imperfecta. Rarely, the cause of a generalized reduction in pulp size in many teeth may be idiopathic, although such cases are usually limited to a few teeth. The same is true of small pulp chambers due to attrition or trauma. Finally, small pulp chambers may be a variant of normal.

82. Name two serious and even potentially fatal conditions that may be detected by dental radiographs before clinical signs or symptoms develop. What are the dental signs and symptoms of these diseases?

Gardner's syndrome and Gorlin-Goltz syndrome have radiographic signs that should alert a vigilant practitioner to the possibility of their presence. **Gardner's syndrome** is characterized by multiple osteomas, which may occur on the mandible; multiple supernumerary teeth, frequently impacted; sebaceous skin cysts; and polyps of the large and occasionally small intestine. The polyps may become malignant. **Gorlin-Goltz syndrome** (multiple basal cell nevoid carcinoma syndrome; basal cells nevus syndrome; bifid rib syndrome) is characterized by the presence of odontogenic keratocysts, basal cell carcinomas, and a host of other potential anomalies, including skin tumors and ocular and neurologic abnormalities, such as calcification of the falx cerebri.

83. What are the radiographic signs of osteomyelitis?

A classic sign of osteomyelitis is a periosteal reaction or periostitis, which is typically seen in the mandible but rarely, if ever, in the maxilla. The periosteum lays down bone on its deep aspect, resulting in new bone, known as an involucrum formation. Cloacae, which are drainage tracts for purulent material, may be visible on radiographs. Sequestra, which are areas of bone separated from adjacent bone, are another typical feature.

84. What radiographic features help to differentiate a malignant lesion from osteomyelitis?

Malignant lesions destroy bone uniformly. In osteomyelitis, areas of radiographically normal-appearing bone are frequently seen between the areas of destruction. Sequestra are not present in malignant lesions. The nature of the periosteal response cannot be used to distinguish between malignancies and infection, with the possible exception of the sun-ray periosteal reaction described in osteogenic sarcoma.

85. What features of a periosteal reaction help to differentiate between infectious periostitis and a periosteal reaction due to malignant disease?

A periosteal reaction by itself does not permit a definitive diagnosis of either an infectious or malignant origin, notwithstanding comments to the contrary. Although some periosteal reactions are more suggestive than others of a particular origin (e.g., the sun-burst appearance of osteogenic sarcoma), none is definitive.

86. Both fluid and a soft tissue mass present as opacification of the maxillary sinus on a Waters view. How can one distinguish radiographically between the two?

Take a second view with patient's head tilted upward, downward, or laterally relative to the position for the first Waters view. If the superior border of the opacity remains the same, one is dealing with soft tissue. If the superior surface changes, one is dealing with fluid because the fluid level changes when the head is tilted (like water in a glass). This technique, of course, does not work when opacification of the sinus is complete. One cannot distinguish between fluid or soft tissue in the sinus on the basis of the degree of opacity on plain films.

87. Sometimes it is difficult to distinguish a tooth or part of a tooth embedded in bone from other opacities in the bone or from opacities in the sinus. What radiographic features are helpful in this predicament?

An opacity surrounded by a thin, relatively uniform radiolucent zone, which in turn is surrounded by a thin radiopaque line or cortex, is of inestimable value. The radiolucent zone and cortex provide conclusive proof that the opacity is not in the sinus. The uniform zone is suggestive of the periodontal ligament space, whereas the cortex is suggestive of the lamina aura. This general appearance is thus reminiscent of a tooth. The presence of a canal in the opacity is also useful. Whether the opacity is in fact tooth depends, among other things, on the density and uniformity of the opacity as well as on its shape and size. An odontoma, for example, has the general features of uniform radiolucent zone, surrounded by a cortex, yet it is a benign tumor. One may not be able to determine with certainty from a periapical view alone whether an opacity is inside or outside the sinus. A Waters view helps to clarify the situation.

88. List the radiographic signs of a fractures.

The radiographic signs of a fracture include a demonstrable radiolucent fracture line, displacement of a bony fragment, disruption in the continuity of the normal bony contour, and increased density (due to overlap of the adjacent fragments).

89. What is the differential diagnosis for early tooth loss?
- Extraction (e.g., for orthodontic reasons, due to caries)
- Periodontal disease (may be nonspecific; a result of conditions such as juvenile periodontitis or Papillon-Lefevre syndrome; or a result of systemic conditions predisposing to periodontal disease, such as diabetes mellitus and Down syndrome)
- Trauma
- Dentinogenesis imperfecta
- Dentinal dysplasia
- Regional odontodysplasia/ghost teeth
- Hypophosphatasia
- Langerhans cell disease/histiocytosis X
- Vitamin D-resistant rickets/hypophosphatemia
- Cyclic neutropenia
- Acrodynia (Pink disease)
- Acatalasia

- Chediak-Higashi syndrome
- Chediak-Steinbrink syndrome
- Vitamin C deficiency
- Cherubism (due to curettage of lesion)
- Neuroblastima (< 5 years of age)

90. What plain film views are of greatest assistance in evaluating the jaws for fractures?

The Waters view provides the single best plain film view of the maxilla. The zygomatic arches are best examined with a basal or submentovertex view. A PA film of the mandible is helpful, as are lateral oblique films. Occlusal views are useful in both the mandible and maxilla. Periapical films provide the greatest detail about a fracture if the fracture line traverses an area that a periapical film is able to cover. A reverse Towne projection shows the condylar necks and condyles, as does the transorbital or periorbital view.

91. What radiographic features help to differentiate between the radicular cyst emanating from a maxillary central incisor and the nasopalatine or incisive canal cyst?

If the lesion crosses the midline, it is far more likely to be a nasopalatine cyst. An intact lamina aura around the teeth is indicative of vital teeth and effectively rules out a radicular cyst. The presence of large restorations on a central incisor supports the diagnosis of a radicular cyst, but this feature is overridden by an intact lamina aura.

92. To what extent do the amount and degree of calcification in a tumor point to its benign or malignant nature?

Calcification has no significance in predicting the benign or malignant nature of a tumor. Both benign tumors (e.g., odontomas, adenomotoid odontogenic tumors, ossifying fibromas) and malignant tumors (e.g., osteogenic sarcoma) produce bone or calcifications. To determine the benign or malignant nature of a tumor, one must look to other features.

93. Which lesions may present with a soap-bubble or honeycomb appearance?

Ameloblastoma	Giant cell lesions
Keratocyst	Hemangioma
Primordial cyst	Calcifying epithelial odontogenic tumor
Aneurysmal bone cyst	Fibrous dysplasia
Cherubism	

94. What are the radiographic features of degenerative joint disease (DJD) or osteoarthritis involving the TMJs?

The changes of DJD include subchondral sclerosis, flattening of the articular surfaces of the condyle, and osteophyte formation. Osteophyte formation occurs in the later stages of the disease process. Small erosions, called Ely cysts, may be seen on the articulating surfaces. A narrowing of the joint space is another common finding. The eminence may be flattened or hollowed and may also show osteophyte formation.

95. Why is it important to visualize both TMJs on radiograph even when a patient has signs and symptoms only on one side?

The unique nature of the TMJs—both are part of a common mandible—often results in functional symptoms on one side even though the osseous pathology may be on the other side. Once the decision to radiograph a joint has been made, both sides should be examined.

96. What common intracranial calcifications may be observed on a radiographic view of the skull, such as a cephalometric view? What intracranial calcifications represent pathology and should be further evaluated?

Physiologic calcifications include those of the pineal gland, choroid plexus, aura (falx cerebri, tentorium, vault), ligaments (petroclinoid, interclinoid), habenular commissure, basal ganglia, and dentate nucleus. Pathologic calcifications include calcifications in tumors (meningioma, craniopharyngioma, glioma), cysts (dermoid cyst), and infections (parasitic, as in cysticercosis; tuberculosis).

BIBLIOGRAPHY

1. Christensen EE: Christensen's Introduction to the Physics of Diagnostic Radiology, 3rd ed. Philadelphia, Lea & Febiger, 1984.
2. Goaz PW, White SC: Oral Radiology Principles and Interpretation. St. Louis, Mosby, 1982.
3. Jaworowski Z: Beneficial effects of radiation and regulatory policy. Austr Phys Engineer Sci Med 20(3): 125–138, 1997.
4. Kasle MJ, Langlais RP: Basic principles of oral radiography. In Exercises in Dental Radiology, vol. 4. Philadelphia, W.B. Saunders, 1981.
5. Kasle MJ, Langlais RP: Intra-oral radiographic interpretation. In Exercises in Dental Radiology, vol 1. Philadelphia, W.B. Saunders, 1981.
6. van der Stelt PF: Principles of digital imaging. Dent Clin North Am 44:237–248, 2000.
7. Visser H, Rodig T, Hermann KP. Dose reduction by direct-digital cephalometric radiography. Angle Orthod 71:159–163, 2001.
8. Webber RL, Horton RA, Tyndall DA, Ludlow JB: Tuned-aperture computed tomography (TACT). Theory and application for three-dimensional dento-alveolar imaging. Dentomaxillofac Radiol 26:53–62, 1997.
9. White SC, MJ: Oral Radiology: Principles and Interpretation. St. Louis, Mosby, 2000.
10. White SC, Heslop EW, Hollender LG, et al: Parameters of radiologic care: An official report of the American Academy of Oral and Maxillofacial Radiology. Oral Surg Oral Med Oral Pathol Oral Radiol Endod 91:498–511, 2001.
11. Wood NK, Goaz PW: Differential Diagnosis of Oral Lesions. St. Louis, Mosby, 1985.
12. Worth HM: Principles and Practice of Oral Radiologic Interpretation. Chicago, Year Book, 1963.

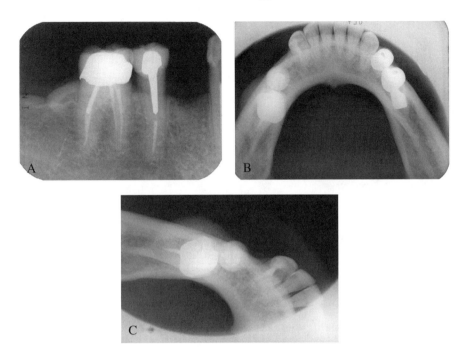

Exostosis. The periapical radiograph (*A*) shows an opacity in the area of tooth 30. Except for the fact that it is slightly distal to the premolar teeth, for all intents and purposes the radiographic appearance is that of a torus. On clinical examination, however, no torus was noted lingually. Instead, a shelf of bone was noted on the buccal aspect. The opposite side looked normal. As a result, the diagnosis of torus was discarded. Occlusal films were taken to evaluate the area further. They show the unilaterality of the condition (*B*), the intact buccal cortex on the right, and the uniformity of the opacity (*B* and *C*). The differential diagnosis includes exostosis, osteoma, and periostitis. The lack of clinical or other radiographic signs and symptoms of infection and the lack of laminations in the opacity make the likelihood of a periostitis very low. The final diagnosis was an exostosis. No biopsy or treatment is necessary. Follow-up for 6–12 moths is reasonable.

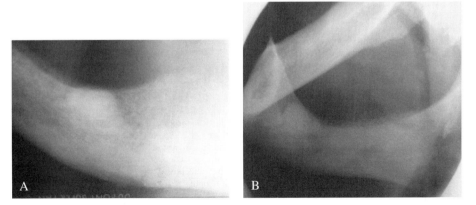

Osteoma. This case also illustrates the need for the radiologist or dentist to do a clinical examination. Portions of the panoramic film (*A* and *B*) show an opacity in the mandibular left posterior quadrant. (*Figure continues on next page*)

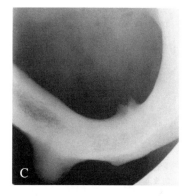

Osteoma. (*continued*) The appearance suggests an area of sclerosis or enostosis. Clinical examination, however, showed a buccal expansion, seen on the occlusal film (*C*). The expanded area consists of cancellous bone. The interpretation was osteoma.

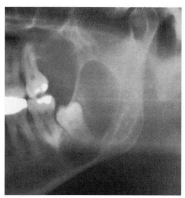

Odontogenic keratocyst. The panoramic film above shows a radiolucency in the mandibular left posterior quadrant of a 35-year-old man. The mandibular left third molar is impacted. The lucency is well defined and corticated. It has spread more in the length of the bone (mesiodistally) than in the superoinferior dimension. Note how the canal has been displaced inferiorly. The differential diagnosis of a radiolucency with this appearance in this location in a 35-year-old man includes dentigerous cyst, odontogenic keratocyst (OKC), and ameloblastoma. Careful examination shows the follicle space around the impacted molar to be within normal limits, thus excluding a dentigerous cyst. OKCs are more likely than ameloblastomas to grow in the length of the bone. They are also more likely to have all of their cortical borders intact. This combination of findings makes the interpretation of OKC the most likely option—a diagnosis that was confirmed histologically.

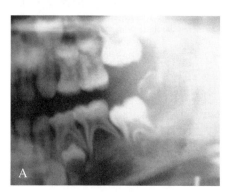 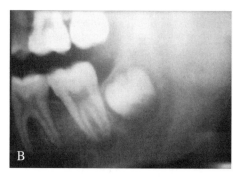

Leukemia. Note the enlargement of the dental papillae at the apices of mandibular left first molar and the destruction of the lamina dura that normally surround the papillae (*A*). The cortex surrounding the crypt of the developing second molar is also destroyed. The most common cause of destruction of the lamina dura in particular or cortices in general is infection. In this case, however, none is evident radiographically, nor did the patient have any clinical signs or symptoms of such. In the absence of infection, destruction of cortices is an ominous sign, raising the specter of malignancy. In this case the developing second molar also has the appearance of "floating in space," another sign of malignancy. The patient was diagnosed with leukemia. This case also raises the question of the differential diagnosis of an enlarged follicle space. If the follicle is enlarged but has a cortex, the more common entities in the differential include hyperplastic follicle, dentigerous cyst, adenomatoid odontogenic tumor, and ameloblastic fibroma or ameloblastic fibroodontoma. If the cortex is absent, more serious conditions, such as leukemia or other blood dyscrasias and the storage diseases (e.g., Hurler disease, Gaucher disease), should be considered. A similar, albeit slightly more subtle, case of leukemia is seen in *B*. Note what looks like a frank periapical radiolucency on the mandibular left second molar, an intact tooth. Additionally, the cortex surrounding the crypt of the developing third molar is destroyed except for the coronal portion.

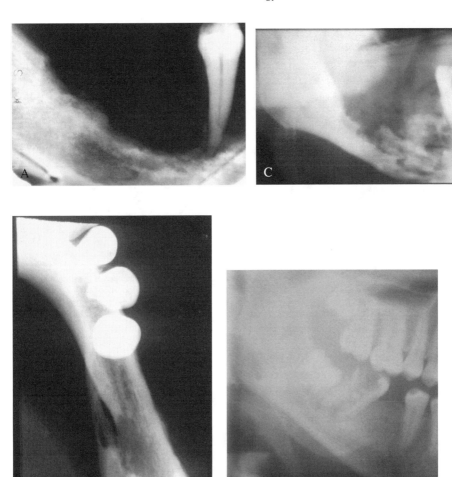

Malignancy and osteomyelitis. The images above contrast well the classical radiographic presentations of a malignancy (*A* and *B*) and osteomyelitis (*C*). The periapical film (*A*) shows the typical "tooth-standing-in-space" appearance so characteristic of malignancy. Note the complete destruction of bone, as though the tumor is following a scorched earth policy, and the irregular outline, so aptly described by Worth as consisting of "bays" and "promontories." The lack of resorption of the premolar is also more in keeping with malignant than a benign lesion. The occlusal radiograph (*B*) shows destruction of the lingual cortex. By contrast, the panoramic film (*C*) shows bone destruction, but with areas of bone intervening. These areas of bone, separated from the bulk of the mandible, are sequestra and constitute the radiographic hallmark of osteomyelitis. Another sign of infection is a periosteal reaction (*D*). By itself, a periosteal reaction is not pathognomonic of osteomyelitis or even of infection, although the latter is its most common case.

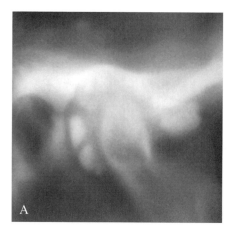
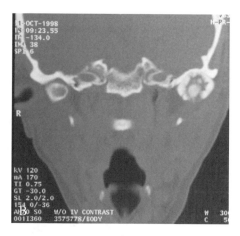

Synovial chondromatosis. In the above case sagittal tomogram of the temporomandibular joint (*A*), the most striking feature in is the presence of a number of opacities within the joint space, both anterior and posterior to the condyle. The opacities are also seen on the coronal CT scan (*B*). The case raises the question: what is the differential diagnosis of opacities, especially multiple ones, in and around the condyle? The answer includes synovial chondrometaplasia (osteochondrometaplasia), pseudogout (chondrocalcinosis), avascular necrosis, osteochondritis dissecans, and even rheumatoid arthritis and degenerative joint disease.

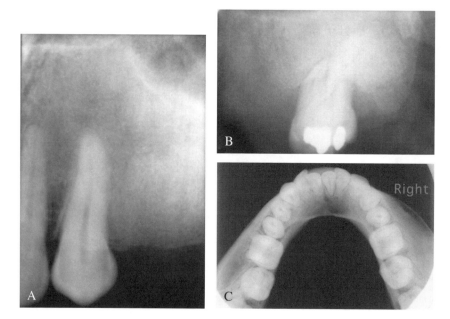

Fibrous dysplasia. Periapical films (*A* and *B*) of the posterior maxilla show a difference in the quality of the bone compared with normal appearance. Note the relative lack of marrow spaces and the granularity of the bone. The radiographic picture is virtually pathognomonic of fibrous dysplasia. An occlusal film (*C*) from a different patient shows the buccal expansion of the mandible on the right side and the granular nature of the bone in this area. In general, the differential diagnosis in such cases includes fibrous dysplasia, Paget's disease, chronic sclerosing sclerosing osteomyelitis, and enostosis/dense bone.

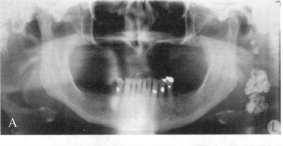

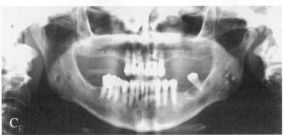

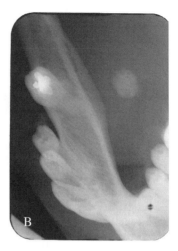

Lymph node calcification. Panoramic view (*A*) shows multiple, discrete radiopacities in the soft tissues posterior to the vertical ramus. Soft tissue opacities in and round the jaws fall into the following general categories: tooth, calcification, bone, and foreign body. Under these categories, especially that of calcifications, falls a long list of items. The most common calcifications, however, constitute a somewhat short list: sialoliths, lymph node calcification, tonsilloliths, phleboliths, acne scars, parasitic larva (e.g., cysticercosis), osteoma cutis, injection granulomas (e.g., gold injections for arthritis), pseudogout, increased parathormone secretion, CREST syndrome, and Ehlers-Danlos syndrome. This case shows lymph node calcifications. Among the most common calcifications that the dentist must distinguish are lymph node calcification vs. sialoliths. Classical lymph node calcifications are described as having a cauliflower appearance (as seen in *A*). Sialoliths, by contrast, appear as smooth, more or less uniform opacities (*B*). Sialoliths in the submandibular gland or duct are located lingual to the mandible. Another common calcification (*C*), overlying the left vertical ramus, is the tonsillolith.

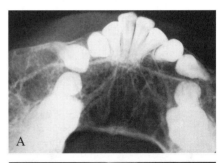

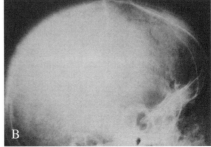

Thalassemia. The occlusal film (*A*) shows a marked variation from normal in the trabecular pattern. The trabeculae are larger and coarser, and the marrow spaces are larger than usual. The jaw is markedly expanded. The radiographic picture is consistent with an attempt by the body to increase the amount of marrow in order to produce more red blood cells. Although a number of conditions, such as sickle cell and other anemias, may give rise to the radiographic appearance, the changes are usually more pronounced in thalassemia, from which this patient suffered. On occasion, one may also see a hair-on-end appearance in thalassemia (*B*).

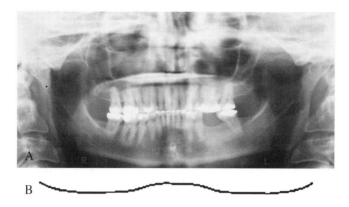

Panoramic technique. Identify three technical errors that were made in taking the above panoramic film (*A*). Answers: (1) The left vertical ramus is much wider than its right counterpart. Although an asymmetry may account for this finding, note how much larger (mesiodistally) the remaining mandibular left molar is than the molars on the right side. Teeth rarely differ in size from side to side, implying that the difference in the size of the rami is due to incorrect side-to-side positioning of the patient. In this case, the patient was positioned off-center to the right side. (2) The occlusal plane should be in the form of a straight line or, more correctly, that of a slight smile. The patient was positioned with the chin too high up, resulting in an occlusal plane as depicted in *B*. (3) The anterior teeth look smaller than they should. The patient was positioned too far forward—that is, with the anterior teeth too close to the film as it moved past these teeth.

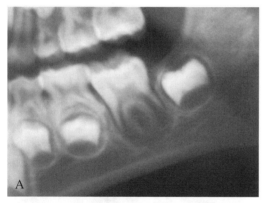

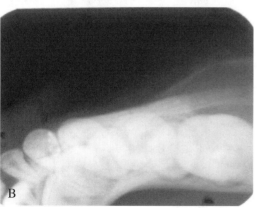

Mandibular infected buccal cyst. The cropped panoramic radiographic (*A*) shows a lucency over the mandibular left first molar. The lucency starts at or about the furcation area and somewhat beyond the apices. Note that, unlike the leukemia case, the lucency retains its cortex, albeit a very thin one at its most inferior aspect. The radiographic picture is highly suggestive of a buccal bifurcation cyst, also known as a mandibular infected buccal cyst. An occlusal film (*B*) shows a buccal expansion. Note how the roots of the first molar have been pushed into the lingual cortex. This latter feature virtually clinches the diagnosis. Other disorders to consider in a differential diagnosis include conditions that may produce a periosteal response on the buccal surface (a radicular cyst). A dentigerous cyst should be readily distinguishable.

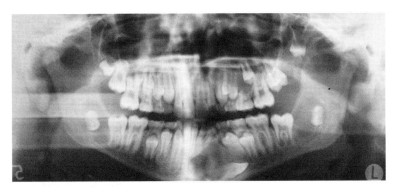

Gorlin-Goltz syndrome. The panoramic image shows radiolucencies around or associated with the crowns of the mandibular left and right third molars, as well as of the mandibular left canine. Closer examination reveals that the maxillary left third molar has been displaced superiorly, suggesting the presence of a lesion here too. The maxillary left second bicuspid also has a pericoronal radiolucency. The differential diagnosis for multiple, well-defined and, in this case, pericoronal radiolucencies includes dentigerous cysts and odontogenic keratocysts. Multiple dentigerous cysts have been reported but are uncommon. This patient suffers from Gorlin-Goltz syndrome. Other causes of multiple pericoronal radiolucencies include the storage diseases (e.g., Hurler disease, Gaucher disease), but in such cases the lucencies are more likely to be noncorticated.

6. PERIODONTOLOGY

Joseph P. Fiorellini, D.M.D, D.M.Sc.

FUNDAMENTALS OF THE PERIODONTIUM

1. What fibers are normally found in a healthy periodontium?
The fibers are described classically in histologic position as the dentogingival, dentoperiosteal, alveologingival, circular, and transseptal.

2. What is the major blood supply to the periodontal ligament? Adjacent gingival tissue?
The blood supply to the periodontal ligament derives from arteries and arterioles within the supporting bone (e.g., inferior alveolar artery) to the socket and periodontal ligament. Adjacent tissue is supplied by other superficial vessels.

3. What cell type is most frequently found in the periodontal ligament?
The predominant cell type is the fibroblast.

4. What immunologic cells are typically found in the healthy periodontium?
Immunologic cells typically found in the healthy periodontium include polymorphonuclear neutrophils (PMNs), mast cells, macrophages, and lymphocytes. The prevalence of these cell types shifts depending on the disease state.

5. What is the major macromolecular component of the cementum, alveolar bone, and periodontal ligament?
Collagen.

CLASSIFICATION AND ETIOLOGY OF PERIODONTAL DISEASES

6. What are the etiologic agents in periodontal disease?
The primary cause of periodontitis is bacterial plaque—specifically, gram-negative bacteria.

7. Does the presence of gram-negative bacteria predispose the patient to periodontal disease?
The bacteria are a critical element of the periodontal disease process; however, the host response to these bacteria is also a major component.

8. What is the chief component of plaque?
Bacteria. Approximately 90–95% of the wet weight of plaque is bacteria. The other 5–10% consists of a few host cells, an organic matrix, and inorganic ions.

9. What are the basic types of plaque? How do they differ in composition?
The basic types of plaque are supragingival and subgingival. Supragingival plaque consists mostly of aerobes and facultative bacteria (mostly gram-positive), whereas subgingival plaque consists mostly of anaerobic bacteria (frequently gram-negative).

10. What type of plaque is associated with caries?
Naturally the supragingival plaque is associated with caries—predominantly the gram-positive cocci and rods (e.g., *Streptococcus mutans*).

11. What coating is responsible for the adherence of plaque to the enamel?
The salivary pellicle.

12. What are the basic types of subgingival plaque?
The three basic types of subgingival plaque are hard tissue, soft tissue, and loose plaque, all of which differ in composition. Hard tissue plaque adheres to the cementum, dentin, and enamel; soft tissue plaque adheres to the epithelial cells; and loose plaque floats in-between. Loose plaque has come under a great deal of investigation because of its possible role in attachment loss. The soft tissue plaque that adheres to the epithelial lining of the pocket has also sparked interest because of the potential involvement of the organisms in tissue invasion.

13. What is the major factor in determining the different bacteria in supragingival and subgingival plaque?
The major factor is oxygen. The redox potential of the gingival sulcus greatly influences the bacterial composition.

14. Do cariogenic bacteria promote colonization by periodontal pathogens?
On the contrary, the cariogenic bacteria tend to inhibit the gram-negative rods associated with periodontal disease.

15. What is the major mechanism by which cariogenic bacteria inhibit gram-negative periodontal pathogens?
Gram-positive cariogenic bacteria produce bacteriocins and other substances that inhibit gram-negative bacterial growth.

16. What is calculus? How is it basically formed?
Calculus is mineralized plaque. It is formed by bathing of the plaque in a supersaturated solution of Ca^{2+} and PO_4^- saliva.

17. Why is calculus frequently a dark color (e.g., black, brown, gray)?
After the plaque has been solidified to calculus and an inflammatory response has occurred, localized bleeding ensues. Red blood cells adhere to and permeate the calculus, hemolysis follows, and the hemoglobin/iron colors the calculus.

18. What terms are used to describe healthy gingiva?
Healthy gingiva has scalloped, knifelike margins and a firm, stippled texture. In Caucasians it is salmon-pink in color.

19. What terms are used to describe inflamed gingiva?
The key word is inflammation, and the cardinal signs of inflammation are calor, rubor, tumor, and dolor. All may apply to inflamed gingiva. The margins are described as rolled, the gingiva as erythematous and edematous. The stippling is absent, and the gingiva is frequently described as boggy.

20. What is gingivitis? What bacterial groups are generally associated with gingivitis?
Gingivitis is inflammation of the gingiva. The bacterial groups associated with gingivitis are spirochetes, *Actinomyces* spp. (gram-positive filament), and *Eikenella* spp. (gram-negative rod).

21. What other terms are used in the clinical description of gingivitis?
Other terms describe severity (mild, moderate, severe), location (marginal or diffuse), and presence or absence of ulceration (desquamative), suppuration, and hemorrhage. Other terms describing the architecture also may apply, such as blunting papilla and clefting.

22. What term is used to describe HIV gingivitis? How does it appear clinically?

Linear gingival erythema (LGE) is frequently used to describe HIV gingivitis. As the name implies, the gingival margin has a distinct red band, and the tissue may bleed easily.

23. Is gingivitis a forerunner of periodontitis?

No. Gingivitis is not necessarily a forerunner of periodontitis. Chronic gingivitis may exist for long periods without advancing to periodontitis.

24. Does periodontitis occur without gingivitis?

To the purist, the answer is yes. This situation may be particularly true in the case of localized juvenile periodontitis, in which negligible gingival inflammation may be accompanied by active periodontal disease. However, most patients with routine adult periodontitis also exhibit gingivitis.

25. What causes the transition from gingivitis to periodontitis?

The exact cause of the progression is most likely multifactorial, including a pathogenic combination of bacteria and an abnormal host response.

26. What are the histologic characteristics of the initial periodontal lesion?

Basically vasculitis of the vessels is accompanied by an increase of gingival exudate from the sulcus. PMNs migrate into the sulcus and junctional epithelium. The most coronal portion of the junctional epithelium is altered, and some perivascular collagen is lost.

27. What histologic changes are associated with the early periodontal lesion?

Many of the changes are a continuation of the initial lesion. PMNs continue to migrate into the epithelium, and other lymphocytes follow. The collagen network continues to break down, and the junctional epithelial cells proliferate.

28. What are the histologic features of the established periodontal lesion?

A key component of the established lesion is the predominance of plasma cells in the connective tissue with the production of antibodies, continued loss of connective tissue substance, and proliferation of junctional epithelium with or without apical migration.

29. What are the key histologic features of the advanced periodontal lesion?

Many of the features are similar to the established lesion. The advanced lesion extends to the periodontal ligament and alveolar bone with pocket formation and goes through periods of exacerbations and remission. There are more extensive cellular changes due to inflammation.

30. What are the clinical signs of necrotizing ulcerative gingivitis (NUG)?

NUG is an acute, recurring infection of the gingiva characterized by necrosis of the papilla (leading to blunting), spontaneous bleeding, pain, and fetor oris. It has been theorized that the disease is stress-related (e.g., taking the National Dental Board examinations, practical examinations, being on death row at Alcatraz).

31. What bacteria are associated with NUG?

The bacteria associated with NUG are a fusospirochetal complex—fusiform bacteria and spirochetes.

32. What bacteria are associated with gingivitis of pregnancy? Why?

Bacteria associated with gingivitis of pregnancy are the black-pigmenting *Bacteroides* spp., which utilize steroid hormones for their own metabolism. Therefore, pregnancy essentially selects for these bacteria. Patients who use birth control pills or receive steroid therapy (chronic autoimmune diseases) are also at risk.

33. What general terms are used to describe periodontitis?

Mild, moderate, and advanced or severe are commonly used. Additonal terms include local-ized, generalized, refractory, chronic, and aggressive.

34. How is periodontitis classified?

The disease is classified according to its severity by the American Dental Association:

Type I   Gingivitis
Type II   Mild periodontitis
Type III   Moderate periodontitis
Type IV   Severe or advanced periodontitis

These categories are based on clinical criteria such as the amount of bone loss, pocket depth, and mobility.

35. Describe HIV periodontitis.

HIV periodontitis involves severe pain, bleeding, rapid loss of bone and soft tissue, exposure of bone, sequestration, and tooth loss.

36. What bacteria are generally associated with chronic periodontitis?

The bacteria most frequently cultured from active adult periodontal lesions include *Prophyoromonas gingivalis, Actinobacillus actinomycetemcomitans, Campylobacter recta (Wolinella recta), Fusobacterium nucleatum, Provetella intermedia, Bacteroides forsythus, Eikenella cor-rodens,* and *Treponema denticola.*

37. Describe the clinical features of localized aggressive periodontitis.

The periodontal destruction is localized to the first permanent molars and/or the permanent central incisors. Clinical signs of inflammation are less acute than would be expected from the severity of destruction. Other features include familial pattern, paucity of plaque, onset during the circumpubertal period, and preponderance of *A. actinomycetemcomitans* when the sites are cultured.

38. What bacteria are associated with generalized aggressive periodontitis?

P. gingivalis	*Bacteroides capillus*
P. intermedia	*E. corrodens*

39. What bacteria are associated with refractory chronic periodontitis?

The major infectious agents are *B. forsythus, F. nucleatum, Streptococcus intermedius, E. corrodens,* and *P. gingivalis.* Although the diseases listed above have clinically distinct man-ifestations, many of the same types show up in cultural studies again and again. When the diag-nosis of refractory or rapidly progressive periodontitis is made, the patient's medical and family history should be thoroughly investigated. There may be underlying systemic medical problems. Do not hesitate to use the clinical medical laboratory and to refer the patient for a complete med-ical examination.

40. What is the first cellular line of defense of the body against the periopathogens?

Other than the epithelial cell barrier, the first line of defense is the PMN.

41. Which periodontal diseases may involve bacterial invasion of the connective tissue?

• Localized aggressive periodontitis
• NUG

42. What bacteria may be associated with tissue invasion?

For localized aggressive peridontitis the answer is again *A. actinomycetemcomitans.* For gin-givitis and NUG the culprits are spirochetes.

43. In what type of plaque are these organisms frequently cultured?

Because these organisms are associated with tissue invasion, they are most commonly isolated from soft tissue plaque and loose plaque in a periodontal pocket.

44. What is meant by a burn-out lesion in a patient with localized aggressive periodontitis?

At one point the patient with localized aggressive periodontitis had an infection with periodontal lesions in which the chief etiologic agent was *A. actinomycetemcomitans*. The body responds with an immunologic response and controls the infection, but the bony defect remains. The deep pocketing now becomes inhabited with bacterial flora more characteristic of chronic periodontal lesions.

45. What bacteria are associated with HIV-related gingivitis and periodontitis?

Studies indicate that the bacteria complexes associated with HIV-related gingivitis (LGE) and periodontitis are similar and include *A. actinomycetemcomitans, P. intermedia, P. gingivalis, C. recta*, and yeasts (*Candida albicans*). A major difference may be the number of *C. recta* that are isolated. Concentrations of *C. recta* tend to be higher in HIV-related periodontitis. Enteric bacteria also may be isolated.

46. Patients with deep periodontal pockets and heavy deposits of plaque and calculus may develop an acute periodontal abscess after scaling. Why?

After scaling and root planing of deep sites the coronal tissue heals (contracts and reattaches), but there may be infective material below. The process is analogous to tightening a pursestring.

47. What is a perioendo abscess?

A perioendo abscess is a combined lesion in which periodontal and endodontic problems occur simultaneously. Symptoms may vary, but as a general rule the lesion demonstrates radiographic involvement of the periodontium and periapex with significant probing depths, percussion sensitivity, and pulpal sensitivity. Treatment may include scaling, root planing, periodontal surgery, and root canal therapy.

48. What treatment is frequently used for a periodontal abscess?

Initial treatment may consist of the establishment of drainage and the removal of the etiologic agents (incision and drainage, scaling, root planing, irrigation), followed first by a course of antibiotic therapy and then by surgical treatment.

49. When is it safe to treat a pregnant woman's nonacute periodontal problem?

In general, the second trimester is the window of treatment for most dental procedures. If antibiotics or other medications are indicated, consult with the obstetrician and *Physicians' Desk Reference*.

50. Which periodontal disease most nearly fulfills Koch's postulates?

Koch's postulates state that a pathogenic bacterium causes a disease, that the disease is transmissible through the bacteria, and that if you eliminate or control the bacteria, you eliminate the infection. Localized aggressive periodontitis, caused by *A. actinomycetemcomitans*, most nearly fulfills Koch's postulates.

51. Why do most periodontal infections not fulfill Koch's postulates?

The answer lies in the preceding question. Most periodontal infections may be described as mixed anaerobic infections.

52. What is the paradox regarding an acute dental abscess?

The paradox basically pertains to bone loss associated with the lesion. An acute infection may involve rapid, extensive bone loss, but after the infection is eradicated, the lesion has great potential to heal completely.

53. What bacterial group is associated with root caries?
Root caries may be a problem for patients with gingival recession and xerostomia (whether induced by drugs, radiation, or some other agent). The bacteria associated with root caries are gram-positive rods and filaments, particularly *Actinomyces viscosus.*

CONCEPT OF DISEASE ACTIVITY

54. What is meant by active destructive disease?
Active destructive disease indicates a loss of periodontal attachment.

55. How is disease activity measured?
Classically disease activity (attachment loss) is measured by using a periodontal probe and a fixed reference point, such as the cementoenamel junction (CEJ). The change in the probing depth, excluding any changes in the gingival height due to inflammation, determines disease activity.

56. What is the classic definition of the presence of periodontal disease?
Radiographic evidence of bone loss.

57. How is the radiographic evidence of bone loss determined?
In health, the crestal bone levels are 2–3 cm below the CEJ. In periodontitis, crestal bone is below this level.

58. Which radiographs tend to be most accurate in the determination of bone loss?
The bitewings because of the parallelism. Vertical bitewings are useful to assess bone in severe cases.

59. What is bone sounding?
Sounding is used to provide the clinician with additional information about the amount of bone loss. The area in question is anesthetized, and a probe is forced through the epithelium until it strikes bone. Sounding may facilitate flap design.

60. How is periodontal disease activity described?
Patterns of periodontal disease activity include random burst and slow continuous processes. Clinical studies indicate that active diseae may have an 0.1 mm per year rate of progress.

61. What is the nonspecific plaque hypothesis?
The hypothesis simply states that it is the quantity and not the quality of the plaque that causes periodontal disease. The specific plaque hypothesis states the converse.

62. What is meant by a shift in flora in comparing a healthy or diseased periodontal site?
The healthy periodontal site is characterized by a preponderance of gram-positive organisms and fewer gram-negative organisms. In the diseased state the opposite holds true.

63. What bacteria are associated with active destructive periodontal disease (chronic periodontitis)?
The bacteria associated with destructive periodontal disease include *P. gingivalis, E. corrodens, F. nucleatum, C. recta, B. forsythus*, and *A. actinomycetemcomitans.*

64. What traditional clinical markers (other than a great change in attachment loss) may be significant in determining active periodontal disease?
One may think that the classic signs of inflammation (tumor, calor, rubor, and suppuration) are predictors of pending attachment loss. Data demonstrate the sensitivity and specificity only of

calor (temperature) for predicting attachment loss. However, it is difficult to leave inflamed gingiva untreated.

65. What two inflammatory mediators may be indicators of disease activity?
Interleukin l-beta and tumor necrosis factor alpha may indicate disease activity.

PERIODONTAL DIAGNOSIS

66. What is periodontal pocketing?
A pathologic fissue from the crest of the gingiva to the base of the pocket.

67. What sites are routinely probed during a thorough periodontal examination?
Six sites are commonly checked: the mesio-, mid-, and distobuccal sites as well as the corresponding lingual/palatal sites. Most periodontists sweep the probe continuously through the sulcus to get a better feel for the pocket depths as a whole.

68. What is periodontal pseudopocketing?
Pseudopocketing is a condition in which pocketing occurs without attachment loss. A classic example is phenytoin (Dilantin) hyperplasia.

69. Which is more important: attachment loss or periodontal pocketing?
Attachment loss is much more significant because supportive structures are destroyed. Pocketing may increase or decrease, depending on the severity of gingival inflammation, without attachment loss. Frequently, extensive attachment loss and gingival recession, with poor prognosis for the tooth, may be accompanied by shallow periodontal pocketing.

70. What are the two most significant clinical parameters for the prognosis of a periodontally involved tooth?
The two most significant clinical parameters are mobility and attachment loss.

71. What is gingival hypertrophy?
Gingival hypertrophy indicates that the gingivae have increased in size and not number. Hypertrophy indicates inflammation, whereas hyperplasia may not.

72. What causes gingival recession?
The major causes are tooth brush or floss abrasion, parafunctional habits, periodontal disease, and orthodontics (if the bands are improperly placed).

73. Which area of the oral cavity has the least amount of attached gingiva?
The buccal mandibular premolar area commonly has the least amount of attached tissue.

74. What is a long junctional epithelium?
After a periodontal pocket has been scaled, root planed, and curetted, a soft tissue reattachment to the root surface may occur. This reattachment is called a long junctional epithelium. Pocket reduction is due to a gain in attachment, not to a decrease of inflammation.

75. What is the term for gingival cells that attach to the root cementum? How do they attach to the root?
The term is junctional epithelium; the cells attach by hemidesmisomes.

76. What is a mucogingival defect?
Mucogingival defects are defined by periodontal pocketing that extends beyond the mucogingival junction.

77. What are the major risk factors for periodontitis?

Major risk factors for periodontal disease include increased age, poor education, neglect of dental care, previous history of periodontal disease, tobacco use, and diabetes.

78. Is periodontal disease a risk factor for other disease?

Some epidemiologic evidence indicates that periodontal disease and other chronic infective diseases may be associated with coronary artery disease and stroke.

79. What is the crown-to-root ratio in a healthy dentition?

As a general rule, the crown-to-root ratio in a healthy dentition is 1:2 (for each tooth).

80. What root shapes generally have a more favorable prognosis?

As the preceding question suggests, the crown-to-root ratio is very important. Long, tapering roots are usually sturdier than short, conical roots.

81. What is the clinical significance of crown-to-root ratios?

Teeth with poor crown-to-root ratios tend to have a worsened prognosis, especially if mobility is significant.

82. Define fenestration.

Fenestration refers to a window in the bone. Bony fenestrations are frequently treated surgically with grafts, with or without guided tissue regeneration.

83. What is a bony dehiscence?

A dehiscence is a V-shaped defect in the supporting bone—buccal or lingual plates. These defects are difficult to treat.

84. What is positive bony architecture?

In the healthy state the bone contours follow the gingival contours, a pattern that is usually described as scalloping. Negative architecture, although not always unavoidable, may result in re-formation of the periodontal pocket.

85. What is negative bony architecture?

As described above, the bony architecture usually follows the gingival tissue. Negative bony architecture denotes intrabony defect(s). Many periodontists believe that when osseous surgery is performed, it is necessary to recreate positive bony architecture, even at the expense of healthy supporting bone. Growing evidence suggests, however, that the recreation of positive bony architecture does not improve the periodontal prognosis.

86. What are the basic classifications of bony defects?

Bony defects are generally classified according to the number of bony walls that remain. For example, a one-wall defect has only one remaining wall of bone, two-wall defects have two remaining walls, and so on.

87. Which bony defect is most likely to repair or fill naturally after treatment?

Three-wall periodontal defects are most likely to repair naturally after therapy.

88. Why are three-wall defects most likely to repair after treatment?

Three-wall defects tend to be narrow, and three walls may contribute regenerative cells. Two- and one-wall defects lack that luxury.

89. Name the microbiologic methods of assessing bacterial plaque.

There are numerous ways to assess bacterial plaque. General categories include cultural, microscopic, enzymatic, and genetic methods.

90. How are furcations classified?

Furcations are classified according to probing. Class I furcations are found at the onset of probing: class II, approximately halfway into the furcation; and class III, throughout the furcation.

91. What periodontal pathology do diabetes, Papillon-LeFevre, and Chediak-Higashi disease have in common?

With all of these diseases the normal cellular immunologic response is impaired. The white cells (PMNs) do not function properly. Therefore, patients are susceptible to periodontal infections. Watch for abscesses.

92. What is gingival crevicular fluid (GCF)?

GCF is an ultrafiltrate of serum. Therefore, it contains many of the components of serum, particularly complement and antibody. The flow rates of GCF have been used in attempt to predict disease activity. Furthermore, investigators have been interested in GCF for other markers of periodontal breakdown (e.g., beta-glucuronidase, interleukin, collagenase).

93. What genetically based techniques are used to assess bacterial plaque?

Most of these techniques are based on DNA/RNA homologies. DNA/RNA probes specific for a suspected periodontal pathogen are used to analyze plaque.

94. Do links to specific genetic alleles predict a risk for periodontitis?

Variation in the IL-1 beta allele may indicate a risk for periodontitis. This variation has been shown to be especially important in smokers.

95. Do current smokers have the same levels of periodontitis as nonsmokers?

Generally, smokers have more attachment loss than nonsmokers.

96. What is the healing response of current smokers?

Typically, the response to nonsurgical and surgical therapy is lower in smokers.

97. What happens to the risk of periodontitis and the healing response if a patient stops smoking?

When a patient becomes a past smoker, the risk for periodontitis decreases and the healing response improves.

ADJUNCTIVE PERIODONTAL THERAPY

98. What antibiotics are used frequently to treat a periodontal abscess?

After the establishment of drainage, whether it be via the sulcus or incision and drainage (I&D), penicillin or amoxicillin (500 mg every 6 hr) provides adequate antibiotic coverage.

99. What antibiotics may be well advised for the treatment of adult periodontitis?

For adult periodontitis, with high concentrations of *P. gingivalis*, doxycycline (50–100 mg 2 times/day) provides adequate coverage. *P. gingivalis* tends to be more sensitive to doxycycline than to tetracycline.

100. What is the appropriate response to refractory periodontitis?

Systemic or local administration of antibiotics with or without conventional therapy may be indicated. Systemic broad-spectrum antibiotics include clindamycin or amoxicillin/clavulanic acid or metronidazole. Combination antibiotic therapy may also be used. Local administration of a doxycyline- or tetracycline-based device can be used to treat specific areas.

101. How is localized aggressive periodontitis treated?

Localized aggressive periontitis has a preponderance of *A. actinomycetemcomitans* and is sufficiently treated with tetracycline (250 mg every 6 hr).

102. In a patient who is allergic to penicillin and erythromycin, what is the next antibiotic to be used for prophylaxis for a heart murmur?

Clindamycin, 600 mg 1 hour before treatment.

Note: The American Heart Association has recently revised the dosage of antibiotics required for prophylaxis. Refer to Chapter 3 (Oral Medicine).

103. Why are third-generation cephalosporins frequently contraindicated for the treatment of a periodontal abscess?

Frequently the spectrum of a third-generation cephalosporin becomes so specific that it does not provide adequate antimicrobial coverage. Penicillins should be the first choice; erythromycin or clindamycin may be is used in penicillin-allergic patients.

104. What complication may occur with broad-spectrum antibiotics?

A major problem is the development of pseudomembranous colitis, which is caused by the overgrowth and toxin production of *Clostridium difficile*.

105. Why are tetracyclines used commonly in the treatment of periodontal disease?

Tetracycline is used primarily for antibiotic coverage, but it has advantages over other antibiotics because it concentrates at levels 2–4 times higher in the GCF than in the serum, binds to the root surface and can be released over a prolonged time, prevents bacterial reattachment to the root surface, promotes reattachment of fibers to the root surface, and inhibits collagenolytic activity.

106. What are some of the common guidelines or precautions that should be given to a patient in prescribing tetracyclines?

Use of any antibiotic involves the potential to upset the natural bacterial flora. Gastrointestinal distress, including nausea, vomiting, and diarrhea, is possible. Women must be advised of the potential of yeast infections. Other side effects include tinnitus, vertigo, and photosensitivity.

107. Are tetracyclines safe and effective for women who are taking birth control pills?

In general, a woman who is taking birth control pills should avoid the use of tetracyclines. Clinical studies have shown that tetracyclines may cause abnormal breakthrough bleeding during the menstrual cycle.

108. If a patient is not sure whether she is pregnant, should tetracyclines be used to treat an acute periodontal infection?

Tetracyclines exert their bacteriostatic effect by inhibiting protein synthesis at the ribosome. They also cross the placenta and inhibit fetal protein synthesis. Avoid tetracyclines in pregnant patients.

109. What directions should be given to the patient in prescribing oral tetracyclines?

Tetracyclines should be taken between meals (on an empty stomach) with a tall glass of water. Foods and antacids containing relatively high concentrations of calcium and iron should not be taken with tetracycline. Tetracycline acts as a chelator with these divalent cations, thereby interfering with its own intestinal absorption. Therapeutic dosages, therefore, are not achieved.

110. What are the major advantages and disadvantages of using doxycycline or minocycline in the treatment of periodontal disease?

The spectrum of doxycycline and minocycline may be slightly better, particularly in covering *P. gingivalis*. Other advantages include less photosensitivity, less chelating, and better patient compliance. Because both antibiotics are more fat-soluble, the dose is reduced to 50 or 100 mg 2 times/day. A significant disadvantage is cost. Doxycycline and minocycline are much more expensive.

111. What is the major problem with the use of metronidazole?

When prescribing metronidazole, you should advise patients that they must refrain from alcohol or they may become violently ill from the combination (Antabuse effect). Patients should always be advised not to mix any medicine with alcohol.

112. Why is metronidazole effective in treating a periodontal infection?

Metronidazole is most effective in treating anaerobic infections.

113. What is localized drug delivery? How does it apply to periodontal therapy?

Localized drug delivery is being developed to administer drug directly to the site of infection, the periodontal pocket. The advantage of such devices includes the elimination of many of the side effects associated with systemic delivery.

114. What are the typical indications for locally administered antibiotics?

These systems are generally used in periodontal pockets that measure greater than 5 mm and that bleed on probing.

115. What preparation is required before administering locally delivered antibiotics?

Teeth should be scaled and root planed.

116. What pathway do nonsteroidal anti-inflammatory drugs (NSAIDs) block?

NSAIDs block the cyclooxygenase metabolism of arachidonic acids.

117. Which mouth rinse appears to be most effective in the control of bacterial plaque?

Chlorhexidine gluconate is the most effective oral rinse for controlling bacterial plaque, particularly because it leaves the greatest residual concentration in the mouth after use.

118. What is sanguinaria? How is it used?

Sanguinaria, an extract from the blood root plant that exhibits antimicrobial properties, has been formulated into various dentifrices and mouthwashes. A major problem with sanguinaria is that it is easily washed from the oral cavity so that the antimicrobial effects are short-lived.

119. What is triclosan? How does it work?

Triclosan is a compound that has broad-spectrum antimicrobial properties. Therefore, it is effective against many of the gram-positive and gram-negative organisms involved with oral disease. Triclosan has recently been approved for use in dentifrices.

120. HIV-positive patients frequently manifest a condition called hairy leukoplakia in their oral cavity. What microbe is commonly associated with hairy leukoplakia? What is the treatment for this condition?

Candida albicans (yeast) is frequently associated with hairy leukoplakia and should be treated with antifungal medication, including nystatin or fluconazole. Chlorhexidine rinses should be included, because chlorhexidine is also effective against *C. albicans*.

121. What is the primary symptom of root sensitivity?

In general, the primary symptom is sensitivity to cold.

122. What is the cause of root sensitivity?

Root sensitivity is believed to be caused by the movement of fluid in the dentinal tubules, which stimulates the pain sensation (the hydrodynamic theory).

123. What factors may contribute significantly to dentinal sensitivity?

Tooth brush abrasion, periodontal and orthodontic treatment, gingival recession, acidic foods, and bruxism.

124. How is root sensitivity treated?

Treatment of root sensitivity usually involves seal-coating of the root. Substances routinely used are fluoride mouth rinses, fluoride toothpastes, desensitizing toothpaste, application of composite monomer, and iontophoresis.

125. How do root desensitizers work?

A number of methods are used, including protein precipitants (e.g., strontium chloride), dentinal tubule blockers (e.g., fluorides, oxalates), nerve desensitizers (potassium nitrate), and physical agents such as burnishing the root, composites, monomers, and resins.

OCCLUSAL TREATMENT

126. What is the role of occlusion in periodontal disease?

As a primary player, occlusion has little significance in the etiology of periodontal disease, but it may act as a contributing factor.

127. What are primary and secondary occlusal trauma?

Primary occlusal trauma refers to excessive force applied to a tooth or teeth with normal supporting structures. Secondary occlusal trauma refers to excessive force applied to a tooth or teeth with inadequate support (periodontal disease).

128. Define fremitus.

Fremitus is occlusal trauma associated with centric occlusion and may indicate a slight occlusal discrepancy. On examination, the patient is asked to open slightly and close. Tooth movements can be detected visually or by digital palpation.

129. When is a nightguard indicated?

A nightguard is indicated whenever the signs or symptoms of bruxism occur.

130. What are the clinical signs of bruxism?

Signs of bruxism may include faceting, temporomandibular joint (TMJ) symptoms, masticatory muscle soreness, fractured teeth or restorations, and widened periodontal ligament spaces (on radiographs). These signs may occur in various combinations.

131. What criteria should be followed in constructing a nightguard for the treatment of bruxism?

A nightguard should have four characteristics: (1) it should be made of hard acrylic; (2) it should snap gently over the occlusal surfaces of the maxillary teeth; (3) it should occlude evenly with the mandibular teeth; and (4) it should have even contacts in excursion and be comfortable so that the patient will wear it.

132. When should the splinting of teeth be considered?

Splinting of teeth is performed basically for patient comfort. Little evidence suggests that splinting improves the prognosis of periodontal mobile teeth. In fact, it may worsen the prognosis by limiting oral hygiene access.

133. What types of splints may be fabricated?

A wide range of splints may be provided from the simple to the elaborate. Examples include interproximal application of composite, composite with mesh reinforcement, Maryland bridge, and other fixed prostheses.

134. What do widened periodontal ligament spaces indicate?

Widened periodontal ligament spaces are indicative of occlusal traumatism (no underlying medical problems). Bone loss patterns include vertical and furcation defects.

135. What situation may be considered to be controlled occlusal trauma?

Orthodontic tooth movement may be considered to be controlled occlusal trauma.

INITIAL TREATMENT OF PERIODONTAL DISEASE

136. What is scaling? Root planing? Curettage?

Scaling is the removal of hard and soft deposits (plaque and calculus) from tooth surfaces. Root planing is the smoothing of the root surfaces with a scaler or curette. The objective of root planing is to remove additional deposits as well as affected cementum in an attempt to achieve soft-tissue attachment. Curettage is the removal of the lining of the periodontal pocket. This procedure is frequently performed with root planing to promote soft tissue attachment.

137. What is the goal of initial therapy?

The primary objective of initial therapy is to reduce the bacterial levels associated with periodontitis.

138. Can antibiotics be used as component of initial therapy?

Bacterial levels can be reduced by combining mechanical and antibiotic therapy. Antibiotics including metronidazole can be used.

139. When do bacterial populations reach pretreatment levels?

Typically, bacteria repopulate the periodontal pocket as soon as 4–6 weeks. The use of antibiotics can extend this time.

140. What is the treatment routinely used for NUG?

Treatment consists of debridement (scaling and root planing) with an antibiotic. Penicillin V/K, 260–500 mg 4 times/day for 7 days, should be sufficient. Pain relievers are prescribed if needed. Instructions for oral hygiene should be stressed.

141. What is the treatment for acute suppurating gingivitis?

The treatment is the same as that for NUG. If the patient does not respond, you may consider changing the antibiotic. If the second antibiotic does not work, you may want to examine systemic factors; for example, diabetics are prone to this type of periodontal problem.

142. What is nonsurgical therapy for periodontal disease?

Nonsurgical therapy is centered on maintenance. Scaling and root planing are performed with greater frequency than in a normal recall schedule.

SURGICAL TREATMENT OF PERIODONTAL DISEASE

143. What are the advantages of periodontal surgery over nonsurgical treatment?

The most important reason for performing periodontal surgery is access. It gives you the opportunity to visualize the roots so that calculus may be removed more completely.

144. What are additional objectives of periodontal surgery?

Other objectives include pocket reduction and promotion of gingival reattachment.

145. Name the major complications that may be associated with periodontal surgery.

As with any form of surgery, there may be associated risks of pain, fever, swelling, infection, and bleeding. In addition, gingival recession, root caries, and root sensitivity may occur.

146. When is gingivectomy indicated?

Gingivectomies are indicated when there are copious amounts of attached tissue and no intrabony defects. The most common application is treatment of drug-induced hyperplasia.

147. What drugs may cause gingival hyperplasia?

Common causative drugs include phenytoin, nifedipine, and cyclosporine A. These medications stimulate proliferation of gingival fibroblasts, causing an overgrowth of the gingiva. Other drugs that may cause gingival hyperplasia include calcium channel blockers (verapamil, felodipine, nisoldipine, diltiazem, amlodipine), antiepileptics (lamotrigine and mephenytoin), the immunosuppressive mycophenolate, the antidepressant sertraline, the antipsychotic pimozide, and interferon alpha$_2$ beta.

148. How may pocket depth be indicated before performing a gingivectomy?

After the tissue has been anesthetized, a probe may be inserted to the depth of the pocket, and a second probe may be used to perforate the gingiva at that depth, creating a bleeding point (Black procedure). A series of bleeding points provides a guide for the amount of tissue to be excised.

149. What instruments are commonly used to perform a gingivectomy?

Instruments may include the Buck and Kirkland knives, dental burs, and scalpel blades.

150. What is a modified Widman flap?

A Widman flap is also known as open or flap curettage. Sulcular or submarginal incisions are made initially, and full-thickness flaps are elevated for debridement, scaling, and root planing. Flaps are then closed with sutures.

151. What is a full-thickness periodontal flap? A partial-thickness periodontal flap?

After the incision is made, a full-thickness flap involves elevation of the entire soft tissue, whereas a partial-thickness flap involves the splitting (dissection) of the gingival flap, leaving the periosteum adherent to the bone.

152. Why are inverse bevel incisions frequently used in flap surgery?

Inverse bevel incisions facilitate degranulation by thinning the flap. Furthermore, the thinning of the flap may promote reattachment of the gingiva to the root by placing connective tissue elements against the root when the flap is closed.

153. What is an apically positioned flap? When is it most frequently performed?

After the flap has been elevated and the necessary treatment has been performed, the gingiva is positioned at the crest of bone. This procedure is most frequently performed after osseous surgery (e.g., positive architecture, crown lengthening) and usually requires vertical releasing components.

154. What is osteoplasty? What is ostectomy?

Osteoplasty is the reshaping or recontouring of nonsupportive bone. An example is the recontouring and ramping of interproximal bone. Ostectomy is the removal of supporting bone. This procedure is usually performed to create positive architecture or to increase the clinical crown length.

155. What is cementoplasty? Where is it commonly applied?

Cementoplasty is the reshaping and smoothing of the root cementum. Teeth with developmental grooves in the roots, such as the premolars and maxillary lateral incisors, may develop localized periodontal defects as bacterial plaque and calculus run apically down the groove.

156. When is a crown-lengthening procedure indicated?

The procedure is indicated when the clinical crown length is inadequate for the placement of a dental restoration. Generally, there should be 4–6 mm between the preparation and the crest of bone. This measurement maintains a proper biologic width.

157. What types of tissue are removed during a crown-lengthening procedure?

Soft tissues with or without bone are removed to provide the proper biologic width.

158. How are furcations routinely treated?

The treatment of furcations depends on the extent of bone loss. Therapy ranges from scaling and root planing to curettage or guided tissue regeneration with or without grafting material.

159. What is a distal wedge procedure? Where is it commonly found clinically?

As the name implies, in the distal wedge procedure a block of tissue is removed from the distal aspect of a tooth to reduce the pocket depth. Distal wedge procedures are frequently the sequel to the extraction of a third molar. After the third molar is extracted, the bone fill is poor, leaving a periodontal defect.

160. What is a palatal/lingual curtain procedure? Where is it frequently used? Why?

The palatal/lingual curtain procedure is a surgical procedure commonly carried out in treating the maxillary anterior teeth. Deep, interproximal buccal incisions are made to free the palatal tissue; the buccal flap is not elevated. After the palatal/lingual flap is elevated, debridement, scaling, and root planing are carried out from the palatal. The rationale behind this procedure is to maintain the buccal gingival architecture to minimize esthetic changes.

161. What is crestal anticipation?

This term is commonly used to describe flap design when surgery is performed, particularly when it is extremely difficult to position the gingival flap apically at the crest of bone. (In palatal and lingual gingiva, vertical releasing incisions are difficult or contraindicated.) Basically an inverse bevel gingivectomy to the crest is carried out.

162. When is a root amputation indicated?

Obviously the procedure applies only to multirooted teeth. In general, a root amputation may be performed when periodontal involvement of a single root is severe. Endodontic and prosthetic considerations also must be taken into account.

163. Which teeth are most frequently involved in root amputation procedures?

The requirement of multirooted teeth limits the number of candidates. A vast majority of root amputations involve the maxillary first and second molars.

164. Why are the maxillary first and second molars frequent candidates for root amputation?

Because of the convergence of the distobuccal root of the first molar and the mesiobuccal root of the second molar as the roots move apically, the first and second molars are commonly involved periodontal sites.

165. What surgical procedure is performed as adjunctive therapy for orthodontic tooth rotation? How successful is it?

Routinely a fiberotomy is performed to prevent relapse of the tooth rotation. In general, a fiberotomy is not enough. The rotated tooth still requires some type of stabilization.

166. What medications may affect salivary flow? How may they affect periodontal health?

Many medicines may influence salivary flow. Prime suspects are tricyclic antidepressants and antihypertensives. Decreased salivary flow diminishes the natural cleansing of the oral cavity, thus increasing the incidence of periodontal disease and caries. Watch for both supra- and subgingival root caries.

MUCOGINGIVAL SURGERY

167. When should a soft-tissue graft be considered as an appropriate treatment of gingival recession?

Soft tissue mucogingival surgery should be considered in patients with an inadequate attachment or and/or keratinized tissue.

168. What types of graft procedures are used to repair a mucogingival defect?

The most common grafting procedures are connective tissue and free gingival grafts. Other grafting procedures include the pedicle or lateral sliding flap.

169. How is bleeding controlled after the palate has been used as the donor site for a free gingival graft?

There are a number of ways to control bleeding at the donor site, including (1) pressure with a moistened gauze, (2) pressure with a tea bag, (3) vasoconstriction (epinephrine in the local anesthetic), (4) suturing (tie off the bleeders), (5) collagen with or without stent, (6) topical thrombin, and (7) chemical/electrical cautery. If bleeding continues, it may be prudent to assess prothrombin time (PT), partial thromboplastin time (PTT), and platelet count.

170. What is the primary reason for failure of a free gingival graft?

The chief reason that a free gingival graft fails is disruption of the vascular supply before engraftment. The second most common reason is infection.

171. What is meant by necrotic slough of a free gingival graft?

After a free gingival graft has been placed, the healing involves revascularization of the graft. The superficial layers of the graft are the last to be revascularized; therefore, the layer dies off, producing a necrotic slough. Pedicle grafts take their vascular supply with them; hence, no necrotic slough.

172. What type of flap is used at the recipient site of a connective tissue or free gingival graft?

Partial-thickness flaps are used so that the periosteum remains attached to the bone. The reason is that the periosteum is the blood supply for the graft.

173. Why is it difficult to place a free gingival graft in the buccal area of the mandibular premolars?

This procedure can be especially problematic when extensive recession has caused a mucogingival defect. The problem lies in the fact that you may encroach on the mental nerve/vascular bundle with the graft and cause problems with these structures.

174. When is a frenectomy indicated?

In general, frenectomy is indicated whenever a frenum is causing a problem. For example, a high attachment of a frenum may cause the crestal gingiva to pull away during phonation (ankyloglossia) and mastication, thus opening the pocket for food impaction. This situation frequently arises in the premolar areas.

175. What procedure may be performed in conjunction with a frenectomy to prevent recurrence?

A frenum also may cause a problem in the area between the maxillary central incisors, thus contributing to a diastema. The fibers of the frenum cross the height of the maxilla to the incisive papilla. The papilla may blanch when the frenum is pulled. A free gingival graft is performed in conjunction with the frenectomy to prevent recurrence of fiber attachment to the papilla.

176. What classification system is used to characterize mucogingival defects?

Miller classifications from class I–IV, depending on the width, depth, and location relative to the mucogingival junction.

177. Which Miller defect responds best to mucogingival surgery?

Miller class I and II defects can have excellent results when treated with a connective tissue graft.

REGENERATIVE PROCEDURES

178. What are the basic types of bone-grafting materials used in the treatment of perio-dontal defects?

Grafts include autografts (intraoral and extraoral), allografts, alloplasts, and xenografts. The autografts may be harvested from the patient's hip and rib (extraoral) or from a healing extraction socket, the chin, maxillary tuberosity, or retromolar areas (intraoral). Allografts consist of freeze-dried bone and freeze-dried decalcified bone from another source (usually cadaver bone). Alloplasts are synthetic materials; the most commonly used are tricalcium phosphate, calcium carbonate, and hydroxyapatite. Xenografts are typically bovine-based and particulate.

179. What is bone/blood coagulum? Where is it used?

Bone/blood coagulum is another type of grafting material, normally obtained with a chisel or file during osseous surgery. The bone/blood shavings are collected and then packed into the defect in an attempt to promote new bone formation. Because the bone is predominantly cortical, the results are not predictable.

180. What is bone swagging?

Swagging is the bending and breaking of the bony walls into the periodontal defect. It, too, has poor predictability and is not used with great frequency.

181. When should an intraoral autograft from an extraction site be harvested?

As a general guideline, the intraoral autograft should be harvested 6–8 weeks after extraction. This gives the extraction site enough time to become organized with osteogenic components.

182. What sequelae may occur with autogenous bone grafts?

Possible sequelae include root resorption and ankylosis.

183. What are connective tissue grafts for soft tissue ridge augmentation?

Connective tissue grafts are commonly used to augment a site that is now concave.

184. What sites are commonly used to harvest connective tissue for grafting?

Common sites include the hard palate, maxillary tuberosity, and retromolar area.

185. What growth factors may potentially be used to stimulate osseous regeneration?

The purpose of this question is to inform you of one of the new hot spots in periodontal research. Some day, after the etiologic agents have been removed and the inflammation is under control, growth factors may be applied to regenerate the periodontium. Three growth factors that appear to have a great deal of potential are bone morphogenic protein, platelet-derived growth factor, and insulinlike growth factor.

186. What is guided tissue regeneration (GTR)? Where is it most successful?

GTR involves the placement of a membrane (usually Gore-Tex) over a bony defect during periodontal surgery. A second surgical procedure is needed 6–8 weeks after initial surgery to retrieve the membrane. Defects amenable to this type of treatment are shallow furcations and narrow intrabony defects. GTR also may be applied to ridge augmentation procedures. A resorbable membrane is now commercially available. Therefore, no second surgery is needed to remove the membrane.

187. What is the purpose of the membrane?

The membrane prevents apical migration of the epithelium, which causes repocketing and prevents bone regeneration.

188. What surgical techniques may be used for ridge augmentation?

Common techniques use GTR membrane fixation or titanium mesh. In both cases, autogenous and/or allograft bone is placed and secured with these materials.

189. What are the indications for ridge augmentation?

Basically it is used whenever more bony mass is indicated. Examples include future placement of an implant and filling a concavity after tooth extraction for esthetic reasons. More extensive augmentation is indicated when the bone becomes too atrophic for a prosthesis.

PERIODONTAL MAINTENANCE

190. What does the typical periodontal maintenance procedure involve?

Generally, the appointment involves charting of clinical indices, scaling, root planing, polish, and reinforcement of oral hygiene instruction. Radiographs also may be indicated.

191. After periodontal therapy is completed, what should be the recall interval?

The recall interval should be individualized. Usually a 3- to 4-month interval is recommended.

192. How important is periodontal maintenance?

Regular periodontal maintenance is extremely important to the long-term prognosis of the dentition. If patients fail to adhere to routine maintenance, their periodontal status will worsen.

193. What clinical parameters are generally used to indicate periodontal breakdown?

Periodontal pocket depth and full-mouth bleeding sores are typically used, along with radiographs.

194. How many patients return for periodontal maintenance?

Typically compliance is poor. Approximately one-third of patients return.

DENTAL IMPLANTS

195. What are the two basic types of implant placement?

The two basic types of implant placement are submerged and nonsubmerged. Submerged implants require a second surgical procedure to uncover the fixture.

196. Define osseointegration.

Osseointegration is defined as bone-to-implant contact at the light microscopic level. At the clinical level, a healthy dental implant is characterized as stable.

197. In which region of the jaws are dental implants the most successful?

Dental implants in the anterior mandible have the highest success rate. The highest rate of failure is in the posterior maxilla.

198. What parameter usually indicates a failing implant?

Radiographic bone loss is the primary parameter to evaluate the status of a dental implant.

199. What considerations are important during surgical placement of implants?

During the surgery, the implant site should be cooled during drill. In addition, the implant should have primary stability (no movement).

200. What bacteria are associated with peri-implantitis?

Many of the same species associated with periimplantitis are also associated with adult periodontitis, including *A. actinomycetemcomitans, P. gingivalis*, and *P. intermedia*. Other species frequently detected by cultural methods are *Capnocytophaga* species, *C. recta*, and *E. corrodens*.

201. What can cause a dental implant to fail?

Dental implant failure can result from occlusal overload and/or peri-implantitis.

202. How are implants maintained?

Implants require maintenance, much like crowns and bridges and natural teeth. The maintenance instruments are usually plastic-tipped so that the surface of the implant is not scratched. Floss, superfloss, and braided floss are also handy.

BIBLIOGRAPHY

Classification of Periodontal Diseases and Etiologies

1. Haffajee AD, Socransky SS, Dzink JL, et al: Clinical, microbiological and immunological features of subjects with refractory periodontal diseases. J Clin Periodontol 15:390, 1988.
2. Kornman KS, Loesche WJ: Effects of estradiol and progesterone on *Bacteroides melaningogenicus* and *Bacteroides gingivalis*. Infect Immun 35:256–263, 1982.
3. Listgarten MA: The role of dental plaque in gingivitis and periodontitis. J Clin Periodontol 15:485–487, 1988.
4. Mandell ID, Gaffar A: Calculus revisited. J Clin Periodontal 13:249–257, 1986.
5. Moore WEC, Moore LH, Ranney RR, et al: The microflora of periodontal sites showing active progression. J Clin Periodontol 18:729–739, 1991.
6. Newman MN, Socransky SS: Predominant microbiota of periodontosis. J Periodontol Res 12:120–128, 1977.
7. Sooriyamoorthy M, Gower DB: Hormonal influences on gingival tissue: Relationship to periodontal disease. J Clin Periodontol 16:201–208, 1989.
8. Tanner ACR, Haffer C, Brathall GT, et al: A study of the bacteria associated with advancing periodontitis in man. J Clin Periodontol 6:278, 1979.
9. Zambon JJ, Reynolds HS, Genco RJ: Studies of the subgingival microflora in patients with acquired immunodeficiency syndrome. J Clin Periodontol 61:699–704, 1990.

Concepts of Disease Activity

10. Jandinski JJ, Stashenko P, Feder LS, et al: Localization of interleukin l-beta in human periodontal tissue. J Penodontol 62:36–43, 1991.
11. Lindhe J, Haffajee AD, Socransky SS: The progression of periodontal disease in the absence of periodontal therapy. J Clin Periodontol 10:433–442, 1983.
12. Rossomando EF, Kennedy JE, Handjmichael J: Tumor necrosis factor alpha in gingival crevicular fluid as a possible indicator of periodontal disease in humans. Arch Oral Biol 35:431–434, 1990.
13. Socransky SS, Haffajee AD, Goodson JM, Lindhe J: New concepts of destructive periodontal disease. J Clin Periodontol 11:21–32, 1984.

Periodontal Diagnosis

14. Cochran DL: Bacteriological monitoring of periodontal disease: Cultural, enzymatic, immunological, and nucleic acid studies. Curr Opin Dent 1:37–44, 1991.
15. Goultschin J, Cohen HDS, Donchin M, et al: Association of smoking with periodontal treatment needs. J Periodontol 61:364–367, 1990.
16. Grbic JT, Lamster IB, Celenti RS, Fine JB: Risk indicators for future clinical attachment loss in adult penodontitis: Patient variables. J Periodontol 62:322–329, 1991.
17. Savitt ED, Keville MW, Peros WJ: DNA probes in the diagnosis of periodontal microorganisms. Arch Oral Biol 35(Suppl):153S–159S, 1990.
18. Schlossman M, Knowler WC, Pettitt DT, Genco RJ: Type 2 diabetes mellitus and periodontal disease. J Am Dent Assoc 121:532–536, 1990.

Adjunctive Periodontal Therapy

19. Bonesville P: Oral pharmacology of chlorhexidine. J Clin Periodontol 4:49–65, 1977.
20. Ciancio SA: Antibiotics in periodontal care. In Newman MG, Kornman KS (eds): Antibiotic/Antimicrobial Use in Dental Practice. Carol Stream, IL, Quintessence, 1990, pp 136–147.
21. Goodson JM: Drug delivery. In Perspectives on Oral Antimicrobial Therapeutics. Chicago, American Academy of Periodontology, 1987, pp 61–78.
22. Southard GL, Boulware RT, Walborn DR, et al: Sanguinarine: A new antiplaque agent. Compend Cont Educ Dent 5(Suppl):72–75, 1984.

23. Williams RC: Non-steroidal anti-inflammatory drugs in periodontal disease. In Lewis AJ, Furst DE (eds): Non-steroidal Anti-inflammatory Drugs. New York, Marcel Dekker, 1987, pp 143–155.

Initial Treatment of Periodontal Disease

24. Drisko CL, Killoy WJ: Scaling and root planing: Removal of calculus and subgingival organisms. Curr Opin Dent 1:74–80, 1991.
25. Hirshfeld L, Wasserman B: A long term survey of tooth loss in 600 treated periodontal patients. J Periodontol 49:225–237, 1978.
26. Pihlstrom B, McHugh RB, Oliphant TH, Ortiz-Campos C: Comparison of surgical and non-surgical treatment of periodontal disease. J Clin Periodontol 10:524–541, 1983.

Surgical Treatment of Periodontal Disease

27. Becker BE, Becker W, Caffesse R, et al: Three modalities of periodontal therapy: 5-year final results. J Dent Res 69:219, 1990.
28. Kalkwarf KL: Surgical treatment of periodontal diseases: Access flaps, bone resection techniques, root preparation, and flap closure. Curr Opin Dent 1:87–92, 1991.
29. Ramfjord SP, Morrison EC, Kerry GJ, et al: Four modalities of periodontal treatment compared over five years. J Clin Periodontol 14:445–452, 1987.
30. Ramfjord SP, Nissle RR, Shick RR, Cooper H: Subgingival curettage versus surgical elimination of periodontal pockets. J Periodontol 39:167–175, 1968.
31. Robertson PB: The residual calculus paradox. J Periodontol 61:65–66, 1990.
32. Tarnow DP, Fletcher P: Root resection vs. maintenance of furcated molars. NY State Dent J 55:34, 36, 39, 1989.

Mucogingival Surgery

33. Allen EP: Use of mucogingival surgery to enhance esthetics. Dent Clin North Am 32:307–330, 1988.
34. Lang NP, Loe H: The relationship between the width of keratinized gingiva and gingival health. J Periodontol 43:623–627, 1972.
35. Miller PD: Regenerative and reconstructive periodontal plastic surgery: Mucogingival surgery. Dent Clin North Am 32:287–306, 1988.
36. Prato GPP, De Sanctis M: Soft tissue plastic surgery. Curr Opin Dent 1:98–103, 1991.

Regenerative Procedures

37. Becker BE, Becker W: Regenerative procedures: Grafting materials, guided tissue regeneration, and growth factors. Curr Opin Dent 1:93–97, 1991.
38. Branemark Pl, Zarb GA, Albrektsson T: Tissue-integrated prostheses. In Osseointegration in Clinical Dentistry. Carol Stream, IL, Quintessence, 1985.
39. Lynch SE, Williams RC, Polson AM, et al: A combination of platelet-derived growth factors enhances periodontal regeneration. J Clin Periodontol 16:545–548, 1989.
40. Magnusson I, Batch C, Collins BR: New attachment formation following controlled tissue regeneration using biodegradable membranes. J Periodontol 59:1–6, 1988.

7. ENDODONTICS

Steven P. Levine, D.M.D.

DIAGNOSIS

1. What is the proper role of the pulp tester in clinical diagnosis?

The pulp tester excites the nervous system of the pulp through electrical stimulation. However, the pulp tester suggests only whether the tooth is vital or nonvital; the crucial factor is the vascularity of the tooth. The pulp test alone is not sufficient to allow a diagnosis and must be combined with other tests.

2. What is the importance of percussion sensitivity in endodontic diagnosis?

Percussion sensitivity is a valuable diagnostic tool. Once the infection or inflammatory process has extended through the apical foremen into the periodontal ligament (PDL) space and apical tissues, pain is localizable with a percussion test. The PDL space is richly innervated by proprioceptive fibers, which make the percussion test a valuable tool.

3. Listening to a patient's complaint of pain is a valuable diagnostic aid. What differentiates reversible from irreversible pulpitis?

In general, with **reversible pulpitis** pain is elicited only on application of a stimulus (i.e., cold, sweets). The pain is sharp and quick but disappears on removal of the stimulus. Spontaneous pain is absent. The pulp is generally noninflamed. Treatment usually is a sedative dressing or a new restoration with a base. **Irreversible pulpitis** is generally characterized by pain that is spontaneous and lingers for some time after stimulus removal. There are various forms of irreversible pulpitis, but all require endodontic intervention.

4. What are the clinical and radiographic signs of an acute apical abscess?

Clinically an acute apical abscess is characterized by acute pain of rapid onset. The affected tooth is exquisitely sensitive to percussion and may feel "elevated" because of apical suppuration. Radiographic examination may show a totally normal periapical complex or a slightly widened PDL space, because the infection has not had enough time to demineralize the cortical bone and reveal a radiolucency. Electric and thermal tests are negative.

5. Discuss the importance of inflammatory resorption.

Resorption after avulsion injuries depends on the thickness of cementum. When the PDL does not repair and the cementum is shallow, resorption penetrates to the dentinal tubules. If the tubules contain infected tissue, the toxic products pass into the surrounding alveolus to cause severe inflammatory resorption and potential loss of the tooth.

6. After a luxation injury, ankylosis and replacement resorption can occur. How does this process take place?

After extensive dental trauma that affects a large part of the root surface, an acute inflammatory response ensues. Because of the inflammatory response, the root surface loses its cementum. The cells that repopulate the root surface are often bone cells instead of periodontal ligament cells, which migrate more slowly. Thus, the migratory precursor bone cells produce bone that forms where cementum was and directly contacts the root without any attachment complex such as the PDL. This bone ingrowth, which continually forms and resorbs the root, is characteristic of replacement resorption.

Andreasen JO: Etiology and pathogenesis of traumatic dental injuries. Scand J Dent Res 78:273, 1970.

7. A patient presents with a "gumboil" or fistula. What steps do you take to diagnose the cause or to determine which tooth is involved?

All fistulas should be traced with a gutta percha cone, because the originating tooth may not be directly next to the fistula. Fistulas positioned high on the marginal gingiva, with concomitant deep probing and normal response of teeth to vitality testing, may have a periodontal etiology.

8. Why is it often quite difficult to find the source of pain in endodontic diagnosis when a patient complains of radiating pain without sensitivity to percussion or palpation?

Teeth are quite often the source of referred pain. Percussion or palpation pain may be lacking in a tooth in which the inflammatory process has not reached the proprioceptive fibers of the periodontal ligament. The pulp contains no proprioceptive fibers.

9. What is the anatomic reason that pain from pulpitis can be referred to all parts of the head and neck?

In brief, nerve endings of cranial nerves VII (facial), IX (glossopharyngeal), and X (vagus) are profusely and diffusely distributed within the subnucleus caudalis of the trigeminal cranial nerve (V). A profuse intermingling of nerve fibers creates the potential for referral of dental pain to many sites.

10. Is there any correlation between the presence of symptoms and the histologic condition of the pulp?

No. Several studies have shown that the pulp may actually degenerate and necrose over a period of time without symptoms. Microabscess formation in the pulp may be totally asymptomatic.

11. Describe the process of internal resorption and the necessary treatment.

Internal resorption begins on the internal dentin surface and spreads laterally. It may or may not reach the external tooth surface. The process is often asymptomatic and becomes identifiable only after it has progressed enough to be seen radiographically. The etiology is unknown. Trauma is often but not always implicated. Resorption that occurs in inflamed pulps is characterized histologically by dentinoclasts, which are specialized, multinucleated giant cells similar to osteoclasts. Treatment is prompt endodontic therapy. However, once external perforation has caused a periodontal defect, the tooth is often lost.

12. How can one deduce a clinical impression of pulpal health by examining canal width on a radiograph?

Although not a definitive diagnostic tool, pulp chamber and root canal width on a radiograph may give a suggestion of pulp health. When compared with adjacent teeth, very narrowed root canals usually indicate pulpal pathology, such as degeneration due to prior trauma, capping, or pulpotomy or periodontal disease. Conversely, root canals that are very wide in comparison to adjacent teeth often indicate prior pulp damage that has led to pulpal necrosis.

13. What is the significance of the intact lamina aura in radiographic diagnosis?

The lamina aura is the cribiform plate or alveolar bone proper, a layer of compact bone lining the socket. Because of its thickness, an x-ray beam passing through it produces a white line around the root on the radiograph. Byproducts of pupal disease, passing from the apex or lateral canals, may degenerate the compact bone; its loss can be seen on a radiograph. However, this finding is not always diagnostic, because teeth with normal pulps may have no lamina aura.

14. Which radiographic technique produces the most accurate radiograph of the root and surrounding tissues?

The paralleling or right-angle technique is best for endodontics. The film is placed parallel to the long axis of the tooth and the beam at a right angle to the film. The technique allows the most accurate representation of tooth size.

15. What is the definition of a true combined lesion?

A true combined lesion is due to both endodontic and periodontal disorders that progress independently. The lesions may join as the periodontal lesion progresses apically. Such lesions, if any chance of healing is to occur, require both endodontic therapy and aggressive periodontal therapy. Usually, the prognosis is determined more by the extent of the periodontal lesion.

16. What is the reason that radiographic examination does not show periapical radiolucencies in certain teeth with acute abscesses?

One study showed that 30–50% of bone calcium must be altered before radiographic evidence of periapical breakdown appears. Therefore, in acute infection apical radiolucencies may not appear until later, as treatment progresses.

17. Why do pulpal-periapical infections of mandibular second and third molars often involve the submandibular space?

Extension of any infection is closely tied to bone density, the proximity of root apices to cortical bone, and muscle attachments. The apices of the mandibular second and third molars are usually below the mylohyoid attachment; therefore infection usually spreads to the lingual and submandibular spaces; often the masticator space is also involved.

18. A patient presents with a large swelling involving her chin. Diagnostic tests reveal that the culprit is the lower right lateral incisor. What factor determines whether the swelling extends into the buccal fold or points facially?

A major determining factor in the spread of an apical abscess is the position of the root apex in relation to local muscle attachments. In this particular case, the apex of the lateral incisor is below the level of the attachment of the mentalis muscle; therefore, the abscess extends into the soft tissues of the chin.

19. A middle-aged woman has been referred for diagnosis of multiple radiolucent lesions around the apices of her mandibular incisors. The patient is asymptomatic, the teeth are normal on vitality tests, no cortical expansion is noted, and the periodontium is normal. Medical history and blood tests are normal. What is your diagnosis?

The most likely diagnosis is periradicular cemental dysplasia or cementoma. This benign condition of unknown etiology is characterized by an initial osteolytic phase in which fibroblasts and collagen proliferate in the apical region of the mandibular incisors, replacing medullary bone. The teeth remain normal to all testing. Eventually, cementoblasts differentiate to cause reossification of the area. Treatment is to monitor over time.

Torabinejad M, Walton R: Periradicular lesions. In Ingle JI (ed): Endodontics, 4th ed. Baltimore, Williams & Wilkins, 1994, pp 434–457.

CLINICAL ENDODONTICS (TREATMENT)

20. What is the current thinking on use of the rubber dam?

The dam is an absolute necessity for treatment. It ensures a surgically clean operating field that reduces chance of cross-contamination of the root canal, retracts tissues, improves visibility, and improves efficiency. It protects the patient from aspiration of files, debris, irrigating solutions, and medicaments. From a medicolegal standpoint, use of the dam is considered the standard of care.

21. What basic principles should be kept in mind for proper access opening?

Proper access is a crucial and overlooked aspect of endodontic practice. The root canal system is usually a multicanaled configuration with fins, loops, and accessory foramina. When possible, the opening must be of sufficient size, position, and shape to allow straight-line access into the canals. Access of inadequate size and position invites inadequate removal of caries, compromises proper instrumentation, and inhibits proper obturation. However, overzealous access leads to perforation, weakening of tooth structure, and potential fracture.

22. What are the current concepts on irrigating solutions in endodontics?

The type of irrigant is of minor importance in relation to the volume and frequency. The crucial factor is constant irrigation to remove dentinal debris, to prevent blockage, and to lessen the chance of apical introduction of debris. Several studies have shown the efficacy of saline, distilled water, sodium hypochlorite, hydrogen peroxide, combinations of the above, and many other agents. The results show no advantage to chemomechanical preparation of the root canal system.

23. Of what material are endodontic files currently made?

Hand-operated instruments, including broaches, H-files, K-files, reamers, K-flex files, and S-files, are made of stainless steel as opposed to carbon steel, which was used in the past. Stainless steel bends more easily, is not as brittle, is less likely to break compared with carbon steel, and can be autoclaved without dulling. In addition, hand and rotary files are now being made of nickel-titanium.

24. What are the characteristics of a K-file?

The K-file is made by machine grinding of stainless steel wire into a square shape (some companies produce a triangular shape). The square wire is then twisted by machines in a counterclockwise direction to produce a tightly spiraled file.

25. What are the characteristics of a reamer?

The reamer is made by machine twisting of a triangular stainless steel stock wire in a counterclockwise direction but into a less tightly spiraled instrument than the K-file.

26. How does the K-flex file differ?

The K-flex file is produced from a rhomboid or a diamond-shaped stainless steel stock wire twisted to produce a file. However, the two acute angles of the rhombus produce a cutting edge of increased sharpness and cutting efficiency. The low flutes made from the obtuse angles form an area for debris removal.

27. How does filing differ from reaming?

Filing establishes its cutting action upon withdrawal of the instrument. The instrument is removed from the canal without turning. Thus it uses basically a push-pull motion. Reaming is done by placing the instrument in the canal, rotating, and withdrawing.

28. What is the recommended use for Gates-Glidden and Reeso drills?

These two types of engine-driven instruments, especially the Gates-Glidden drills, are useful in the new recommended instrumentation technique of step-down preparation. They are efficient in initial coronal preparation of the canal, thereby allowing easier, more efficient, and less traumatic apical preparation.

29. What is RC-prep? How is it used?

RC-prep is composed of ethylene diamine tetraacetic acid (EDTA) and urea peroxide in a carbwax base. Its use as a canal lubricant is also enhanced by combination with sodium hypochlorite, which produces much bubbling action, allowing enhanced removal of dentinal debris and permeability into the tubules.

30. Why is nickel-titanium becoming a material of choice for endodontic hand and rotary instruments?

The new instruments made from nickel-titanium have excellent flexibility and strength after repeated sterilization, are quite anticorrosive, and resist fracture well. The nickel titanium alloy has good elastic flexibility because of its low elastic modulus. The alloy is approximately 55%

nickel and 45% titanium by weight, and its superelastic behavior allows the files to return to their original shape after the load during use is removed.

31. What is the Tooth Slooth?

Diagnosis of tooth fractures is often difficult. This simple but highly effective and well-designed instrument allows biting force to be applied one cusp at a time into an indentation (the cusp receptacle on the "Slooth"), thereby selectively examining each cusp separately in an attempt to locate a weakness due to fracture.

32. What types of hand-operated implements for root canal instrumentation are currently available?

A detailed discussion of the various properties and differences in file-reamer types is beyond the scope of this chapter. K-type files and reamers are still widely used because of their strength and flexibility. H-type Hedstrom files are quite popular because of their aggressive ability to cut dentin. S-files are highly efficient for cutting dentin on the withdrawal stroke and for filing and reaming. Flex-it files are a new modification with a noncutting tip design. This design allows guidance of the tip through curvatures and reduces the risk of ledging, perforation, and transportation of the apex. For an excellent discussion of instrumentation devices and techniques, the reader is referred to Cohen S, Burns RC (eds): Pathways of the Pulp, 6th ed. St. Louis, Mosby, 1994.

33. What is the current status on acceptability of root canal obturation materials?

Gutta percha remains the most popular and accepted filling material for root canals. Numerous studies have demonstrated that it is the least tissue-irritating and most biocompatible material available. Although differences occur among manufacturers, gutta percha contains transpolyisoprene, barium sulfate, and zinc oxide, which provide an inert, compactible, dimensionally stable material that can adapt to the root canal walls.

N-2 pastes and other paraformaldehyde-containing pastes are not approved by the Food and Drug Administration (FDA). Several studies have shown conclusively that such root-filling pastes are highly cytotoxic in tissue culture; reactions to bone include chronic inflammation, necrosis, and bone sequestration. Compared with gutta percha, the pastes are highly antigenic and perpetuate inflammatory lesions. For these reasons they are not considered the standard of endodontic care.

34. What is the proper apical extension of a root canal filling?

The proper apical extension of a root canal filling has been discussed extensively for years, and the debate continues. In the past recommendations were made to fill a root canal to the radiographic apex in teeth that exhibited necrosis or areas of periapical breakdown and to stop slightly short of this point in vital teeth. Currently, however, it is generally recommended that a root canal be filled to the dentinocementum junction, which is 0.5-2 mm from the radiographic apex. Filling to the radiographic apex is usually overfilling or overextending and increases the chance of chronic irritation of periapical tissues.

35. Describe the walking bleach technique.

The walking bleach technique is used to bleach nonvital teeth with roots that have been obturated. The technique involves the placement of a thick white paste composed of sodium perborate and Superoxol in the tooth chamber with a temporary restoration. Several repetitions of this procedure, along with the in-office application of heat to Superoxol-saturated cotton pellets in the tooth chamber, work quite well.

36. Several authors report extensive cervical resorption after bleaching of pulpless teeth with the walking bleach technique using Superoxol, sodium perborate, and heat. What is the cause?

In approximately 10% of all teeth, defects at the cementoenamel junction allow dentinal tubules to communicate from the root canal system to the PDL. These tubules remain open, without sclerosis, if the tooth becomes pulpless at a young age. It is thought that the bleaching agents may leach through the open tubules to cause the resorption. Therefore, a barrier of some type is recommended, such as zinc, phosphate cement, or some type of light canal bonding agent.

Rothstein CD: Bleaching and vital discolored teeth. In Cohen S. Burns RC (eds): Pathways of the Pulp, 7th ed. St. Louis, Mosby, 1998, pp 674–691.

37. List four useful tools in the diagnosis of a vertical crown-root fracture.

1. Transillumination with fiberoptic light
2. Persistent periodontal defects in otherwise healthy teeth
3. Wedging and staining of defects
4. Radiographs rarely show vertical fractures but do show a radiolucent defect laterally from sulcus to apex (which can be probed).

38. Describe the crown-down pressureless technique of root canal instrumentation.

With the crown-down pressureless technique the canal is prepared in a coronal to apical direction by initially instrumenting the coronal two-thirds of the canal before any apical preparation. This technique, popularized by Marshall-Pappin, minimizes apically extruded debris and eliminates binding of instruments coronally, thereby making apical preparation more difficult.

39. What is the balanced-force concept of root canal instrumentation and preparation?

The balanced-force concept, proposed by Roane and Sabala, is based on the idea of balancing the cutting forces over a greater area of the canal and focusing less force on the area where the file tip engages the dentin. The technique is done with the Flex-it file with a noncutting tip and a triangular cross-section. By using this type of file in a counterclockwise reaming motion, ledging is minimized, more inner canal curvature is accomplished, and less zipping of the apex occurs.

Roane JB, Sabala C, Duncanson M: The "balanced force" concept for instrumentation of curved canals. J Endod 11:203, 1985.

40. What is the frequency of fourth canals in mesial roots of maxillary first molars?

In an extensive study of maxillary first molars, 51% of the mesiobuccal roots contained either a larger buccal and smaller lingual canal or two separate canals and foramina. This finding shows the importance of searching for a fourth canal to ensure clinical success.

Pineda: Roentgenographic investigations of the mesiobuccal root of the maxillary first molar. Oral Surg 36:253, 1973.

41. What is the current thinking about the manner of storage of an avulsed permanent tooth and its relationship to postreplantation success?

After 15–12 minutes of extraoral exposure, the cell metabolites in the periodontal ligament have been depleted and need to be reconstituted before replantation. Research by Cvek has shown that soaking the tooth in a physiologic solution for 30 minutes before replanting reduces the chance of postreplant resorption. The media of choice are Hank's balanced salt solution (found in Save-A-Tooth) and Viaspan (used for storage of transplant organs). If neither is available, milk or saline may be used, but not as successfully.

42. What is the current guideline for the length of time to splint an avulsed tooth, with and without alveolar fracture?

The current recommendation is to splint an avulsed tooth for 7–14 days (3–5 weeks with alveolar fracture). If an avulsed tooth is replanted fairly quickly (within 1 hour) and some of the fibroblasts of the periodontal ligament (PDL) and cementoblasts of the root surface remain viable, initial PDL repair may occur in 7–14 days.

43. When an avulsed tooth is replanted, what are the current recommendations concerning rigid or functional splinting?

Recent studies show that early functional stimulus may improve the healing of luxated teeth. It is advantageous to reduce the time of fixation to the time necessary for clinical healing of the periodontium, which may take place in a few weeks. Andreasen has shown that prolonged rigid immobilization increases the risk of ankylosis; thus the splint should allow some vertical movement of the involved teeth.

Andreasen J: Effect of masticatory stimulation on dentoalveolar ankylosis after experimental tooth replantation. Endod Dent Traumatol 1:13–16, 1985.

Andreasen J: Periodontal healing after replantation of traumatically avulsed human teeth: Assessment by mobility testing and radiography. Acta Odontol Scand 33:325–335, 1975.

44. What is the physiologic basis for the use of calcium hydroxide pastes for resorptive defects or avulsed teeth?

The theory behind the use of calcium hydroxide pastes is that areas of resorption have an acidic pH of approximately 4.5–5. Such areas are more acidic than normal tissue because of the effects of inflammatory mediators and tissue breakdown products. The basic pH of calcium hydroxide neutralizes the acidic pH, thereby inhibiting the resorptive process of osteoclastic hydrolases.

Tronstad L, et al: pH changes in dental tissues after root canal with calcium hydroxide. J Endod 7:17, 1981.

45. What is the current thinking on the use of medicaments in endodontic practice?

Formerly, medicaments were in wide use in endodontics to kill bacteria in the canal. However, current thinking stresses thorough debridement of canals and the use of irrigating solutions to clean canals. Medicaments are not stressed, because all have been shown to be cytotoxic in tissue culture. In addition, several medicaments have been shown to elicit immunologic reactions in animal studies. Mechanical canal cleaning sufficiently lowers microbial levels to allow the local defense mechanisms to heal endodontic periapical lesions.

46. Discuss the variations of postoperative pain in one-visit vs. two-visit endodontic procedures.

Several studies show no difference in postoperative pain in one-visit vs. two-visit endodontic procedures. In fact, one study found that single-visit therapy resulted in postoperative pain approximately one-half as often as multiple-visit therapy.

47. What is the treatment of choice for an intruded maxillary central incisor with a fully formed apex?

Repositioning or surgical extrusion should be done immediately with splinting for 7–10 days. Because pupal necrosis is the usual outcome, pulpectomy within 2 weeks and placement of calcium hydroxide are recommended. Close observation every few months is needed.

48. What is the desired shape of the endodontic cavity (root canal) for obturation in both lateral and vertical condensation techniques?

The canal should be instrumented and shaped so that it has a continuously tapering funnel shape. The narrowest diameter should be at the dentinocemental junction (0.5–1 mm from apex) and the widest diameter at the canal opening.

49. Are electronic measuring devices for root canal of any clinical value in everyday endodontic practice?

Yes. Electronic measuring devices have been shown by several investigators to be quite accurate. In general, they work by measuring gradients in electrical resistance when a file passes from dentin (insulator) to conductive apical tissues. They are quite useful when the apex is obscured on a radiograph by sinus superimposition, other roots, or osseous structures.

50. What is the accepted material of choice for pulp-capping procedures?

The literature has reports of many drugs, medicaments, and antiinflammatory agents used for pulp capping, but the material of choice remains calcium hydroxide. Calcium hydroxide, applied to the pulp tissue, seems to cause necrosis of the underlying tissue, but the continuous tissue often forms calcific bridges.

51. Describe the process of apexification.

Apexification involves the placement of agents in the pulpless permanent tooth, with an incompletely formed apex, to stimulate continued apical closure. Calcium hydroxide pastes are the accepted agents for use in the canals.

52. What is the accepted treatment for carious exposures in primary teeth?

For carious exposures in primary teeth in which the tissue appears vital and the inflammation is only in the coronal pulp, the formocresol pulpotomy is still widely accepted. When a carious exposure shows total pulpal degeneration (necrosis), full pulpectomy is indicated with placement of a resorbable zinc oxide-eugenol (ZOE) paste.

53. What is the role of sealer-cements in root canal obturation?

Sealer-cements are still widely recommended for use with a semisolid obturating material (gutta percha). The sealers fill discrepancies between the root filling and canal wall, act as a lubricant, help to seat cones of gutta percha, and fill accessory canals and/or foramina apically.

54. What biologic property is shared by all sealer-cements used in endodontics?

Studies of biocompatability have shown that all sealer-cements are highly toxic when freshly mixed, but the toxicity is reduced on setting. Chronic inflammatory responses, which usually persist for several days, are often cited as a reason not to avoid apical overextension of the sealer. Several studies have recommended the use of sealers that are more biocompatible, such as AH-26 and the newer calcium hydroxide-based sealers (Sealapex and CRCS).

55. In using Cavit as an interappointment temporary seal, what precautions must be taken?

Cavit, which is a hygroscopic single paste containing zinc oxide, calcium and zinc phosphate, polyvinyl and chloride acetate, and triethanolamine, requires placement of at least 3 mm of material to ensure a proper seal and fracture resistance.

56. What materials or devices are of use in removing gutta percha for retreatment?

Initial removal should be done with endodontic drills (Gates-Glidden or Peezo) or by using a heated plugger to remove the coronal portion of the gutta percha. This procedure allows space in the canal for placement of solvents to dissolve remaining material. Solvents include chloroform, xylene, methyl chloroform, and eucalyptol. Chloroform is the most effective, although it has been used less because of reported carcinogenic potential. Xylene and eucalyptol are the least effective. Once the remaining gutta percha has been softened, it often can be removed by files or reamers.

Wennberg A, Orstavik D: Evaluation of alternatives to chloroform in endodontic practice. Endod Dent Traumatol 5:234,1989.

57. What are the cause, histologic characteristics, and treatment for internal resorption?

The exact cause is unknown, but internal resorption is often seen after trauma that results in hemorrhage of vessels in the pulp and infiltration of chronic inflammatory cells. Macrophages have been shown to differentiate into dentinoclastic-type cells. With this proliferation of granulation tissue, resorption can occur. Treatment is to remove the pulpal tissues as soon as possible so that tooth structure is not perforated.

58. How can you diagnose the difference between internal and external root resorption?

Often it is difficult to definitively tell the difference between the two. One of the best techniques is often radiographic:

- External resorption defects move away from the pulpal space as the radiographic angle changes. With an internal defect, it does not change.
- Internal defects do not involve bone; thus, the lucent defect involves only the root. External resorption also includes bone resorption adjacent to the root.

- Periodontal probing is often a useful aid. A resorption defect at the level of the attachment apparatus often creates a periodontal defect that can easily be probed.

Cohen S, Barns RC (eds): Pathways of the Pulp, 7th ed. St. Louis, Mosby, 1998.

59. Does preparation of the post immediately on obturation have a different effect on the apical seal of a root canal filling from delayed preparation?

Dye leakage studies have shown no difference and no effect on the apical seal whether post preparation is immediate or delayed.

Madison S, Zakariasen K: Linear and volumetric analysis of apical leakage in teeth prepared for posts. J Endod 10:422–427,1984.

60. What temperature and immersion time are needed to sterilize endodontic files in a bead sterilizer?

At the proper temperature of 220°C (428°F) in the bead sterilizer, an endodontic file should be immersed for 15 seconds. However, because of the potential for a wide variation of temperatures in the transfer medium (beads or salt), this technique should be secondary to other, more reliable techniques of sterilization.

61. What is the best and easiest technique for sterilization of gutta percha cones?

Immersion of the cone in a 5.25% solution of sodium hypochlorite for 1 minute is quite effective in killing spores and vegetative organisms.

Senia SE, et al: Rapid sterilization of gutta percha cones with 5.25% sodium hypochlorite. J Endod 1: 136, 1975.

62. What simple techniques should be used to avoid apical ledging and perforation?

Overly aggressive force should not be used in the apical area. A light touch with a precurved file to negotiate apical curvature is necessary to maintain proper canal curvature.

63. Recently a new material called MTA has gained acceptance as a root-end filling material and a perforation repair material. Describe its properties and benefits.

Mineral trioxide aggregate (MTA) is a powder composed mainly of tricalcium oxide, tricalcium aluminate, and tricalcium silicate, along with silicate oxide, which crystallizes in the presence of moisture. It is easy to mix and place in root ends or perforations, is quite hydrophilic, and in leakage studies is quite favorable compared with amalgam and Super EBA, which are other commonly used materials for the same purpose.

Torabinejad, et al: Physical and chemical properties of a new root-end filling material. Endod 21:349, 1995.

64. Which type of file is the strongest and cuts least aggressively?

K-files are the strongest of all files. Because they cut the least aggressively, they can be used with quarter-turn pulling motion, rasping, or clockwise-counterclockwise motions.

65. List four criteria that must be met before obturation of a canal.

1. The patient must be asymptomatic; the tooth in question must not be sensitive to percussion or palpation.
2. No foul odor should emanate from the tooth.
3. The canal should not produce exudate.
4. The temporary restoration should be intact, i.e., no leakage has contaminated the canal.

66. How does preparation of the canal for filling techniques that use injection of gutta percha differ from that for conventional techniques?

All injection techniques require a more flared canal body and a definite apical constriction to prevent flow of softened gutta percha into periapical tissues.

67. What is the treatment of choice for a primary endodontic lesion in a mandibular molar with secondary periodontal involvement (including furcation lucency) in a periodontally healthy mouth?

Treatment generally consists solely of endodontic therapy. Necrotic pulpal tissue that causes furcation and lateral root or apical breakdown also may cause periodontal pockets through the sulcus, but these are actually fistulas rather than true pockets. Endodontic therapy alone often heals this secondary periodontal involvement.

68. What is the current thinking on the prognosis of pulp capping and partial pulpectomy procedures on traumatically exposed pulps?

In a study of traumatically exposed pulps, including both mature teeth and teeth with immature apices, Cvek found that pulp capping or partial pulpectomy procedures were successful in 96% of cases. In all teeth the superficial pulp in the traumatized area was carefully excised. Cvek and others agree that such procedures are generally more successful in vital teeth with immature root formation.

Cvek M, Lundberg M: et al: Histological appearance of pulps after exposure by a crown fracture: Partial pulpotomy and clinical diagnosis of healing. J Endod 9:8–11, 1983.

69. Several articles and case reports have recently described the "one-shot" apexification procedure. Do they have clinical and scientific merit?

The goal of apexification is to promote the formation of a calcified apical tissue. Most studies show that in the context of a pulpless open apex in permanent teeth, the Hertwig epithelial root sheath is not present. Calcium hydroxide is usually used to cause a differentiation of connective tissue cells adjacent to the open root end into specialized cells to deposit calcified material to close the root end partially or completely. This biologic process can take weeks, if not months. The claims of one-shot procedure are false and not grounded on scientific reality. Placing mineral trioxide aggregate into the open apex situation is placing an artificial "closure," which may not work over the long term and is certainly not speeding up a normal biologic closure process.

Cohen S, Burns RC (eds): Pathways of the Pulp, 7th ed. St. Louis, Mosby, 1998.

70. What is the current thinking on ideal treatment for carious exposure of a mature permanent tooth?

There is general agreement that carious exposure of a mature permanent tooth generally requires endodontic therapy. Carious exposure generally implies bacterial invasion of the pulp, with toxic products involving much of the pulp. However, partial pulpotomy and pulp capping of a carious exposure in a tooth with an immature apex have a higher chance of working.

71. You have elected to perform partial pulpotomy and to place a calcium hydroxide cap on a maxillary permanent central incisor with blunderbuss apex in a young boy. What follow-up is necessary?

Close monitoring of the tooth is necessary. First, it is important to see whether any pathology develops. If necrosis occurs with apical pathology, extirpation with apexification is needed. On the other hand, if vitality is maintained in such teeth, root formation continues, along with dystrophic calcification.

72. What is the recommended technique for the access opening in endodontic therapy for maxillary primary incisors?

A facial approach is generally recommended for such teeth, which need pulpectomy with a filling of zinc oxide-eugenol paste. Because of esthetic problems and the difficulty in bleaching, endodontic therapy is followed by composite facial restoration.

73. Can infections of deciduous teeth cause odontogenesis of the permanent teeth?

In one study, local infections of deciduous teeth for up to 6 weeks did not influence odontogenesis of the permanent central incisors. However, longstanding infections may have a profound effect on permanent teeth buds because of direct communication between the pulpal and periodontal vasculature of the deciduous tooth and the plexus surrounding the developing permanent tooth.

74. Describe the characteristics of the Profile Rotary Instrumentation Series.

This series of nickel-titanium rotary files has a rounded, guided tip and a U-shaped flute for collecting debris. It is available in a .04 and .06 taper series; the .06 taper is used in a sequential series, allowing for a crown-down preparation.

75. Thermafil endodontic obturators are now widely used. What is the basic methodology?

Prenotched stainless steel files coated with alpha-phase gutta percha are used to obturate the canal. Selection of the Thermafil device depends on the last carrier and condenser for the thermally plasticized alpha-phase gutta percha. Alpha-phase rather than the more common beta-phase gutta percha is used because, when heated, it has superior flow properties and adheres well to the metal carrier.

76. What is the major difference between the two main thermoplasticized gutta percha techniques on the market?

In the Obtara II system, gutta percha heated to 160°C is injected through a silver needle tip at a temperature of about 65°C. The Ultrafil system is a low-temperature technique that heats the gutta percha to 70°C for injection. Both techniques stress the importance of maintaining constriction at the cementodentinal junction to prevent flow of gutta percha beyond the apex.

77. What is the "dentin-chips apical-plug filling technique"?

This technique consists of filling the last 1–2 mm of the apex of the canal with dentin chips to seal the apical foremen. Above this is placed a seal of gutta percha. This so-called biologic seal of dentin chips should be made only after proper debridement of the canal to avoid apical placement of infected chips. The efficacy of this technique is controversial.

78. During instrumentation of a mandibular first molar, you separate the tip of an 0.06 series Profile nickel-titanium rotary file in the distal root. What steps should you take to rectify the situation and to deal with any future problems?

The initial step is to try to remove the separated instrument. Currently, the best techniques to do so are with the aid of a microscope. Ultrasonics is often used with success to remove instruments that are lodged in canals. In addition, several instrument systems are available to aid in removal if ultrasonic tips are not successful. One of the most popular is the Cancellier system, which uses canulas glued onto the separated instrument tip in the canal, then attached to a threaded hand canula, which hopefully will remove the instrument. If all this fails, the canal is debrided and obturated to the best of your ability. The patient should be made aware of the fact that a portion of a sterile instrument separated in the canal space and was incorporated into the root canal filling. The tooth should be restored, and there is a need for periodic follow-up. If any clinical or radiographic signs of failure occur, apical surgery with retrograde filling is required.

79. In treating a maxillary lateral incisor, what particular care must be taken in instrumenting the apical portion?

The apical root portion usually curves toward the distal palatal space; this configuration must be negotiated carefully.

80. Should the smeared layer of dentinal debris be removed from canal walls?

Yes. Removal of the smeared layer is recommended because of the possibility that it harbors bacteria.

81. What is considered the most reliable technique to remove the smeared layer of organic and inorganic dentinal debris from canal walls?

The recommended technique is the use of a chelating agent, such as EDTA with sodium hypochlorite, during instrumentation.

82. What is the single most important factor in determining the degree and severity of the pulpal response to a tooth preparation (cutting) procedure?

Research has shown that the remaining dentin thickness between the floor of the cavity preparation and the pulp chamber is the most crucial determinant of the pulpal response. In general, a 2-mm thickness of dentin provides a sufficient degree of protection from the trauma of high-speed drills and restorative materials. With a thickness less than 2 mm, the inflammatory response in the pulp seems to increase dramatically. Neither age nor tooth size has as significant an effect.

Swerdlow H, Stanley HR: Reaction of human dental pulp to cavity preparation. J Prosthet Dent 9:121, 1959.

83. In restoring a tooth with a deep carious lesion, clinicians often excavate the caries and place a temporary sedative restoration to allow symptoms to subside. What is the rationale behind this procedure in relation to pulpal physiology?

A deep carious lesion produces an inflammatory response in the pulp tissue adjacent to the dentinal tubules in the area of the caries. Removal of the irritation to the pulp and placement of a sedative filling allow new odontoblasts to differentiate and to produce a reparative dentin in the involved area. This process usually requires approximately 20 days for odontoplastic regeneration and 80 days for reparative dentin formation.

Stanley HR: The rate of tertiary dentin formation in the human tooth. Oral Surg 21:100, 1966.

84. What is the most common reason for failure of root canals?

Although an endodontically treated tooth may fail for various reasons, including fracture, periodontal disease, or prosthetic complication leading to one of the above, the most common cause of failure is incompletely and inadequately debrided and disinfected root canals. The time-honored saying that what you take out of the canal is not as important as what you put in has much merit. The chemomechanical debridement of the root canal system, which is necessary to remove all irritants to the surrounding apical and periodontal tissues, is still the crucial aspect of root canal treatment.

PULP AND PERIAPICAL BIOLOGY

85. What is the dental pulp? Describe in a brief paragraph the ultrastructural characteristics of this remarkable tissue.

The dental pulp is a matrix composed of ground substance, connective cells and fibers, nerves, a microcirculatory system, and a highly specialized and differentiated cell called the odontoblast. The dental pulp is similar to other connective tissues in the body, but its ability to deal with injury and inflammatory reactions is severely limited by the mineralized walls that surround it. Therefore, its ability to increase blood supply during vasodilation is impaired.

86. The odontoblast is a remarkable and unique cell. Briefly describe its major characteristics.

The odontoblast is a highly differentiated cell that forms a pseudostratified layer of cells along the periphery of the pulp chamber. It is a highly polarized cell with synthesizing activity in its cell body and secretory activity in the odontoblastic process, which forms the predentin matrix. Because it is the main cell for dentin formation, injury by caries or restorative procedures may affect this activity.

87. Give a brief description of the most accepted theory about the mechanism of dentin sensitivity.

The most plausible theories are based on the fact that the dentinal tubule acts as a capillary tube. The tubule contains fluid, or a pulpal transudate, that is displaced easily by air, heat, cold, and explorer tips. This rapid inward or outward movement of fluid in tubules may excite odontoblastic processes, which have been shown to travel within the tubules, or sensory receptors in the underlying pulp.

Brannstrom M, Astrom A: The hydrodynamics of the dentine: Its possible relationship to dental pain. Int Dent J 22:219–227, 1972.

88. A 45-year-old woman presents for consultation. She is asymptomatic. Radiographs reveal a radiolucent lesion apical to teeth 24 and 25 with no swelling or buccal plate expansion. The dentist diagnosed periapical cemental dysplasia. How is this diagnosis confirmed?

Periapical cemental dysplasia or cementoma presents as a radiolucent lesion in its early stages. It is a fibroosseous lesion developing from cells in the periodontal ligament space. The teeth involved respond normally to vitality testing.

89. What is the effect of orthodontic tooth movement on the pulp?

In progressive, slow orthodontic movement, the minor circulatory changes and inflammatory reactions are reversible. However, with excessively severe orthodontic forces, disruption of pulpal vascularity may be irreversible, leading to disruption of odontoblasts and fibroblasts and possible pulpal necrosis. Rupture of blood vessels in the periodontal ligament also may affect pulpal vascularity. In addition, orthodontic tooth movement is associated with excessive root resorption and blunted roots, both of which may occur with continued vitality.

90. Inflammatory mediators cause vasodilation of blood vessels. How does vasodilation in the pulp differ from that in other tissues?

Vasodilation in all tissues is a defense mechanism, controlled by various inflammatory mediators, to allow tissue survival during inflammation. The pulp responds differently, with an increase in blood flow followed by a sustained decrease. This secondary vasoconstriction often leads to the demise of the pulp.

Kim S: Regulation of blood flow of the dental pulp. J Endod 15(9):1989.

91. Is it possible to differentiate a periapical cyst from a periapical granuloma on the basis of radiographic appearance alone?

No. Radiographic appearance is not diagnostic. Often a sclerotic border may be present, but its absence does not preclude cystic formation. An exhaustive study indicates that lesions greater than 200 mm^3 are usually cystic in nature.

Natkin E, Oswald RJ, Carnes LI: The relationship of lesion size to diagnosis, incidence and treatment of periapical cysts and granulomas. Oral Surg Oral Med Oral Pathol 57:82–94, 1984.

92. A patient presents with a maxillary central incisor that has a history of trauma. The patient is asymptomatic, and the radiograph is normal. Because the tooth gives no response to an electric pulp tester, you elect to do endodontic therapy without anesthesia. However, with access and instrumentation the patient feels everything. Explain the inconsistency.

The electric pulp tester excites the Aδ fibers in the tooth. The pulp contains Aδ and C nociceptive fibers; the Aδ fibers have a lower stimulation threshold than the C fibers. The C fibers are more resistant to hypoxia and can function long after the Aδ fibers are inactivated by injury to pulp tissue. The electric pulp tester does not stimulate C fibers.

93. List six normal changes in pulp tissue due to age.

(1) Decrease in size and volume of pulp, (2) increase in number of collagen fibers, (3) decreased number of odontoblasts (4) decrease in number and quality of nerves, (5) decreased vascularity, and (6) overall increase in cellularity.

Bernick S: Effect of aging on the nerve supply to human teeth. J Dent Res 46:694, 1967.

94. What is the meaning of the term *dentinal pain*?

Dentinal pain is due to the outflow of fluid in dentinal tubules that stimulates free nerve endings, most likely Aδ fibers. Dentinal pain is usually associated with cracked teeth (into the dentin),

defective fillings, or hypersensitive dentin. The pain produced by such stimulation does not usually signify that the pulp is inflamed or the tissue injured, whereas pulpal pain is due to true tissue injury associated with stimulation of C fibers.

95. Do the odontoblastic processes extend all the way through the dentin?

This controversial topic has been studied extensively by several investigators. The process is
basically an extension of the cell body of the odontoblast. It is the secretory portion of the odontoblast and contains large amounts of microtubules and microfilaments. Light microscopic studies have generally shown odontoblastic processes only in the inner one-third of dentin; this finding agrees with scanning electron microscope studies and transmission electron microscope
studies, which showed processes mainly in the inner one-third of dentin. However, one series of
studies suggested that processes go all the way through dentin. More elaborate techniques with
immunofluorescent antibody labeling against microtubules also showed staining the entire length
of the dentin, suggesting that the processes extend the entire length of the dentinal tubule.

Brannstrom M: The dentinal tubules and the odontoblast processes. Acta Odontol Scand 30:291, 1972.
Gunji T, et al: Distribution and organization of odontoblast processes in human dentin. Arch Histol Jpn
46:213, 1983.
Sigal MJ: The odontoblast process extends to the dentinoenamel junction: An immunocytochemical
study of rat dentine. J Histochem Cytochem 32:872, 1984.
Thomas HF: The extent of the odontoblast process in human dentin. J Dent Res 58:2207, 1979.

96. Describe briefly the circulatory system of the dental pulp.

The pulp contains a true microcirculatory system. The major vessels are arterioles, venules,
and capillaries. The capillary network in the pulp is extensive, especially in the subodontoblastic
region, where the important functions of transporting nutrients and oxygen to pulpal cells occurs
and waste products are removed. The pulpal microcirculation is under neural control and also under the influence of chemical agents, such as catecholamines, that exert their effects at the alpha
and beta receptors found in pulpal arterioles.

Cohen S, Burns RC (eds): Pathways of the Pulp, 6th ed. St. Louis, Mosby, 1994.

97. Have immunoglobulins and immunocompetent cells been found in the dental pulp?

Yes. Numerous studies have demonstrated that the pulp and periapical tissues are able to
mount an immune response against injury to the pulp and apical tissues. All classes of im-
munoglobulins have been identified in the dental pulp, and microscopic examination of damaged
pulpal tissue reveals the presence of leukocytes, macrophages, plasma cells, lymphocytes, giant
cells, and mast cells.

MICROBIOLOGY AND PHARMACOLOGY

98. Which two drugs are the latest of the macrolide class to be available for oral use?

The macrolide class, which includes the erythromycins, has not had additions since the 1950s.
Recently, two new antibiotics have been developed in this class and are available for oral use:
azithromycin (Zithromax) and clarithromycin (Biaxin). Both drugs are part of the antibiotic prophylactic regimen for SBE prevention by the American Heart Association (AHA). Both drugs are
absorbed well from the GI tract when taken orally and are available for use in the AHA regimen
for penicillin-allergic patients.

99. What types of bacteria are the predominant pathogens in endodontic-periapical infec-
tions?

Many well-done studies have shown definitively the predominant role of gram-negative obligate anaerobic bacteria in endodontic-periapical infections. Earlier studies generally implicated
facultative organisms (streptococci, enterococci, lactobacilli), but improved culturing techniques
established the predominance of obligate anaerobes. A recent study further demonstrated the im-

portant role of *Porphyromonas endodontalis* (formerly *Bacteroides endodontalis*) in endodontic infections.

Van Winkelhoff, et al: Porphyromonas endodontalis: Its role in endodontic infections. J Endod 18:431, 1992.

100. What is considered the antibiotic of choice in treatment of orofacial infections of endodontic origin?

In light of all the new microbiologic research implicating the predominance of obligate anaerobes, drug sensitivity tests still show the penicillins to be the drugs of choice. Penicillin is highly effective against most of the obligate anaerobes in endodontic infections, and because the infections are of a mixed nature with strict substrate interrelationships among various bacteria, the death of several strains has a profound effect on the overall population of an endodontic-periapical infection.

101. What antibiotics are considered most effective in treatment of orofacial infections of endodontic origin that do not respond to the penicillins?

For infections not responding to the penicillins, clindamycin is often recommended. It produces high bone levels and is highly effective against anaerobic bacteria, but it must be used with caution because of the potential for pseudomembranous colitis. A second choice is metronidazole, which also is quite effective against gram-negative obligate anaerobes.

102. A patient presents to your office for endodontic therapy on a lower right first molar. The molar is extremely "hot," and you anticipate the need for intraligamentary anesthesia and potential instrumentation beyond the apex. Because of the patient's medical history, which is significant for mitral valve prolapse with regurgitation, antibiotic prophylaxis for endocarditis prevention is necessary. In addition, the patient has been on Biaxin, 500 mg 2 times/day for 2 weeks, for a respiratory infection. Does the fact that the patient has been on this antibiotic obviate the need for additional prophylaxis?

The current recommendation by the AHA committee on antibiotic prophylaxis for the prevention of SBE is that the above patient should go to another class of antibiotic before endodontic therapy to prevent endocarditis. After 2 weeks of Biaxin therapy resistant organisms may be growing, and procedures such as ligamentary anesthesia and endodontic therapy, which can cause bacteremias, may allow resistant organisms to seed on a susceptible site, vegetate, and cause endocarditis. Therefore, the patient should premedicate with another class of antibiotics, such as amoxicillin or clindamycin, before the endodontic procedure.

Dajani AS, Taubert KA, Wilson W et al: Prevention of bacterial endocarditis: Recommendations by the American Heart association." JAMA 7:1794–801, 1997.

103. What is the current status of culturing and sensitivity testing for endodontic-periapical infections?

Culturing and sensitivity testing have been a controversial topic in endodontic practice for years. According to current thinking, if the proper clinical guidelines are followed, including use of rubber dam, proper chemomechanical cleaning of the root canal system, and proper use of correct antibiotics as indicated, culturing and sensitivity testing are not required. Proper culturing for both facultative and anaerobic bacteria is expensive, time-consuming, and not cost-effective, given the high success rate of properly done endodontic therapy.

104. The role of gram-negative anaerobic bacteria is an established fact in the pathogenesis of endodontic lesions. What role does the bacterial endotoxin play?

Endotoxins are highly potent lipopolysaccharides released from the cell walls of gram-negative bacteria. They are able to resorb bone via stimulation of osteoclastic activity, activation of complement cascades, and stimulation of lymphocytes and macrophages. Various studies have demonstrated their presence in pulpless teeth (with necrotic tissue) and apical lesions.

105. What three types of bacteria have recently been implicated in a large percentage of failed endodontic cases?

Recent investigations have especially implicated *Enterococcus faecalis, Actinomyces* spp., and *Streptococcus anginosus* in cases of endodontic failure. These bacteria seem to be able to adhere to dentinal walls and to dentinal debris forced through the apex and to colonize the dentinal tubules of pulpless, necrotic teeth.

Sundqvist, et al: Microbiologic analysis of teeth with failed endodontic treatment and the outcome of conservative retreatment. Oral Surg Oral Med Oral Pathol Endod 85:86–93, 1998.

106. What is the significance of the above mentioned bacteria, which are commonly found in cases of endodontic failure?

For years it has been assumed that gram-negative bacteria are associated with symptomatic endodontic disease, and much evidence supports this assumption. However, recent findings show that gram-positive bacteria are more often associated with persistent infections in cases of endodontic failure.

- *Enterococcus faecalis,* which is occasionally found in primary root canal infections, is found in almost 30–40% of root and failures. *E. faecalis* may be resistant to chemomechanical endodontic procedures and to calcium hydroxide—a common intracanal medication. Increased resistance to antibiotics has been noted in this species.
- *Actinomyces* species, though of low pathogenicity, seem to be able to thrive in necrotic pulpal tissues and chronic periapical tissues for long periods without causing a host response. Low pathogenicity and ability to invade host tissues to set up a chronic infection is prevalent in therapy-resistant lesions.
- The *Streptococcus anginosus* group (*S. intermedius, constellatus,* and *anginosus*) is part of the normal oral flora, prevalent in purulent infections, and highly prevalent in acute and chronic endodontic-periapical infections. This group is usually found in symbiotic relationships with other bacteria.

Siqueira, et al: J Endod 28:181–184, 2002.

107. What is the current recommendation for antibiotic prophylaxis for patients with a joint prosthesis?

Even though there is no definite antibiotic prophylactic regimen for patients with prosthetic joints, bacteremias during dental procedures are considered to be a major risk factor for a late joint prosthesis infection. For this reason, antibiotic prophylaxis is strongly urged. Consultation with the orthopedist is recommended. Usually, the prophylaxis regimen used for SBE prevention is used for joint prosthetic protection, but variations may be recommended by various orthopedic surgeons.

Antibiotic prophylaxis for dental patients with total joint replacement. J Am Dent Assoc 128:1004–1008, 1997.

108. What roles do nonsteroidal antiinflammatory drugs (NSAIDs) have in endodontic practice?

NSAIDs have a significant role in endodontic practice. Many patients require postoperative medication to control pericementitis, which can be quite painful after pulpectomy and may persist for several days. The NSAIDs are quite effective; their mechanism of action is to inhibit synthesis of prostaglandins. One study showed that ibuprofen, when given preoperatively to symptomatic and asymptomatic patients, significantly reduces postoperative pericementitis.

Dionne RA, et al: Suppression of postoperative pain by preoperative administration of ibuprofen in comparison to placebo, acetaminophen and acetaminophen plus codeine. J Clin Pharmacol 23:37–43, 1983.

109. What is the latest thinking on the role of black-pigmented anaerobic rods in the etiology of infected root canals and periapical infection?

Black-pigmented anaerobic rods have been shown to play an essential role in the etiology of endodontic infections when present in anaerobic mixed infections. The most strongly implicated organism is *Porphyromonas endodontalis*, which, because of its need for various growth factors, is directly related to the presence of acute periapical inflammation, pain, and exudation.

110. A patient presents with swelling, in obvious need of endodontic therapy. His medical history is significant for penicillin allergy and asthma, for which he is taking Theo-Dur. What precautions should you exercise?

By no means should erythromycin be used as an alternative to penicillin. Theo-Dur is a form of theophylline used for chronic reversible bronchospasm associated with bronchial asthma, and erythromycin has been shown to elevate significantly serum levels of theophylline.

111. For years it was taught that any bacteria left behind in an obturated canal would die and therefore cause no problems. What are the latest findings about this controversy?

The most recent electron micrograph studies have shown persistence of bacteria in the apical portion of roots in therapy-resistant lesions. The result is persistent periapical pathosis.

112. What efficacy do the cephalosporins have in treating acute pulpal-periapical infections?

Although the cephalosporins are broad-spectrum antibiotics, their activity is limited in pulpal-periapical infections, which are mixed infections predominantly due to obligate anaerobic - bacteria. The cephalosporins are not highly effective against such bacteria and actually have less activity against many anaerobes than penicillin. For serious infections that are penicillin or erythromycin-resistant, clindamycin is much more effective because of its activity against the obligate and facultative organisms in pulpal-periapical infections.

113. What precautions should be taken in prescribing antibiotics to a female patient who takes birth control pills?

The dentist should warn the patient that oral antibiotics may decrease the effectiveness of birth control pills and that they may be ineffective during the course of antibiotic therapy. The most often implicated antibiotic is the penicillin class, although erythromycin, cephalosporin, tetracyclines, and metronidazole also have been implicated.

114. The quinolone class of antibiotics, which includes ciprofloxacin, is becoming quite popular. Do quinolones have any role in treating alveolar infections?

Very little, if any. Most anaerobes implicated in endodontic-alveolar abscesses are resistant to the quinolones.

ANESTHESIA

115. What is the physiologic basis of the difficulty in achieving proper pulpal anesthesia in the presence of inflammation or infection?

Attaining effective pulpal anesthesia in the presence of pulpal-alveolar infection or inflammation is often quite difficult because of changes in tissue pH. The normal tissue pH of 7.4 decreases to 4.5–5.5. This change in pH due to pulpal-periapical pathology favors a shift to a cationic form of the local anesthesia molecule, which cannot diffuse through the lipoprotein neural sheath. Therefore, anesthesia is ineffective.

116. What is the significance of the mylohyoid nerve in successful anesthesia of the mandibular first molar?

The mylohyoid nerve is often implicated in unsuccessful anesthesia of the first molar. This nerve branches off the inferior alveolar nerve above its entry into the mandibular foremen. The mylohyoid nerve then travels in the mylohyoid groove in the lingual border of the mandible to the digastric and mylohyoid muscles. However, because it often carries sensory fibers to the mesial root of the first molar, lingual anesthetic infiltration may be required to block it.

117. What is the method of action of injection into the periodontal ligament?

Injection into the periodontal ligament is not a pressure-dependent technique. The local anesthetic works by traveling down the periodontal ligament space and shutting off the pulpal microcirculation. To be effective, this technique requires the use of a local anesthetic with a vasoconstrictor.

118. The Gow-Gates block is an effective alternative to the inferior alveolar block. When is it indicated? Briefly describe how it works.

In patients in whom the traditional inferior alveolar block is ineffective or impossible to perform because of infection or inflammation, the Gow-Gates block has a high success rate. It is a true mandibular block that anesthetizes all of the sensory portions of the mandibular nerve. The injection site is the lateral side of the neck of the mandibular condyle; thus, it is effective when intraoral swelling contraindicates the inferior alveolar block.

119. What is the reason for attempting to anesthetize the mylohyoid nerve for endodontic treatment of a symptomatic lower first molar?

The mylohyoid nerve has been shown to supply sensory innervation to mandibular molars, especially the mesial root of first molars. Infiltration of this nerve as it courses along the medial surface of the mandible is often helpful.

120. A drug salesman has convinced you to use propoxycaine hydrochloride as a local anesthetic. Is there any true or absolute contraindication to use of an ester anesthetic?

Yes. Patients who have a hereditary trait known as atypical pseudocholinesterase have an inability to hydrolyze ester-type local anesthetics. Therefore, toxic reactions may result. Only amide anesthetics should be used.

121. A patient presents with an extremely painful lower molar requiring endodontic therapy. You have already used six cartridges of lidocaine with epinephrine to achieve anesthesia. The patient begins to react differently. In brief, what are the signs of local anesthetic toxicity?

Local anesthetic toxicity depends on the blood level and the patient's status. In general, a mild toxic reaction manifests as agitation, talkativeness, and increased vital parameters (blood pressure, heart rate, and respiration). A massive reaction manifests as seizures, generalized collapse of the central nervous system, and possible myocardial depression and vasodilation.

122. The newest local anesthetic available in dental cartridges is called septocaine (Articaine). In brief, what characteristics are making it so popular?

Septicaine (Articaine) as an amide local anesthetic in the same class as lidocaine, prilocaine, and bupivacaine. It comes in a 4% solution with a 1:200,000 concentration of epinephrine. However, because it is the only amide local anesthetic with an additional ester ring and a thiophene ring, it has increased liposolubility, is extremely diffusible, and has a high capability to penetrate tissue. In addition, its plasma protein-binding of 95% is higher than practically all local anesthetics and contributes to its effectiveness.

SURGICAL ENDODONTICS

123. Methylene blue dye is currently a useful adjunct during endodontic surgery. What is its purpose?

During endodontic surgery it is often difficult to determine accurately where the exact root outline is and where pulp tissue exists apically in order to prepare properly the retrograde preparation with ultrasonic tips. The methylene blue dye stains vital tissue, therefore delineating quite nicely the periodontal ligament space and any pulp tissue that is remaining in an isthmus or poorly instrumented and obturated root canal space.

124. What is the purpose of the apicoectomy procedure in surgical endodontics?
Perpetuation of apical inflammation or infection often is due to poorly obturated canals, tissue left in the canal, or quite often an apical delta of accessory foramina containing remnants of necrotic tissue. The removal of this apical segment via apicoectomy usually removes the nidus of infection.

125. A patient presents for apicoectomy on a maxillary central incisor with failed endodontic therapy. A well-done porcelain-to-gold crown is present, with the gold margin placed in the gingival sulcus for esthetic purposes. What flap design is most appropriate?
A full mucoperiosteal flap involving the marginal and interdental gingival tissues may potentially cause loss of soft-tissue attachments and crestal bone height, thereby causing an esthetic problem with the gold margin of the crown. Instead, a submarginal rectangular (Luebke-Ochsenbein) flap that preserves the marginal and interdental gingiva, is recommended.

126. What is the material of choice for root end fillings in surgical endodontics?
Histologic studies have compared several materials, including amalgam, EBA cement, resins, polycarboxylate cements, glass ionomers, and gold foils. Although no study has shown a definitive superiority of one over another, the most commonly used today are amalgam and EBA cements. The type of material is properly secondary in importance to the root resection technique, apical preparation, curettage of the lesion, and technique in placement.

127. What type of scalpel is best used for intraoral incision and drainage of an endodontic abscess?
A pointed no. 11 or no. 12 blade is preferred over a rounded no. 15 blade.

128. In performing apical surgery on the mesial root of maxillary molars, what mistake is commonly made?
It is important to look for unfilled mesiolingual canals in such roots. Therefore, a proper long bevel is necessary to expose this commonly unfilled fourth canal.

129. Numerous studies have addressed the success rates of endodontic surgery. Most agree, however, on certain basic conclusions. Can you name the most common conclusions?
All of the success studies share certain basic conclusions. First, the success of endodontic surgery is closely related to the standard of treatment of the root canal. Second, orthograde (conventional) root fills are preferred, if possible. Thirdly, the success rate is about 20% lower for retrograde fills than for properly done orthograde fills.
Andreasen JO, Rud J: A multivariate analysis of various factors upon healing after endodontic surgery. Int J Oral Surg 1:258–271, 1972.
Rud J, Andreasen JO: Radiographic criteria for the assessment of healing after endodontic surgery. Int J Oral Surg 1:195–214, 1972.

130. What is the recommended surgical approach for apical surgery on palatal roots of maxillary molars?
The palatal approach is recommended; with proper flap design and size, proper reflection is not a difficult procedure. The buccal approach is potentially too damaging to supporting bone of the molar and may actually cause more risk of postoperative sinus problems.

131. Why is a "slot preparation" often recommended in preparation of root end filling for mesial roots of maxillary or mandibular roots?
The slot preparation is a trough-type preparation that extends from one canal orifice to another canal orifice in the same root. This procedure is accomplished with undercuts in the adjacent walls. The slot preparation allows not only sealing of the canal orifices but also small anastomoses between the main canals.

132. Has the ideal retrosurgical material been developed?

No. Many research studies have been published about a myriad of materials. However, the ideal is not yet determined. Most likely the material itself is not as important as the surgical preparation, the depth of the preparation, and how it is placed.

133. After root end resection during endodontic surgery, many practitioners apply citric acid to the exposed dentin surface. What is the rationale behind this practice?

A desired result of root end surgery (apicoectomy) is to achieve, if possible, a functional apical dentoalveolar apparatus with cementum deposition on the root end. However, the resected root end is covered with a smeared layer of dentin from the high-speed bur, which does not allow reattachment of newly deposited cementum. Applying citric acid for 2 or 3 minutes dissolves the smear layer and causes a small degree of demineralization of dentin. This, in turn, exposes collagen fibrils of the dentinal organic matrix and allows a proper area for attachment of collagen fibrils from newly formed cementum.

Polson AM, et al: The production of a root surface smear layer by instrumentation and its removal by citric acid. J Periodontol 55:443–446, 1984.

134. Several studies have shown that resected mandibular molars fail twice as often as resected maxillary molars. What are the major etiologic reasons for failure?

The most common cause of failure is root fracture, followed in order by cement washouts around restorations, undermining caries, and recurrent periodontal pathoses around remaining roots.

Langer B, Wagenberg B: An evaluation of root resections: A ten-year study. J Periodontol 52:719–722, 1981.

Erpensten H: A 3-year study of hemisectioned molars. J Clin Periodontol 10:1–10, 1983.

135. In performing apical surgery, what is the current thinking about the angle of the apical bevel during apicoectomy and how it relates to depth of retrograde fillings?

Recent studies have shown that increasing the angle of the apical bevel increases the potential for apical leaking due to exposure of more dentinal tubules. A bevel as close to zero degrees as possible is ideal. In addition, increasing the depth of retrograde preparation and filling decreases apical leaking by sealing more dentinal tubules.

136. Why, in the past, have the mesial roots of maxillary first molars and mandibular first molars failed so commonly after endodontic surgery?

Before the advent of enhanced illumination and magnification with surgical loupes and the operating microscope, the isthmus between the mesial canals was commonly not prepared. The isthmus may contain necrotic tissue that can perpetuate the apical lesion.

137. Why are ultrasonic techniques becoming the most popular instruments for retropreparation during apical surgery?

The ultrasonic systems available today are a huge improvement over techniques in the past. They allow retropreparations that align properly with the long axis of the tooth, and they can be sufficiently deep to conform to the true shape of the apical root canal system.

138. During apical surgery in the past, teeth with extensive periodontal defects were extracted because of the poor prognosis. Today, however, guided tissue regeneration can save many of these teeth. How does it work?

An inert barrier is placed over the periodontal defects. These membranes allow proliferation of undifferentiated cells of the PDL and surrounding bone to grow across the wound, potentially forming a new attachment, and prevent the downgrowth of epithelial cells to form a junctional epithelium.

139. What is the ultimate goal of apical surgery?

The goal is to eliminate the source of periapical irritation emanating from the root canal, which perpetuates apical infection. In addition, it is important to allow reformation of cementum around the apex, to reestablish a functioning PDL, and to allow alveolar bone repair. If these goals are not possible, we aim at least to allow repair scar tissue, which is less than ideal but still a form of repair.

BIBLIOGRAPHY

1. Cohen S, Burns RC (eds): Pathways of the Pulp, 7th ed. St. Louis, Mosby, 1998.
2. Guttman J, Harrison J: Surgical Endodontics. Cambridge, MA, Blackwell Scientific Publications, 1991.
3. Journal of Endodontics.

8. RESTORATIVE DENTISTRY

Elliot V. Feldbau, D.M.D., and Steven A. Migliorini, D.M.D.

CARIOLOGY

1. How are dental caries classified?

Anatomic site:
> Pit and fissure: class I
> Smooth surface: proximal: class II, III; cervical, root surface: class V

Rate of progression: incipient, acute, chronic, arrested
Hard tissue involved: enamel, dentin, cementum
Etiology: radiation, baby bottle, rampant

2. Outline the caries susceptibility of teeth in the dental arches.

Maxillary > mandibular arch

Tooth type: first molars (upper and lower) > second molars (upper and lower) > second bicuspids (upper) > first bicuspids (upper) and second bicuspids (lower) > central and lateral incisors (upper) > canine (upper) and first bicuspids (lower) > lower anteriors

Tooth surface: occlusal >> mesial > distal > buccal > lingual

3. List the key risk factors associated with dental caries.

- Susceptible tooth surface that can maintain plaque and bacteria
- Presence of acidogenic bacteria
- Steady supply of dietary fermentable carbohydrates
- Inadequate salivary flow or buffering capacity
- Low exposure to topical/dietary fluoride

4. What organisms are responsible for caries formation?

Streptococcus mutans and *lactobacilli* are the most cariogenic with contributions from *S. sanguis* and *S. salivarius*. These organisms metabolize sucrose to form acidic byproducts destructive to enamel surfaces. Root surface caries are initiated by *Actinomyces viscus* on accumulated plaque deposits.

5. What are the properties of cariogenic bacteria?

Specifically unique are their ability to survive at low pH and to metabolize simple sugars to form acid byproducts. During the process, extracellular polysaccharides are produced which aid in adhesion within the plaque biofilms.

6. What is the role of saliva in caries susceptibility?

- Adequate flow reduces plaque accumulation on tooth surface and rate of clearance of carbohydrates.
- Diffusion of the salivary components calcium, phosphate, hydroxyl, and fluoride ions into plaque can reduce the solubility of enamel and promote remineralization of early carious lesions.
- The bicarbonate buffering capacity of saliva can reduce or limit the fall in pH when bacteria metabolize sugars.
- Salivary proteins form the protective acquired pellicle, which retards the flow of ions out of enamel.
- The salivary components of secretory IgA, lysosomes, lactoperoxidase, and lactoferrin have antibacterial activity.

7. Describe the role of fluoride in preventing dental caries.
- The anticaries effects of fluoride are primarily topical for children and adults.
- Fluoride inhibits demineralization at enamel crystal surfaces inside tooth
- Fluoride enhances the remineralization of the enamel crystal surface after demineralization and increases acid resistance.
- The systemic benefits of fluoride are minimal.

8. Express the caries risk factors in a functional relationship.

Functional Relation In Dental Caries

$$C_A \cong f\left\{[(\text{Bacteria}) \times (\text{CHO})] \times \left[\frac{1}{(S)(F)}\right]\right\}$$

C_A = Caries Activity

Bacteria = S. Mutans/Lactobacillus Activity

CHO = Fermentable Carbohydrate Substrate

F = Fluoride availability

S = Saliva (Flow/Buffering capacity/Components)

Dental caries occurs when the process of demineralization is faster than the process of remineralization and there is a net loss of tooth mineral into the environment. If the acid production is reduced by removing plaque accumulation or reducing dietary sugar substrates, tooth mineral dissociation will cease (decrease in CA). The presence of topical fluoride increases enamel resistance to dissolution (forming fluorapatite) and enhances remineralization. It also inhibits bacterial metabolism. Thus increases in fluoride relates inversely to C_A. Finally, high salivary buffering capacity decreases caries activity, while low flow rates tend to increase C_A.

9. What are the three main tooth mineral complexes and their relative solubilities?
The enamel and dentin of a tooth are composed of tiny crystals embedded in a protein/lipid matrix. The mineral formed during tooth germination is a highly substituted carbonated apatite. It is related to hydroxyapatite but is more acid soluble, as well as calcium-deficient (replaced by sodium, magnesium, and zinc) and contains 3–6% carbonate replacing phosphate ions in the crystal lattice. During demineralization carbonate is preferentially lost, and during remineralization, it is excluded and replaced by OH or F ions, thereby decreasing the acid solubility. This is the maturation cycle. Mature enamel is mostly hydroxy or fluoro-apatite.

Tooth Mineral
Carbonated apatite (most soluble)
$Ca_{10-x}(Na)_x(PO_4)_{6-y}(CO_3)_z(OH)_{2-u}(F)_u$

Hydroxy apatite (less soluble)
$Ca_{10}(PO_4)_{10}(OH)_2$

Fluorapatite (least soluble)
$Ca_{10}(PO_4)10(F)_2$

10. What is a Stephan plot?
The classical experimental measurement of pH changes on tooth enamel surfaces during exposure to fermentable carbohydrates in the presence of acidogenic bacteria (in plaque) over time is called a Stephan plot. It demonstrates the acid production of bacteria (pH decrease) with a glucose swallow and the gradual rise due to salivary buffering.

11. What is the critical pH for enamel dissociation?
The critical pH for enamel (hydroxyapatite) is 5.3–5.5; fluoroapatite 4.5. Carbonated beverages (Coke, Pepsi) have a pH at about 3.5.

12. What is the term for the earliest observable enamel caries lesion?
The term *white spot lesion* is applied to the earliest visually observable or macroscopic lesion in enamel. It represents dissolution of the surface structure with increased porosity and takes on a dull appearance when air-dried because of the differences in light scattering (refractive index) from the surrounding enamel. These lesions may maintain their surface integrity, become stained and arrested, or progress to frank cavitation lesions.

13. What are the differences in the mechanisms of *enamel* and *dentinal* caries?
Enamel caries is primarily an acidogenic or physiochemical progression of tooth mineral dissolution, whereas dentinal caries involves acid decalcification followed by proteolytic or enzymatic degeneration of the organic matrix.

14. What is the current thought about treating early enamel caries or the incipient lesion?
Most early enamel lesions are capable of reminerlization, or arresting, if the risk factors are reduced and there is adequate fluoride content in the microenvironment. Risk factor assessment (including diet, bacterial, and salivary analysis) followed by fluoride supplements in the form of topical sources is thus the first line of therapy.

15. What clinical tests are available to determine caries susceptibility?
Proprietary kits from Ivoclar and Viadent provide the essential components to culture and grade levels of *S. mutans* and *lactobacilli* in saliva as well as to measure salivary pH , flow rates, and buffering capacity.

16. Describe the progression of caries in dentin.
Because dentin is a vital tissue, it shows reactivity with bacterial invasion. Caries generally spreads laterally along the dentoenamel junction (DEFJ), involving dentinal tubules. At the **infected layer** of dentine, bacteria enter the dentinal tubules and decalcify the matrix by acid and proteolytic dissociation (microscopic liquefaction foci and clefts are present). The inner **affected layer** is demineralized, but contains few bacteria. The damage here is reversible if the bacterial metabolism is halted by excavation of the infected layer. Under the affected layer is the **sclerotic** or microscopically termed **translucent layer,** followed by a layer of **reparative or reactionary dentine** produced by odontoblasts at dentopulpal boundary.

17. Clinically, how are the different types of carious dentin treated?
All infected dentin must be removed for successful tooth viability. Because affected dentin has undergone only early demineralization removal may not be necessary. Topical bonded dentin sealants containing fluoride effect a barrier under restorations.

18. Explain the differences between smooth and pit/fissure caries.
Because **smooth surface caries** (interproximal or cervical) have a wide enamel surface pattern that converges with the anatomic form of the enamel rods toward the DEJ, fewer dentinal tubule are affected, enamel undermining is generally less, and the rate of progression is slow. These lesions have a high success of remineralization with adequate fluoride exposure and reduction in risk factors.

Pit and fissure caries are narrow at the enamel surface and spread widely as the caries progresses to the DEJ, involving many dentine tubules and creating extensive undermining. The progression is often more rapid than that of smooth surface caries. Because of the anatomic sheltering of bacterial plaque, remineralization is not easy, and use of fissurotomy followed by sealants is necessary for early lesions.

19. Develop a decision tree for the management of pit and fissure tooth surfaces.

From Summit JB: Conservative cavity preparations. Dent Clin North Am 46(2):174, 2002, with permission.

20. How may caries be diagnosed?

Caries may be detected by a combination of techniques. The most commonly accepted criteria for identifying infected tooth structure are (1) discolored softened tooth structure, (2) frank cavitation, and (3) areas of radiolucency on radiographs. Direct visual inspection of pits and fissures, root surfaces, and interfaces of restorations and tooth with a sharp explorer and air-drying with use of magnification are the first steps of examination. This procedure is supplemented by evaluating properly angulated bitewing and periapical radiographs. Finally, the use of transillumination from a visible light curing wand can reveal shadowing and discoloration on occlusal and interproximal tooth surfaces.

21. Describe two high-tech methods of diagnosing dental caries.

1. **Quantitative light-induced fluorescence** (QFL) measures the scattering of light induced by the degree of enamel demineralization. KaVo's DIAGNOdent probe uses red laser light to assess pit and fissure lesions (www.kavousa.com).

2. **Digital imaging fiberoptic transillumination** (DIFOTI) (www.difoti.com), provides a highly sensitive method of diagnosis occlusal and interproximal carious lesions. Images of transilluminated visible light are captured by a digital CCD camera and sent to a computer where analysis of the decreased densities due to demineralization are shown as images. This methods is claimed to be twice as sensitive in detecting interproximal caries and three times more sensitive in occlusal caries than current x-rays.

22. What are the objectives of operative treatments in carious teeth?
1. To remove bacterially infected enamel and dentin
2. To protect the dental pulp
3. To preserve healthy tooth structure and restore missing structure
4. To remove the sources of cariogenic bacteria by facilitating plaque control
5. To provide minimal fluoride concentrations in the microenvironment

23. List logical steps to stabilize dentition with active and multiple caries.
1. Thorough medical and dental history and examination to assess the caries risk factors.
2. Initiation of appropriate preventive measures.
3. Planned extraction of nonsalvageable teeth (*Note:* This step may be resequenced in the apprehensive patient until full trust and compliance are achieved because extractions may be too traumatic as an initial treatment phase.)
4. Evaluation of caries in teeth that are vital and protection with pulp-capping agents such as $Ca(OH)_2$ sealed with bonded and Flowable resins or resin-reinforced glass ionomers. Use glass ionomer build-up materials for the temporary filling.
5. In frank pulpal exposures, removal of the pulpal tissues is advisable to prevent potential pain, followed by temporization with a suitable glass ionomer material and endodontic treatment.
6. In very deep carious lesions, whether symptomatic or not, where pulpal exposure is to be expected, it is probably best to go directly to endodontic treatment rather than try an intermediate step of excavation and temporary stabilization.
7. Finalize a treatment plan with permanent restorations for the existing teeth and suitable provisions for replacement of missing teeth.

24. What are caries detector solutions? How are they used?
Caries detector solutions are usually a colored dye (red, green, blue) in a propylene glycol base; they help to distinguish between infected and affected dentin. The dye bonds to the denatured collagen in the infected dentin that is part of the decay process. The affected dentin, which may be slightly softer than sound dentin, is not infused with bacteria and is not stained but still may show a dye-stained haze ("pink haze" with red dye). This dentin should not be removed. The caries detector solution is applied for 10 seconds and then rinsed off. Any deeply stained tooth structure is then removed. The materials also help identify cracks in tooth structure. Example products are Seek (Ultradent) and Snoop (Pulpdent). *Note:* Some products may decrease the bond strength to dentin and careful consideration in use is necessary when high bonding requirements are needed.

25. Are cavity disinfectants useful?
Some current thought reflects the goal of cleaning a preparation before bonding or placing a restoration with the addition of a bactericidal agent to reduce sensitivity and bacterial growth under a restoration. It is thought that bacteria reaching the pulp may contribute to sensitivity. Current products contain either benzalkonium chloride and EDTA or 2% chlorhexidine gluconate.

26. What supplemental sources of topical fluoride may be used for caries prevention?
- Public water supplies: 1ppm sodium fluoride (NaF)
- Toothpaste: OTC over-the-count regular brands contain 0.10–0.15% NaF
  Prescription: PreviDent 5000 Plus, 1.1% NaF
- Mouth rinses: Act, FluoriGuard, Prevident Rinse, 0.2–0.5% NaF
- Brush-on gels/fluoride trays: Prevident, 1.1% NaF neutral pH

27. What is a contraindication to the use of acidulated or stannous fluoride preparations?
0.4% stannous fluoride (pH of 3.0) = 0.2% sodium fluoride (pH of 7.0)
Acidulated fluoride (APF) solutions and topical 0.4% stannous gels (Gel-Kam, Colgate) remove the glaze from porcelain, glass ionomer, and composite restorations. It is best to use neutral pH supplements if these restorations are present. Always check the product specifications.

28. What are some indications for fluoride gel applications using a custom tray?

Patients who exhibit high caries incidence, root caries or cervical caries and who might fit into one or more of the following groups:

- High consumption of carbonated beverages (pH of 3.2–3.5) or citric fruits: (e.g., lemons, limes)
- Bulimic patients (10% female adolescents)
- Elderly and nursing home patients
- Gastric reflux patients
- Chemotherapy and radiation-treated patients

29. What is tooth attrition?

Attrition is the physiologic wear of tooth structure resulting from normal tooth-to-tooth contact over time.

30. What is erosion? What are its possible causes?

Erosion is the loss of tooth structure by a chemical process that does not involve bacterial action. It is generally caused by the consumption of foods that contain phosphoric or citric acid, such as fruits, fruit juices, and carbonated or acidic beverages. Excessive exposure to gastric acids due to vomiting also contributes.

31. What is the theory of tooth abfraction?

Abfraction is defined as the pathologic loss of tooth substance caused by biomechanical loading forces. The loss of structure is usually seen as wedged-shaped cervical lesions at the DEJ that may not be carious. This theory is used as an alternative explanation for areas that historically have been attributed to toothbrush abrasion.

32. List generally accepted principles for cavity preparation.

1. Cavity preparations should be governed by tooth anatomy, the tooth position in the dental arch, extent of the carious lesion, and physical properties of the filling material.
2. Gingival margins should be ended on enamel whenever possible.
3. Cavity preparations margins should be supragingival whenever possible.
4. Margins of posterior cavity preparations should not end directly in occlusal contact areas. Contact areas should be composed of one material to allow even wear. Uneven wear results if two materials meet at the contact area, thereby producing open margins.
5. Weakened and unsupported tooth structure should be removed.
6. Maintaining a dry work field with the use of a rubber dam always enhances the consistent quality of restorations.

33. Describe the principles of cavity preparation for composite resins and amalgam alloy.

The classic cavity preparations, according to Black's principles, are generally not needed for contemporary bonded retained composite and amalgam restorations. Dovetails, retention grooves, and extension into uninvolved occlusal groves are generally not needed. Maximizing tooth structure dominates design with sealants replacing groove extensions.

34. How do the basic principles of operative microdentistry differ from those of traditional operative dentistry, as advocated by Black?

The Black approach to operative dentistry tends toward the destruction of healthy tooth structure to remove smaller amounts of unhealthy tooth structure (extension for prevention). The concept of microdentistry seeks to diagnose unsound tooth structure that is a threat to the tooth and remove that threat with minimal encroachment on the surrounding healthy tooth structure.

35. What is a fissurotomy procedure? What are its applications?

A fissurotomy involves the conservative preparation of occlusal pits and fissures using either air abrasion or special burs designed for this purpose; the Fissurotomy Kit by Ivoclar North America is one example. This procedure is used to treat pits and fissures with incipient decay. Preparations are typically narrow, long, and irregularly deep so that they are often restored with flowable composites. Hybrid composites, although stronger and more wear-resistant than flowables, may be clinically more difficult to place into such preparations without the incorporation of voids.

36. What are the advantages of the fissurotomy procedure over pit and fissure sealants?

It is often difficult to determine caries activity in pits and fissures, particularly with conventional means. Concerns arise about the placement of sealants over undiagnosed caries. Questionable occlusal grooves, particularly in fluoridated communities, that are covered with a sealant may mask more extensive subsurface caries activity. The fissurotomy offers better access and is a conservative technique for maximizing the retention of healthy tooth structure while ensuring certain removal of all decay.

37. Describe the "tunnel preparation."

The tunnel preparation is a conservative approach to restoring class II caries in teeth with relatively small interproximal lesions. It conserves the proximal marginal enamel by using only the occlusal or a buccal or lingual access and then angulating either mesially or distally until the external tooth enamel is perforated. Usually application of a matrix band beforehand protects the adjacent tooth wall. The tooth cavity is then packed from the access dimension.

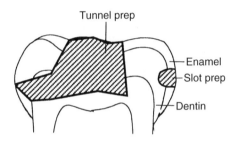

38. What is a slot preparation?

Any narrow access to reach interproximal caries can be called a slot preparation. The access may be from the buccal or lingual as in a class III lesion, or from the occlusal aspect. The ideal is to conserve tooth structure by removing only caries and a minimal amount of tooth structure.

39. Define micro-air abrasion, When is it used?

This technique uses pressurized delivery of abrasive powders (aluminum oxide) to prepare teeth for restoration. The claimed advantages are less trauma and a less invasive, heatless procedure often not requiring local anesthesia. It is ideally suited for pit and fissure sealant preparations and conservative class I and V preparations using flowable composites. Disadvantages include the need for special high speed evacuation equipment and high cost of the units.

40. Describe the principle behind air abrasion for cavity preparation.

Air abrasion is based on kinetic energy. Abrasive particles, typically 27–50 micron aluminum oxide, are propelled at high velocity to remove tooth structure. By varying the speed of the particles, the rate of time to remove tooth structure and often the level of sensitivity can be controlled.

41. What are the various sources of propellant for air abrasion units?

Depending on the type of unit and the manufacturer, the propellant can range from compressed air or nitrogen tanks to operatory compressed air lines or units with built-in air compressors.

42. What dental procedures are well suited for the use of air abrasion? Are any procedures contraindicated?

All classes of cavity preparation may be performed with air abrasion. Some operators may use a high-speed handpiece to gain initial access to deep grooves. pits, marginal ridges, and hard-to-reach areas. Although air abrasion units have the ability to remove dental amalgam, some questions remain about the amount of mercury released by air abrasion vs. removal with conventional high-speed handpieces.

43. Why is air abrasion considered well suited to the application of microdentistry?

Treatment goals of microdentistry include preservation of sound occlusal enamel with minimally invasive occlusal preparations and the use of tunnel or slot preparations to treat primary interproximal caries. Air abrasion is much more selective in the structure it cuts, thereby removing very little sound tooth structure relative to high-speed handpieces. Additionally, the vibration from high-speed handpieces can cause enamel fractures that air abrasion cannot.

Air Abrasion Systems

COMPANY	PRODUCT NAME	MODEL TYPE	ABRASIVE PARTICLE SIZE	TYPE OF ABRASIVE	PROPELLANT	MAXIMUM PROPELLANT PRESSURE	BUILT-IN COMPRESSOR
Air Techniques	Air Dent II CS	Chairside	27 and 50 micron	Aluminum oxide	High-pressure compressor	160 psi	No
Bisco, Inc.	Accu-prep Deluxe	Chairside	50 micron	Aluminum oxide	Air	40 psi	No
Danville Enginering	PrepStart	Tabletop	27 and 50 micron	Aluminum oxide	Air or bottled gas	145 psi	No
Dentsply Gendex	AirTouch	Tower, Desktop	27 and 50 micron	Aluminum oxide	Carbon dioxide, compressed air	120 psi	Yes
J. Morita USA, Inc.	AdAbrader Plus	Tabletop	50 micron	Aluminum oxide	Compressed air	100 psi	No
Lares Research	MicroPrep Director	Cart	27 micron	Aluminum oxide	Compressed air	120 psi	Yes

DENTAL ADHESIVES

44. What are dental adhesives?

Dental adhesives are products that allow the predictable adhesion of restorative material to dentin and enamel. They are based on multiple agents to prepare the surface, bond to the tooth surface and act as a substrate to which the restorative material bonds. In general they are technique-sensitive and constantly evolving in the marketplace.

45. What are the goals of dental bonding?

- Eliminate or minimize the contraction gap of composite polymerization
- Sustain thermal expansion and contraction cycles
- Create 20–30 MPa bond strengths to enamel and dentin
- Eliminate microleakage

46. What are signs of microleakage?

Stains, sensitivity and pulpal symptoms, recurrent caries, and bond failures.

47. What are the components of adhesive systems?

Most current systems are combinations of components. Some are multicomponent, depending on whether they are self-cure or light-cure only or both, whereas others have a single component. Unlike early-generation systems, all of the new bonding agents are hydrophilic to allow compatibility to dentin bonding. The basic components are an acid etchant solution, hydrophilic primer, and resin.

48. What types of adhesive systems are currently available?

Type 1. Etchant applied, washed off to remove smear layer; primer and adhesive resin applied separately as two solutions. Type 1 systems are "all-purpose" types. They generally bond to light, dual, and self-cured composites.

Type 2. Etchant applied and washed off to remove smear layer; primer and adhesive applied as a single solution. Type 2 systems have nearly all-purpose capability.

Type 3. Self-etching primer (SEP) applied to dissolve smear layer and *not* washed off; adhesive applied separately.

Type 4. Self-etching primer and adhesive applied as a single solution to dissolve and treat the smear layer simultaneously.

Dental Adhesives

BRAND NAME	COMPANY	NUMBER OF COMPONENTS	SHEAR BOND STRENGTH MPA, DENTIN	SHEAR BOND STRENGTH, MPA, ENAMEL
Type 1				
All Bond 2	Bisco	4	13.9	12.3
Amalgambond Plus	Parkell	4	17.6	20.5
Scotchbond Multipurpose	3M	3	19.4	18.0
Optibond FL	Kerr	3	20.3	34.1
Type 2				
Excite	Ivoclar	2	16.6	15.1
Fuji Bond LC	GC America	3	10.8	14.3
One-Step	Bisco	2	10.2	24.7
Prime & Bond NT	Dentsply/Caulk	2	10.3	20.0
Optibond Solo Plus	Kerr	2	15.3	19.8
Single Bond	3M	2	16.3	17.8
Type 3				
ClearFill SE Bond	Kuraray	2	21.3	24.0
ClearFill liner Bond	Kuraray	3	21.1	22.8
Type 4				
One-Up Bond	J Morita	2	17.8	16.6
Prompt L-Pop	ESP	1	8.8	22.2

From CRA Newsletter, vol. 24, issue 11, Nov. 2000 p 1.

49. What is the hybrid layer?

The hybrid layer is a multilayered zone of composite resin, and dentin, and collagen. After removing the organic and inorganic debris of the smear layer by etching and some hydroxyapatite from the intertubular dentin down to 2–5 μ, a plate of moist collagen remains on the dentin floor. Priming agents penetrate this moist collagen substrate and migrate into the tubules, lateral canals, and all areas of peritubular dentin. This becomes the hybridization process as the dentin, both collagen and hydroxyapatite crystals, become totally impregnated with bonding resin. The resin further penetrates into the dentin tubules. Light curing produces a mechanically and chemically bonded surface that can polymerize to composite restoratives.

50. What is essential for successful hybrid layer formation?

Supersaturating of the dentin substrate with primer, or wetting agent, is essential. If the etchant time is 15 seconds, the wash should be at least as long. The water is then dispersed to leave the dentin moist. Then multiple coats of priming agent are applied to achieve a glossy surface on air dispersion. Resin is then applied and cured.

51. How is enamel bonding achieved?

Bonding to enamel is micromechanical; a low viscosity resin penetrates the microporosity created by acid etching on the enamel surface. Once the resin is cured, it strongly adheres to the enamel and forms the suitable substrate for composite bonding. Although previously done under dry conditions, contemporary adhesive systems use a wet bond to enamel. If one is bonding only to enamel, it is necessary to use only an unfilled resin without the primer application.

52. How is bonding to dentin achieved?

Dentin is largely composed of organic materials, mostly collagen and water. (Enamel is 86% mineralized, whereas dentin is 45%.) Bonding to dentin can require removal of preparation debris (**smear layer**) and demineralization of the dentin surface by acid etchant. This leaves a lattice of unsupported collagen as long as the surface stays moist. Then hydrophilic primers and resins (applied in solvents of acetone or alcohol) can penetrate this matrix, infusing a micromechanical lock similar to enamel. When cured, this resin-reinforced dentin complex forms the **hybrid layer,** and is a suitable substrate for composite bonding. With newer self-etch primer adhesives (SEP), the etchant and primer are applied and not washed off (the smear layer remains). Then an adhesive is applied separately. The dentin with these latter systems is never denuded, and there may be less technique sensitivity as the concept of leaving dentin damp dry is eliminated.

53. How long should you etch?

Etching dentin demineralizes its surface to a depth of 1–10 μ. If you etch too long, you may create a depth of demineralized collage that is too deep for adhesives to penetrate and thus weaken the bond or actually denature the remaining collagen. The "total etch" of a tooth preparation with 32–40% phosphoric gels should be a **maximum of 15 seconds** (which also works for enamel).

54. Why must the dentin surface be kept wet?

When using type 1 and 2 adhesive systems, the etching step leaves the dentin collagen lattice largely unsupported. If this layer dehydrates, it will collapse and the applied adhesives will not be able to infuse through the collage. The surface should be left moist by only the slightest application of air to eliminate puddles of water—or, even better, blotted with sponge or gauze. Some adhesive systems rehydrate the demineralized zone even if it is over dried.

55. What potential problem may cause an incomplete seal of dentin tubules?

Incomplete placement of the bonding reagents may result in an increase in postoperative pulpal sensitivity. There may be either an incomplete wetting in application of the primer agent or incomplete curing of the bonding agent. One must be sure to place incremental layers of wetting agent until a glossy appearance is observed on gentle air dispersion, and a well-calibrated curing light must be used for sufficient exposure times.

56. What factors contribute to increased pulpal sensitivity even with proper technique?

If the dentin is dried too completely, air emboli may enter the dentin tubules and the dentin-bonding layer may overseal the layer of air. There then exists a potential for mechanical masticatory stresses and a resultant sensitivity on biting on the tooth restoration unit. To best avoid this problem, leave the dentin moist by gentle air dispersion; do *not* use drying. Then the hydrophilic primers will follow fluid down the tubules and fill both intertubular dentin and tubules with resin.

57. How long should you apply the adhesive?

The adhesive must penetrate through the demineralized dentin to form the hybrid layer for maximal bond strength. Some systems are faster than others; thus, following the manufacture's instructions are important. In general, after applying the adhesive, 15–20 seconds should be allowed for penetration. Then air evaporation of the solvent (acetone or alcohol) is followed by curing (visible light-cured generally). This should leave a shiny dentin surface. If this goal is not achieved, reapplication of the adhesive should be performed until a shiny layer appears.

58. Describe the composition of contemporary primers in adhesive systems.

Primers are bifunctional molecules. One end is hydrophobic to bind to the adhesive, and the other end is hydrophilic. The hydrophilic end permeates conditioned dentin and chases the water of the moist surface, assisted by solvents (acetone or alcohol). After this penetration, the solvents need to be evaporated by air drying. Examples of primers are HEMA, 4-Meta, and PENTA. Generally they do not contain any light-curing capabilities.

59. Describe the bonding resin adhesive.

Bonding resins are unfilled BIS-GMA or UDMA. They may be visible light-cured (VLC), auto-cured or dual-cured. The latest generation (fifth generation) of adhesive systems consolidates the primer and adhesive into premixed applications. This results in a time savings. Examples are Prime and Bond NT (Dentsply/Caulk), 3M Single Bond; and OptiBond Solo (Kerr). There is a trend to add fillers to the adhesive bonding agents to enhance their physical properties.

60. What enhancement do fillers contribute to newer adhesive bonding resins?
- Increase the bond strength at the hybrid layer.
- Improve stress absorption at the tooth restoration interface, enabling better retention.
- Lower modulus of elasticity to impart added flexibility and thus relieve contraction stress due to polymerization shrinkage. The adhesive absorbs within itself some of the contraction stress.
- Help adhesive cover the dentin in one application rather than multiple applications.

61. What are the sixth generation adhesive systems?

The latest systems combine the etchant and primer and even the etchant, primer, and adhesive into one all-encompassing step. The advantages are even depth of etch and primer penetration into the demineralized collagen zone of dentin, minimal postoperative sensitivity by efficiently sealing tubules, and saving time. However, these systems are highly technique-sensitive and use only VLC. Furthermore, they are not shown to have enough strength to bond enamel and therefore should be considered mainly as dentin-bonding agents. Product examples are Prompt L-Pop (3M ESPE), Panavia F, Touch and Bond (Parkell), and Clearfil SE Bond (Kuraray).

62. Can you use any adhesive with any composite?

Generally any light-cured composite should bond to any light-cured adhesive. However, self-cured composites such as core pastes are not compatible with most single component adhesives. You must use dual component or self-cure adhesives with self-cure composites.

63. Outline the adhesive procedures for bonding composites and amalgam to tooth structure.
For composite materials

To enamel: Clean surface with pumice; wash; etch 15 seconds; wash; air dry; apply unfilled VLC resin only.

To dentin and enamel: Clean surface; etch 15 seconds; wash; leave moist; use VLC adhesive components in layers before composite; consider filled adhesives.

For amalgam (bonding to dentin only)

Clean surface; etch 15 seconds; wash; use VLC primer to seal tubules; self-cure resin adhesive (two-component system); pack amalgam before resin sets.

COMPOSITES

64. What are the components in composite resins?
- Monomers: BIS-GMA, UDMA
- Diluent monomers: TEG-DMA, MMA
- Inorganic fillers: quartz, glass, zirconium,
- Organic fillers: silica
- Coupling agents: silane
- Iniators: tertiary amines, camphorquinone (CMP), phenyl-dipropanedione (PPD), benzoyl peroxide

- Inhibitors: ether of hydroquinone
- Ultraviolet absorbers: benzophenone

65. Describe the function of each monomer component.

Principal monomers are high-molecular-weight compounds that can undergo free radical addition polymerization to create rigid cross-linked polymers. The most common monomer is BIS-GMA (an aromatic dimethacrylate that is the addition product of bisphenol A and glycidal methacrylate [GMA]). An alternative monomer is urethane dimethacrylate.

Diluent monomers are low-molecular-weight compounds used to reduce the viscosity of the unpolymerized resins to improve physical properties and handling. There are two types: mono-functiuonal (methylmethacrylate) and difunctional (ethylene glychol dimethacrylate or triethylene glychol). The latter are used most often because they form harder and stronger cross-linked composite structures because of a lower coefficient of thermal expansion. They also have less polymerization shrinkage, are less volatile, and have less water absorption.

66. What are the filler particles?

Inorganic filler particles used in composite resins include quartz, glass, and colloidal silica, along with additions of lithium, barium, or strontium to enhance optical properties. These fillers are coated with a silane coupling agent (organosilane) to bond adhesively to the organic resin matrix. Silane bonds to the quartz, glass, and silica particles, whereas the organic end bonds to the resin matrix.

67. Describe the mechanism of silane coupling.

During free radical polymerization of the organic BIS-GMA, covalent bonds are formed between this polymer matrix and the silane coupling agent, commonly gamma methacryloxy-propyltrimethoxy. The coupling agent that coats the filler particles at the silane end thus holds the inorganic and organic phases together. This process further prevents water absorption.

68. What is the mechanism of polymerization in composite resin systems?

Benzoyl peroxide and aromatic tertiary amines are used to initiate polymerization reactions by supplying free radicals. This process is induced by photoactivation with visible light in the 420- to 450-nm range using alpha-diketones and a reducing agent, often a tertiary aliphatic amine. The diketone absorbs light to form an excited triplet state, which together with the amine produces ion radicals to initiate polymerization.

69. Describe the function of polymerization inhibitors.

Inhibitors are necessary to provide shelf life and delay the polymerization reaction, thus allowing clinical placement of composite materials. The dimethylacrylate monomers spontaneously polymerize in the presence of atmospheric oxygen. To this end monomethyl ethers of hydroquinone are used as inhibitors.

70. What are radiation absorbers?

Ultraviolet absorbers provide color stability to composite resins and thus limit discoloration.

71. How are composites classified?

There are a number of classification systems, generally based on filler particle size and the how the fillers are distributed.
- Large-particle (conventional) composites: 20–50 μm in diameter
- Intermediate: 1–5 μm
- Hybrids or blends: 0.8–1.0 μm
- Fine particle and minifilled: 0.1–0.5 μm
- Microfilled: 0.05–0.1 μm
- Homogenous microfilled: organic matrix and directly admixed microfiller particles
- Heterogeneous microfilled: organic matrix, directly admixed microfiller particles, and microfiller-based complexes

72. Which are presently the most commonly used composite materials?
The microfilled and hybrid composites.

73. List major characteristics of hybrid composites.
- Most universal in application, both anterior and posterior usage
- Combine strength and polishability
- Easier to use than thin microfills and more closely match the refractive index of tooth structure
- Composed of several filler particles; a glass in the 1- to 3-μm range plus silica, 0.04 μm
- Hybrids get *darker* when cured; match shade with cured sample
- Fillers are 75–80% by weight

PRODUCT	FILLER % WEIGHT	FILLER % VOLUME	PARTICLE SIZE μ	HARDNESS	DEPTH OF CURE MM 20 SEC HALOGEN
EsthetX (Dentsply/Caulk)	77.5	60	0.7	62	3
Renamel Hybrid (Cosmedant)	75	56	0.7	70.4	2
Point4 (SDS/Kerr)	76	57	0.4	58.8	3
XRV Herculite (SDS/Kerr)	79	59	0.6	64.4	2
Vitalescence (Ultradent)	75	56	0.7	80.1	2

From Reality 2002, Vol. 16, p 316.

74. What are the major properties of microfill composites?
- Allow the most esthetic polishability and mimic porcelain in result
- Used in class III, IV, and V restorations, diasthema closure, hand-sculpted facial veneers
- Resist wear; more elastic than hybrids and may be better suited to abfraction lesions
- Particle size 0.01–0.1 μm
- Get *lighter* when cured; match shade with cured sample
- Fillers are 40–50% by weight

PRODUCT	HARDNESS (KNOOP)	BOND STRENGTH MPA HALOGEN 40 SEC	PLASMA ARC 20 SEC
Renamel (Cosmedent)	33.8	17.5	22.1
Durafil VS (Kulzer)	27.2	20.1	9.9
Heliomolar (Ivoclar Viadent)	41.3	20.4	20.4
Filtek A110 (3M ESPE)	40.1	23.4	24.9
Micronew (Bisco)	64.7	14.8	19.3

From Reality 2002, Vol. 16, p 440.

75. How are hybrids and microfilled composites used together for maximizing strength and esthetics, the so-called "sandwich technique"?
1. A sandwich technique is a layering of materials to create the maximum of desirable properties in a restoration. In a class IV anterior restoration of an incisal angle, for example, first using a hybrid composite to build up the body of underlying dentin provides strength and dentin-like opacity. Then over-laying the final tooth structure with a microfilled composite provides the incisal translucency, the desired reflective characteristics, and the high polishability of a microfill.
2. A layer of hybrid, together with opaquers, may block out undesirable colors prior to using a microfill.
3. All posterior restorations, as well as porcelain repairs and periodontal splinting, benefit from the superior strength of a hybrid.

76. What are packable composites?

Packable composites have a consistency that more closely resembles that of amalgam than conventional composites. They are most commonly used in class I and II restorations. However, they cannot be condensed but are more packable than hybrids. Because they are much more stiff in consistency, there is some ability to sculpt the restoration before curing. Bulk curing, however, is at best to 2–3 mm. Products include Prodigy (SDS/Kerr), Filtek (3M ESPE), Heliomolar HB (Ivoclar Vivadent), SureFil (Dentsply/Caulk), and Solitaire 2 (Heraeus Kulzer).

77. What are composite opaquers or tints? How may they be used?

Opaquers and tints are light-cured, low-viscosity, highly shaded composites used to add esthetic characteristics to restorations. They often match the Vita Shade System and can be brushed on in layers to create life-like matches to natural teeth. They may be applied on a bonded tooth, between layers of the sandwich buildup, or even on the surface to characterize the restoration, (e.g., Renamel Creative Color, Cosmedent).

78. What is a compomer?

A compomer is a polyacid modified composite that incorporates the properties of resin ionomers and composites. Compomers are self-adhesive to dentin because of their acid-base re-action and light curing and release fluoride. They still require a primer/adhesive and may not require etching first for dentin bonding, but etching increases bond strength to enamel. They may be used in carious class V lesions, as a flow application in the gingival wall of a proximal box in class II preparations, and to block out undercuts in inlay-only crown preparations. They are also suitable in all restorations in primary teeth. Dyract (Dentsply/Caulk) is the leading material.

79. Define composite sealant.

Composite sealants are unfilled resins that that are applied to seal microcracks that may be left after finishing and polishing of composite or bonded restorations. They are very thin-filmed and have a minimal air-inhibited layer. Application is done after a 20-second etch; wash; and then allow 20-second light cure.

80. What are flowable composites?

Flowable composites are low-viscosity, visible light-cured, radiopaque, hybrid composite resins, often containing fluoride and dispensed by syringe directly into cavity preparations. They have 37–53% filler by volume (compared with 60% conventional composites). They are claimed to be easy to deliver via a narrow syringe tip, offer flexibility for class 5 preparations, and are able to access small areas. They may be used as a base material under class I and II restorations. Although long-term performance is not known, they seem well suited for the long channels of air abrasion preparations, cementing veneers, dental sealants, margin repairs of all types, inner layer in sandwich techniques, porcelain repairs, and sealing the head of implants. Examples include Aeliteflo (BISCO), Florestore (DenMat), Revolution (Kerr), and Ultraseal XT Plus (Ultradent)

81. How are flowable composites used?

Class V defects: use in abfraction, erosions, and sealing marginal defects.

Minimal class I restorations: Use like a thick sealant for pit and fissure restorations whether prepare with air abrasion or fissurotomy burs.

Gingival wall of class II restorations: Use in the gingival wall of a proximal box has been shown to reduce leakage at this margin in composite restorations. Be sure to cure for a minimum of 40 sec with halogen lights (from buccal and lingual as well).

Blocking out small undercuts: eliminates removing sound tooth structure; fast and simple application.

82. What are the advantages of all-purpose composite resins?

Products such as Geristore (Den-Mat) are termed multipurpose products. They are small-particle composites, fluoride-releasing, are self- or dual-curing; they have high compressive strengths and low viscosity. They have applications as cements, bases and liners, or pediatric restoratives. They bond to dentin, enamel porcelain, amalgam, precious and semiprecious metals, and moistsurfaces. They function as luting materials for crowns (with dentin-bonding systems) and are suitable for Maryland bridge bonding.

83. What is an ormocer?

Ormocer is an acronym for **or**ganically **mo**dified **cer**amic. Ormocers are a class of restorative material that links glass-like inorganic components with organic polymer components that make them nearly as hard as glass but similar to polymer materials in behavior. The prepolymerized filler particles in ormocers are large and tightly packed, which leads to less shrinkage on curing. Admira by Voco GmbH is a commerciallyavailable ormocer-based restorative material. It features low polymerization shrinkage, high biocompatibility, tooth-like thermal expansion and a nonsticky, packable consistency. The technique for placement is direct and similar to that of traditional composites.

84. What is a ceromer?

Ceromer is an acronym for **cer**amic **op**timized poly**mer** and was introduced by Ivoclar as Tetric Ceram.

Other commercial products of this type include BelleGlass by Kerr, Sculpture by Jeneric/Pentron, and Artglass by Heraeus/Kulzer. The formulations of these materials give them many of the ideal properties found in composites and porcelain but with a much higher level of fluoride release. These materials have high strength because of their low modulus of elasticity as well as high flexural strength and fracture toughness. Additionally, their surface hardness is similar to that of enamel, giving them low wear and excellent polishability. These materials can be used for inlays, onlays, veneers, and crowns, using the direct/indirect or indirect techniques.

85. What are "smart" composites?

Smart composites were introduced by Ivoclar Vivadent as Ariston pHc. This material is an ion-releasing composite formulation that releases fluoride, hydroxyl, and calcium ions in response to a drop in the pH in the area adjacent to the material. What makes these composites "smart" is that the greater the drop in pH, which results from plaque, the greater the release of active ions. The effect is a reduction in secondary caries formation by inhibiting bacterial growth and reducing demineralization. The fluoride release from this material is not as high as from glass ionomers but is much higher than from other esthetic materials.

86. Define direct resin, indirect resin, and indirect-direct resin restorations.

Direct resin restorations are the placement of composite resins into class 1, 2, 3, and 5 preparations directly at chairside. They are the most commonly performed.

Indirect resin procedures involve tooth preparation, impressions, and temporization as a first visit. Laboratory fabrication of onlays or inlays of resin or ceramic restorations are cemented on a second visit.

Indirect-direct resin restorations are a single-visit technique using fast-setting die stones to allow preparation, impression taking, chair-side fabrication of the restoration, and delivery of the final inlay or onlay.

87. What are the characteristics of the newer indirect composite resin systems?

These composite resin systems are fabricated in the laboratory from impressions of prepared teeth. They may be fiber-reinforced for crowns and bridges. By treating with heat, high-intensity light, vacuum, nitrogen, and/or pressure, the restoration's physical properties are greatly advanced. They exhibit reduced polymerization shrinkage, increased flexural and tensile strength, resistance to abrasion and fracture, and improved color stability. Examples of current materials are BelleGlass (SDS/Kerr), Sinfony (3M ESPE), and Targis/Vectris (Ivoclar Vivadent).

88. What criteria are used to choose direct placement composite resins in class 2 restorations?

1. The best use in narrow slot-type restorations and smaller restorations of one-fourth to one-third of intercuspal distance.

2. If used in larger, greater than one-third intercuspal distance, weak cusps must be covered, and longevity is not considered long-term.

3. Persons with known metal allergies or patients who wish to avoid metal restorations.

4. Use is contraindicated in bruxers or clenchers or when extensive tooth loss places resin margins in occlusal contact.

89. Discuss the challenges of the class 2 composite restoration.

1. Most current resins wear significantly more than amalgam, gold, or porcelain. To minimize wear, sufficient light curing is suggested (30- to 40-second cures on facial, occlusal, and lingual surfaces with a calibrated light source).

2. They are generally time- and technique-sensitive restorations. Contact areas are harder to establish, and finishing is time-consuming. Use magnification to view; also use thin, dead, soft matrix bands or sectional matrices, well burnished against the proximal tooth, and held tightly with one instrument as the second places composite against the band and curing occurs. Finish dry, with sharp 12-bladed burs and a light touch.

3. Sufficiently light-cure the primer and bonding resins before placing composite to avoid postoperative tooth sensitivity. Apply composite in 2-mm increments.

90. Compare indirect resins with porcelain.

Indirect resins inlays tend to fit better, are easier to adjust and polish introrally, can be repaired with similar materials in the mouth, and most importantly are not as hard or abrasive to the opposing teeth as porcelain. Porcelain restorations may be better for onlays or when restoring multiple cusp and occlusal schemes, but the wear to opposing teeth is significant and the need to adjust occlusion and polish intraorally after cementation requires time and is more difficult.

91. Summarize guidelines for indirect resin and full-coverage ceramic crown preparations.
   Indirect resin preparations:
      1.5-mm reduction on occlusal aspect
      1.5–2.0 mm reduction on cusps
      Rounded internal line angles
      No bevel margins
      Butt-joint or deep chamfer margins
      Divergent walls
   Specialized ceramics full crowns (i.e., Empress or Procera)
      2.0 mm occlusal reduction
      1.5 mm chamfer margin
      1.5–2.0 facial reduction
      No internal preparations with Procera (fill-in)

92. Outline the step-by-step procedure for the direct posterior resin restoration.

1. Apply rubber dam.

2. Remove the defective tooth structure or restoration.

3. Use a caries indicator (i.e., Seek-Ultra crown dent), if desired.

4. Prepare the tooth for the restoration.

5. Place a matrix system (sectional matrix or full-band). Wedge.

6. Wash and clean prep; you may use antibacterial, if desired.

7. Use total etch time of 15 seconds for enamel and a maximum of 10–15 seconds for dentin with phosphoric acid. Do *not* overetch dentin.

8. Rinse etchant off well, and lightly air or blot excessive water; leave surface moist.

9. Apply multiple layers of primer/adhesive to enamel and dentin, leaving for 20 seconds to allow penetration and hybrid layer formation.

10. Air-disperse to evaporate the solvent.

11. Light-cure for 10–20 seconds.

12. Apply a layer (< 2-mm increments) of flowable composite to the pulpal floor in proximal box.

13. Build up with composite (hybrid, packable, reinforced microfill).

14. Sculpt, shape, and gross occlusal adjustment.

15. Remove rubber dam, and adjust occlusion.

16. Apply occlusal resin stains, if desired (Kolor-plus [Kerr]).

17. Polish with points, cups, discs, and wheels.

18. Etch surface; rinse and dry.

19. Apply composite surface sealant and cure for 20 seconds.

93. What methods are used to provisionalize indirect resin restorations?

Take a preoperative polyvinyl matrix in a triple try. Then fill with an acrylic or provisional composite resin and cement with a temporary cement. Use a light-cured flexible resin such as Fermit (Ivoclar) to insert, light-cure, and trim.

94. Outline the cementation technique for resin-bonded inlays/onlays.

1. Remove provisional restoration.

2. Apply rubber dam.

3. Clean prep, rinse, dry; try restoration, checking margins, interproximal contacts, and overall fit.

4. Remove restoration, clean with etch, and rinse; place a silane coupling agent on the internal surface for 1 minute.

5. Etch tooth enamel and dentin for 15 seconds; rinse; light air-disperse moisture.

6. Apply multiple layers of single-component adhesive; air-disperse to evaporate solvent; leave for 20 seconds.

7. Light-cure 20 seconds.

8. Apply thin layer of adhesive to internal surface of restoration

9. Mix dual cure resin cement (i.e., Calibra [Dentsply], Nexus2 [Kerr], and apply into prep; seat restoration

10. While holding restoration, remove as much cement as possible with brush or rubber tip.

11. Spot cure into place 10 seconds from buccal and lingual aspects.

12. Apply floss through contacts.

13. Light-cure finally for 30 seconds on each surface; remove rubber dam and adjust occlusion; finish and polish.

14. Re-etch for 15 seconds, rinse, and dry.

15. Brush on a thin layer of surface sealant and light-cure.

95. Describe the direct/indirect technique for posterior resin restorations.

This combination technique involves taking an elastomeric impression of the prepared teeth and pouring up a die in a fast-setting material such as ultrafast-setting gypsum products. The clinician then generates the restoration in the office lab, light-cures it, and cements it in the same visit.

96. List the advantages and disadvantages of the direct/indirect technique over the indirect laboratory-processed resin restorative technique.

Major advantages

- Decreased chair time
- Decreased laboratory expenses
- No need for temporization

Major disadvantages
- Possible deformation of the restoration, especially if a flexible die material is used
- The restorative material formulations available in the dental laboratory provide better strength and wear resistance
- The processes available in the dental laboratory provide a better cure of the resin polymer material

97. Give examples of lab-processed resin restorative materials. How are they cured compared with in-office resins?

Most lab-processed resins are cured by a combination of light of varying intensities, pressure, and heat. Examples include Cristobal+ by DENTSPLY Ceramco and Sculpture by Jeneric/ Pentron. Another material in this category is belleGlass HP by Kerr Lab, which is processed in a nitrogen environment under heat and pressure. The nitrogen removes any oxygen-inhibiting air from the resin and improves the cure.

98. What cementing materials should be used with indirect resin restorations?

All three of the polymer resin systems mentioned above should be luted with resin cements. Only resin cements possess the ability to bond adequately to both tooth structure and the internal surface of the restoration. All other types of cements are strictly contraindicated. Hybrid-type resin cements are best suited for onlay and full-coverage restorations because of their higher strength. Microfill resin cements are preferred for inlays, because they possess greater wear resistance to occlusal masticatory forces.

99. Why are the polymer resin restorative materials such as belleGlass HP well suited to restoring the occlusal surfaces of implant-supported restorations as opposed to conventional porcelains?

Because porcelain has poor shock-absorbing ability, masticatory energy in implant restorations is transferred almost totally to the interfacial region between the implant and osseous tissue that supports the fixture. In contrast, polymer resins such as belleGlass HP are much more energy-absorbent while still providing excellent resistance to wear on occlusal surfaces.

100. What considerations shall be kept in mind for repair of older composite restorations?

As composites age, it is harder to chemically bond to the surface. There are fewer reactive sites on the resin surface, and impregnated proteins and debris limit the bonding capacity. It is necessary to remove the outer surface with a bur to remove contaminants and increase the surface area. Pumice, followed by etching, proceeds as usual. Then coating with silane allows better bonding to the silica particles. Final application of unfilled resin and curing before placement of the composite should result in predictable bonding.

101. How is a fractured porcelain restoration repaired?

The first step is to determine the cause. Is it a structural weakness or perhaps an occlusal stress-related fracture? Try to resolve any causative factors first. The next step is to create some mechanical hold wherever possible. Roughen and bevel around the defect, because the restorative cannot bond to a glazed surface. Microetch when possible with an air abrasion microetcher, or use a porcelain acid etchant such as 10–12% hydrofluoric acid gel. Then silanate and apply bonding resin, opaquers, and finally the appropriate color of composite restorative.

102. What is the function of a curing light?

Primarily curing lights apply a visible light spectrum (400–700 nm) to photo imitators such as camphorquinone (450–525 nm) and phenyl-dipropanedione (PPD, 430 nm) that allow polymerization on demand of a vast array of dental materials. Output should be at least 300 mW/cm^2, and built-in radiometers are advantageous.

103. List the current basic light types.
Quartz halogen bulb
- Most common; least expensive; reliable
- Wide-spectrum bandwidth: 400–510 nm
- Cures all materials
- Top models: Optilux 501 (Kerr); Spectrum 800 (Dentsply/Caulk)

Plasma arc
- Very fast; expensive; larger than halogen
- May not cure all materials
- Example: Rembrant's Sapphire

Argon laser
- Fast; expensive; larger than halogen
- May not cure all materials
- Example: Arago (Premiere Laser Systems)

Light-emitting diode (LED)
- Cordless; light weight; small; long battery life
- May not cure all materials;
- NRG (Caulk)

104. Why and how should lights be tested and maintained?
The power output of a light is critical to proper curing of a restoration. Any decrease is likely to give inadequate polymerization. The power output should be tested with a radiometer (built-in to many newer lights) when new and weekly thereafter. Any decrease should be checked. Most commonly a deterioration in bulb strength (change the bulb), a dirty wand tip (clean regularly), or a worn light filter or optical guide (replace as needed) can decrease output. When all of these steps fail, return the light to the manufacturer.

105. What constitutes an ideal cure?
- Pack and cure materials incrementally to a 2-mm maximal thickness, with 20- to 40-second cure times.
- Keep light at right angles to the cure material.
- Keep distance from tip to material less than 6 mm.
- Use a proper diameter tip for the curing objective.
- Darker shades and thicker layers need more time.
- There is apparently no difference in ramped, stepped or pulsed delivery of light and final cure results

Composites do not shrink toward the light, but direction is determined by cavity shape and bond quality. The latter is determined by proper adhesive technique

CEMENTS

106. What are resin cements?
Modified low-viscosity composites use to bond ceramic and indirect resin restorations.

107. Summarize the types of resin cements and the indications for each.
Light-cured
Metal-free restorations < 1.5 mm in thickness
Metal-free orthodontic retainers
Metal-free periodontal splints
Product examples: Calibra (Dentsply/Caulk); Nexus2 (SDS/Kerr); RelyX Veneer (3M ESPE).
Dual-cured
Metal free inlays, onlays, crowns and bridges
Any application where a curing light may not reach
Product Examples: RelyX ARC (3m ESPE); Panavia F (Kuraray); Duo-link (Bisco).

Self-cure

    Metal-based inlays, onlays
    Ceramometal crown and bridges
    Full metal crowns and bridges
    Endodontic posts
    Bonded amalgams
    Product examples: Panavia 21(Kuraray); C&B Metabond (Parkell); Post Cement Hi- X (Bisco).

108. What are the advantages of glass ionomer restorative materials?

They bond to tooth structure, have a nearly ideal expansion-contraction ratio and low microleakage, and release fluoride. The light-cured materials are the easiest to work with because they provide extended working times, have rapid on-demand set, and are less technique-sensitive on mixing.

109. How are glass ionomer cements (GICs) classified?

GICs are mixed powder-liquid component systems. The powder consists of a calcium-aluminofluorosilicate glass that reacts with polyacrylic acid to form a cement of glass particles surrounded by a matrix of fluoride elements.

    1. **Hydrous types:** a slower-setting material characterized by a viscous liquid of polyacrylic acid, tartaric acid, itaconic acid, and water plus fluoroaluminosilicate glass powder. Examples: GC Lining cement (GC America), Chelon-Silver (Espe-America).

    2. **Anhydrous types:** flouroaluminosilicate glass, vacuum-dried polyacrylic acid, itaconic acid powder, and a water and tartaric acid solution. These materials have better shelf life. Example: Ketac Chem (Espe-Premiere).

    3. **Hybrid forms:** combination of anhydrous and hydrous forms of glass ionomer powder and liquid. Example: Fuji II (GC America).

    4. **Light-cured glass ionomers:** an acid-base setting material in a photo-initiated liquid. These materials offer extended working times and rapid on-demand set-up and are less technique sensitive on mixing. Examples: Vitrabond (3M) and XR Ionomer (Kerr).

110. What are metal-reinforced GICs?

Metallic silver particles of up to 40% of weight are added to GICs to increase the strength and to speed the setting time. Metal-reinforced GICs may be used for (1) core buildups when at least 50% of tooth structure remains (GICs alone do not have the strength to be a total core); (2) as a temporary filling material; and (3) as a filler or base/liner for undercuts in any cavity preparation. An example is KetecSilver (Espe-Premiere).

111. What are glass ionomer resin cements (GIRs)?

These resin-modified glass ionomers improve the properties of glass ionomers significantly:

    1. They are easy to mix and place.
    2. They are equal or higher in fluoride release.
    3. They have higher retention, higher strength, lower solubility, and lower postoperative sensitivity than glass ionomer or zinc phosphate cements.

    Current brands are Vitremer (3M), Advance (Caulk/Dentsply), and Fuji Plus (GC).

TECHNIQUE TIPS

112. What is considered the most important requisite for successful adhesive dentistry?

The formation of maximal strength bonding requires a clean operating field free of debris and contamination. Whenever possible, this goal is best accomplished with a rubber dam.

113. What is the function of a matrix band? What types are currently available?

Matrix bands establish the foundation for a missing proximal wall of a tooth preparation. They may be metal or plastic and usually have a retainer to keep their form against the axial tooth walls and support tight contacts. The use of a wedge adapts the band fully at the gingival margin, but the wedge should not be placed under too much pressure to avoid unwanted effects on the gingival papilla. The traditional metal band and Tofflemire-type retainers are being replaced by the **sectional types** that are used to form predictable proximal contacts when posterior direct resins are placed. They require an individual matrix for each proximal box (two are used for MODs). The concaved metal form is place interproximally and gently wedged. Then, using a rubber dam or dedicated forceps, the retaining ring is grasped, expanded, and positioned over the proximal line angles. When released, the ring tines grab the matrix and hold it against the tooth. The result is close adaptation of band to tooth to minimize excessive composite at the line angles but also to exert pressure on the band against the adjacent tooth to ensure a tight contact. Product examples are Palodent Plus (Dentsply/Caulk), Omni-Matrix (Ultradent), and Contact Matrix (Danville Materials).

114. How can one achieve a tight interproximal contact in direct class II posterior composite restorations?

1. Use a thin burnished band, well-adapted and wedged, or a prefabricated sectional matrix system.
2. Apply a proximally applied force with an instrument to the band while curing the composite. This technique keeps the restoration tightly against the band and provides optimal contact.

115. What are clinical procedures to may injury pulps of teeth?

1. Dull burs and diamonds can result in increased heat production.
2. Noncentric hand pieces traumatize teeth like mini-jackhammers.
3. Inadequate water delivery causes heat and dehydration.
4. Over-drying tooth preparations dehydrates the pulp causing sensitivity.
5. The acidity of astringent materials such as Hemodent (pH of 1.9) can injure if left in dentin or root contact. Use only minimally on cord or in sulcus.
6. Temporary resin exothermic reactions for provisional restorations may be harmful. Cool with water often during exothermal period.
7. Poor fitting temporary restorations can result in leakage that injures pulps. Margins should fit well.
8. Over contoured restorations can result in trauma from occlusion. Carefully adjust occlusion and check in all excursions.

116. Describe the symptoms generally associated with coronal fracture syndrome (CFS).

Patients who have CFS typically present with pain on chewing, particularly with hard foods and at the correct contact angle on the offending tooth. Additionally there may be some sensitivity to cold and sweets, depending on the extent and nature of the fracture. Symptoms that include lingering temperature sensitivity may indicate that the pulp has undergone irreversible damage as a result of the fracture.

117. What diagnostic tools and methods may be used to determine the location of the fracture in a patient with CFS?

In addition to the customary methods of locating dental pathology, the use of a bite stick or Tooth Sleuth enables you to isolate cusps to see whether pain can be elicited by occlusal stress on a potential offending cusp. The offending cusp often elicits a response on release of the bite on the stick. Intraoral cameras, magnification, and light refraction are also helpful in determining the location and extent of fractures.

118. Describe the use of diagnostic restoration removal in the treatment of coronal fracture syndrome.

Diagnostic restoration removal is the removal of an existing filling material to inspect visually the pulpal floor as well as to evaluate the integrity of the dentin at the base of the cusps. This procedure is performed when a hairline crack is visible externally but its extent and disposition are unclear.

119. What types of restorations should be considered for teeth with CFS?

Generally speaking, restorations that bond and/or provide cuspal reinforcement should be used on CFS teeth. Fractures that have minimal dentin involvement may be restored with direct or indirect resins. Fractures involving significant amounts of dentin or involving one or more cusps should be restored with ceramic or gold onlays and crowns.

120. Describe the clinical relationship between bruxism, tooth wear, and the incidence of CFS.

Bruxism and tooth wear often lead to loss of cuspid guidance, resulting in more of a group function occlusal scheme. This leaves the posterior teeth, especially those that are more heavily restored, prone to fracture.

121. If a patient presents with tooth sensitivity to biting and cold in a clinically normal-appearing molar with an MOD amalgam, what are the possible differential diagnoses? What is the suggested treatment?

First, to confirm the specific tooth, attempt to duplicate the symptoms with a cold spray and when biting on a wet cotton roll. Take a radiograph to rule out recurrent decay, periapical pathology, or periodontal involvement. If there are no positive radiographic findings, we may consider a cracked tooth or a pulp that is hyperemic and may or may not be approaching irreversible change. The best first treatment is to remove all old amalgam and explore the tooth for cracks or decay. Placing a bonded, nonmetallic restoration allows observation to see whether the pulp can resolve. If symptoms subside within 3–6 weeks, a permanent restoration (full-coverage crown or onlay) may be placed. If symptoms persist or at any time worsen, endodontic treatment should begin. If endodontic treatment does not resolve the pain, one may conclude that the fracture proceeds subgingivally or through the furcation. At this time extraction must be considered.

122. What is the biologic width? Explain its relationship to restorative dentistry.

The biologic width is an area that ideally is approximately 3 mm wide from the crest of bone to the gingival margin. It consists of approximately 1 mm of connective tissue, 1 mm of epithelial attachment, and 1 mm of sulcus. As it relates to restorative dentistry, if a restorative procedure violates this zone, there is a higher likelihood that periodontal inflammation will ensue, causing the attachment apparatus to move apically.

123. When it becomes necessary for restorative reasons to impinge on the biologic width, what steps can be taken before final restoration to create a maintainable periodontal environment?

Crown lengthening and orthodontic extrusion are the two most common ways to deal with this problem. Crown lengthening exposes more tooth structure surgically and is in effect surgical repositioning of the biologic width. Orthodontic extrusion is done when crown lengthening would unduly compromise the periodontal health of the adjacent teeth or create an unfavorable esthetic situation, as often can occur in the anterior maxilla.

124. What techniques can be used to achieve marginal exposure and to control hemorrhage in a class V cavity preparation?

If the preparation is < 2 mm below the gingival sulcus, an impregnated retraction cord with a gingival retraction rubber-dam clamp may be effective. If the defect approaches 3 mm or greater, the hemostasis and margin exposure often require surgical exposure (crown lengthening) or excision via electrosurgery.

125. Describe the options for treatment of root surface sensitivity.

Root sensitivity is a common problem and can be adequately resolved in many instances by modifying the patient's tooth-brushing technique and having patients use desensitizing toothpaste such as Sensodyne or fluoride gels. Other desensitizing agents, such as Protect by Butler, use oxalate precipitates to occlude the dentin tubules. Dentin-bonding systems work well to reduce sensitivity as well. Others advocate iontophoresis to apply fluoride to the sensitive surface.

126. Should composite resins be placed to cover exposed root surfaces in a patient with gingival recession?

In the absence of caries, the placement of composite to cover exposed root surfaces should generally be performed with careful consideration. Composites bond only marginally well to cementum and, like all restorative materials, can further promote gingival recession. In addition, if surgical root coverage is performed, success depends on the establishment of a biologic attachment between the grafted tissue and cementum. Grafts do not attach to composites! Root surface coverage may be considered in cases of protracted and extreme root sensitivity or when it is a significant esthetic concern to the patient.

127. Should direct placement composites be placed in bulk or in increments to the cavity preparation?

Opinions vary as to the optimal method of composite placement. Some manufacturers and clinicians advocate bulk placement, but most recommend the layering and curing of material in approximately 2.0-mm increments to allow more thorough curing. Incremental placement also allows the layering of materials of different shades, opacities, and viscosities to achieve better esthetics.

128. What is the relationship between the size and location of the restoration and the potential for failure when direct resins are used on posterior teeth?

The more posterior the composite resin is placed, the greater the occlusal force. This force greatly increases the possibility of fracture, especially when there is an occlusal stop on the resin. Additionally, the larger the restoration, the greater the likelihood that polymerization shrinkage will compromise the integrity of the margins, leading to postoperative sensitivity and failure.

129. Describe the ideal clinical situation for placement of a class II direct resin restoration.

Ideally, a class II resin should be fairly conservative with minimal exposure of dentin, all margins should be in enamel for optimal seal and marginal integrity, and there should be no occlusal stops on the restoration to minimize the likelihood of resin fracture.

130. What are helpful aids in shade-matching for anterior teeth?

Choose the shade with color-corrected or natural light. Match teeth that are moist. Liquid coatings (saliva) alter reflected light. Place a cotton roll behind adjacent teeth to study changes in color, and note incisal shade changes that occur with light and dark backgrounds. Place a small amount of composite on the facial aspect of a tooth and light cure. Hybrid composites turn darker and microfills lighter on curing.

131. Describe recent technologic advances in chairside shade-taking for porcelain restorations.

In the past, shade-taking involved manual shade tabs and the subjective viewpoint of the practitioner. Today digital shade-taking systems such as ShadeVision by X-Rite, ShadeScan by Cynovad, ShadeEye NCC by Shofu, and SpectroShade by MHT International allow dentists to digitally map teeth with all of their variations of hue, value, and chroma. This information can be sent to the lab via e-mail, CD, or Flashcard. The software then calculates the shades of porcelain to be layered to achieve the proper match.

132. List uses of the stainless steel crown (SSC) in adult dentition.

1. Extensive decay in the dentition of young adults may leave a vital tooth with limited structure that requires a crown. If a permanent cast or ceramic restoration is not feasible, one may use the SSC in conjunction with a pin//bonded composite core build-up to stabilize the tooth until a permanent crown is constructed. A typical restoration involves the following steps: (1) complete excavation; (2) application of a glass ionomer liner or dentin bonding; (3) optional placement of pins at the four corner line angles; (4) beveling of the cervical enamel or dentin margin; (5) trial fitting of the SSC with careful adaptation of the cervical margins and checking for occlusal clearance; (6) etching of the preparation; (7) application of a self cure bonding resin; (8) filling of a well-adapted SSC with self-curing composite core material, and (9) seating of the crown. Removal of excessive and expressed composite leaves a well-sealed restoration that may serve for many years. When it is time to prepare the tooth for the permanent crown, slitting the SSC leaves the core buildup ready for final preparation.

2. SSCs may be used to stabilize rampant decay at any age.

3. SSCs may be used as a substitute for the copper band to stabilize a tooth before endodontic treatment. The SSC is more hygienic and kinder to the periodontium when it has been well adapted. Traditional access is through the occlusal dimension.

4. The SSC may be used as a temporary crown when lined with acrylic.

133. Outline design criteria for closing spaces in the anterior dentition.

1. Most commonly, composite bonding and/or porcelain veneers may close the maxillary central diasthema. Careful space analysis with calipers allows the most esthetic result. The width of each central incisor is measured, along with the diasthema space. One-half the dimension of the diasthema space is normally added to each crown unless the central incisors are unequal. Then adjustment is made to create equal central incisors.

2. If the central incisors appear too wide esthetically, one can reduce the distal incisal to narrow the tooth and bond it over to seal any exposed dentin. One then adds to the mesial incisal of the lateral incisor to effect closure of space.

3. A tooth in the palatal crossbite may even be transformed into a two-cuspid tooth by building up the facial aspect to the buccal profile. This bicuspidization is reasonably durable and esthetically pleasing.

4. Peg laterals and congenitally absent laterals replaced by cuspids may similarly be transformed by bonding and/or porcelain veneers. Reduction of protrusive contours, followed by addition to mesial and distal incisal areas, establishes esthetic results.

134. List the indications for the porcelain veneer restoration.

1. Stained teeth or teeth in which color changes are desired
2. Enamel defects
3. Malposed teeth
4. Malformed teeth
5. Replacement for multisurfaced composite restoration when adequate tooth structure remains (at least 30%)

Each patient must be evaluated on an individual basis. A general requirement is excellent periodontal health and good hygiene practices. In the case of stained teeth, prior bleaching (either passive home or in-office) helps to ensure better color esthetics.

135. Describe the basic tooth preparation for the porcelain veneer restoration on anterior teeth.

1. **Vital bleaching** (optional).

2. **Preparation.** Enamel reduction of at least 0.5 mm, which may extend to 0.7 mm at the cervical line angles, is necessary to avoid overcontouring. The only exception may be a tooth with a very flat labial contour and slight linguoversion. Chamfer-type labial preparations can be achieved with bullet-type diamonds, and the use of self-limiting 0.3-, 0.5-, 0.7-mm diamond burs is essential for consistent depth of preparation. The gingival cavosurface margin should be level with the free gingival crest. The mesial and distal proximal margins are immediately labial to the proximal con-

tact area. The contacts are not broken but may be relaxed with fine specialty strips of 10–20–? thickness. This allows placement of smooth metal matrix strips at the time of placement. The incisal margin is placed at the crest of the incisal ridge. Placing retraction cord into the gingival sulcus prior to preparing the gingival cavosurface margin helps in the atraumatic completion of the preparation.

3. **Impressions.** Standard impression techniques use vinyl polysiloxane materials.

4. **Temporization,** if at all possible, should be limited in use; it may be time-consuming and add to the expense of the procedure. One should use fine discs on the labial enamel surface for polishing the rough surface of the diamond-cut preparation to limit the accumulation of stain and debris. If it is necessary to temporize, preconstructed laboratory composite veneers or chairside direct temporization may be used. The techniques are similar. Spot etch two or three internal enamel areas on the labial preparation. Apply unfilled resin and tack-bond the veneer, or place some light-cured composite on the tooth and spread it with a gloved finger dipped in unfilled resin to a smooth finish. The preparation should be light-cured, and one should be able to lift it off relatively easily at the unetched areas and polish down the etched spots.

136. Describe the technique for insertion of porcelain veneers.

1. After isolation, pumicing, and washing, the fragile porcelain veneers are tried on the chamfer-prepared tooth. First, the inside surface of the veneer is wetted with water to increase the adhesion. Margins are then carefully evaluated.

2. Try-in pastes are used to determine the correct color-matching. Water-soluble pastes are the easiest to use. The try-in pastes closely match the final resin cements but are not light-activated.

3. The porcelain veneers are prepared for bonding. Apply a 30-second phosphoric acid etchant for cleaning. Wash and dry. Apply a silane coupling agent, and air-dry. Apply the unfilled light-cured bonding resin, and cure for 20 seconds.

4. To bond the porcelain veneer to the tooth, first clear interproximal areas with fine strips. Pumice and wash thoroughly. Place strips of dead, soft interproximal matrix, and etch the enamel for 30 seconds. Wash for 60 seconds and dry. Apply the bonding resin. Any known dentin areas should be primed (with dentin primer materials) before applying the bonding resin. Any opaquers or shade tints may now be applied. The light-cured resin luting cement is then applied to tooth and veneer. The veneer is carefully placed into position, and gross excessive composite is removed. Precure at the incisal edge for 10 seconds, and remove any partially polymerized material gingivally and proximally. Light-cure fully for 30–60 seconds. Finish the margins with strips, discs, and finishing burst. Check for protrusive excursions. Apply the central incisors first, then the laterals and then the cuspids.

137. What are CAD/CAM restorations?

CAD/CAM stands for computer-aided design/computer-aided manufacturing. The Cerec system, introduced in 1986 by Sirona Dental Systems, fabricates an esthetic restoration using an intraoral camera, software, and a precision milling machine, thus allowing the completion of the restoration in one appointment. In 2000, the Cerec 3 unit was introduced. This latest version has a Windows-based software program with a separate milling unit.

138. Describe the process by which the Cerec 3 CAD/CAM unit fabricates a restoration.

The Cerec 3 intraoral camera is placed over the tooth preparation, and a three-dimensional image of the preparation is generated. The operator then delineates the margins on the computer screen, and the system calculates and proposes the other morphologic contours, which the operator either accepts or modifies. Once the design is accepted, the software directs the modular milling unit to fabricate the restoration from a preselected block of restorative material. When completed, the restoration can be adjusted, if necessary, chairside and can be stained both internally and externally to modify shade.

139. How does the Cerec 3 capture the image of the tooth preparation?

The Cerec 3 has an intraoral camera that captures an optical impression of the prepared teeth. Titanium oxide powder is sprayed in a very thin layer on the surface of the teeth to be imaged.

This powder is needed to make the preparation reflective to the optical impression. Obtaining the optical impression takes the unit less than 0.5 sec.

140. Describe the milling system used in the Cerec 3 CAD/CAM unit.

The Cerec 3 milling unit uses two 1.6-mm diamond burs, one for gross preparation and a cone-shaped bur for production of finer detail. The system provides a warning to the operator when the burs need to be replaced, and changing them is easily done.

141. What restorative materials are currently available for the Cerec 3 unit?

The initial material developed for the Cerec CAD/CAM units was ceramic. Currently, Pro-Cad by Ivoclar Vivadent and Vitablocs Mark II by Vita are the two ceramic materials available for the system. Recently a composite block material, Paradigm MZ 100 by 3M ESPE, was introduced. This composite material has many of the advantages of traditional composites over porcelain counterparts. In particular, the Paradigm material causes much less wear on the milling burs and is much more easily repaired intraorally than porcelain.

142. Describe the classification for dental casting gold alloys.

Dental gold casting alloys are classified as type I to IV according to their composition as it affects surface hardness and strength as measured by their Vickers Hardness Number (VHN).

Type I (soft): VHN 50–90
Type II (medium): VHN 90–120
Type III (hard): VHN 120–150
Type IV (extra hard): VHN 150+

143. What are the benefits of cast gold inlays and onlays?

It is generally accepted that cast gold is the standard against which all other restorative materials are judged. The gold onlay provides cuspal protection as well as the following benefits:

1. Low restoration wear
2. Low wear of opposing teeth
3. Lack of breakage
4. Burnishable and malleable
5. Proven long-term service
6. Bonded cast gold restorations offer improvement in their main weakness, the cementing media.

144. What type of gold is recommended for use in a class II gold inlay?

Type II gold such as Academy Gold by Ivoclar Vivadent, JRVT by Jensen Industries Inc., and High Purity 77 by Argen Corporation should be used.

145. What are the advantages of cast gold onlays over other materials for restoring posterior teeth?

It is generally accepted that cast gold is the standard against which all other restorative materials are judged. Cast gold onlays afford cuspal protection to prevent fracture, have excellent marginal integrity, and, unlike porcelain, are kind to the opposing dentition.

146. Describe two methods to improve the seating of gold onlays and crowns.

1. Die spacers used in the laboratory provide a thin layer of cement and ensures more complete seating of castings.
2. Venting of a gold casting has also been shown to improve seating. The vent hole allows entrapped air and excess cement to escape during cementation. The vent hole is then filled with a cast pin, which is tapped in place and finished down as needed.

147. What is a Captek crown?

Captek stands for capillary casting technology and is a type of porcelain fused to the high noble type of crown. The technique involves the layering of gold by capillary action on a previously placed layer of platinum on a die. This process is followed by the placement of a bonding agent and the application of porcelain.

TOOTH-WHITENING

148. What are the most common methods to lighten vital teeth?

Generally, most tooth-whitening is done with home bleaching kits using custom tray fabrication. In-office techniques are suitable for some patients based on the type and intensity of stain and the temperament and desire of the patient. Home treatment requires compliance and patience, whereas chair-side techniques are faster and often more costly. Direct composite or laboratory porcelain veneers are the next most conservative approach and may be used when bleaching does not produce satisfactory results. Veneers are also useful when the shape, size, or arrangement of teeth is esthetically unacceptable. Finally, full-coverage porcelain and porcelain fused to metal crowns are the most invasive method and may be used when there is a need to replace damaged or missing tooth structure.

149. What factors influence tooth discoloration?

Extrinsic agents either consumed or not subject to removal by proper hygiene can stain and darken teeth. Intrinsic discoloration may be caused commonly by aging (increased yellowing), disease, injury, or certain exposures such as tetracycline.

150. For intrinsic stains, what agent has proved most effective for general use?

Intrinsic stains respond favorably to the chemical oxidation actions of peroxides. In fact, the use of vital bleaching with tray-delivered peroxide-based systems was the fastest growing dental procedure in the 1990s and continues to grow. Over 90% of U.S. dental practices offer this service.

151. What are the peripheral benefits of tooth whitening?

Often patients describe increased self -esteem, improved oral hygiene practices, and increased interest and involvement in dentistry.

152. List appropriate expectations of present bleaching techniques.

1. Natural teeth generally darken with age. Patients over 50 accumulate brown, orange, or yellow stains that are decreased by bleaching. Light yellow or brown shades lighten better than gray shades. External stains respond better than deeper internal stains, such as those from tetracycline staining or staining related to endodontic events.

2. Teeth lighten visibly regardless of the system used (in office or home methods).

3. The degree of lightening is a function of the concentration of active ingredient and the time of contact. In-office techniques use higher concentrations applied for up to 1 hour on isolated teeth, whereas at home methods use lower concentrations applied over several weeks in custom-molded trays constructed with or without reservoirs on the facial surfaces.

4. Generally few side effects are reported, and they tend to be transient.

5. Bleached teeth retain color for up to several years, although some patients request touch-ups at 6- to 12-month intervals. Patients with high consumption of coffee, tea, cola, or red wine, and tobacco users may require more frequent applications.

6. All current tooth-lightening products are generally similar when adjusted for contact time and concentration of reagent. Changes of 2–6 or more shades on the Vita scale are common.

153. How are bleaching procedures currently performed?

Professionally administered chairside. After tooth isolation with latex or paint on rubber dam, a peroxide gel is coated on teeth and usually activated via high-energy lights to shorten the treatment interval. Higher concentrations of peroxide gels in the form of up to 35% carbamide peroxide are used in 1- to 2-hour treatment sessions.

Professionally dispensed systems using custom fabricated trays to deliver 10–20% carbamide peroxide solution in at-home procedures. Trays are worn for 2 hours or over night for periods of 2–3 weeks. Favorable results have been reported even with tetracycline staining with prolonged applications of up to 3–6 months.

Self-administered over-the-counter and professionally dispensed whitening strips (Crest) containing 5–6.5 % hydrogen peroxide (Equivalent to 10% carbamide peroxide) that are adherent to the teeth and worn in two 30 minute intervals daily for 2 weeks or about half the time of tray-delivered systems.

154. What are the active ingredients in bleaching systems?

Hydrogen peroxide (H_2O_2) is the active ingredient in all bleaching systems. In carbamide peroxide formulations, the hydrogen peroxide is stabilized by urea and appears to be more stable than H_2O_2 alone and to produce fewer side effects. A 10% carbamide peroxide solution contains 7% urea and 3% hydrogen peroxide. Formulations are presently available containing 3–50% H_2O_2. Formulations are based in viscous gels to avoid side effects and to maximize the retention to teeth. They are buffered to near neutral pH.

155. Describe the mechanism of action of hydrogen peroxide in lightening teeth.

Hydrogen peroxide oxidizes and removes interprismatic organic matter within the tooth to lighten the shade.

156. Describe "energized" in-office methods to speed the lightening of teeth.

The application of a curing light or laser is claimed by manufacturers to shorten the lightening process; generally less than 1–2 hours in-office will equal 2 weeks at home. This is due to much higher peroxide concentrations delivered on properly isolated teeth and does not seem to be due to the method of energizing. Higher in-office concentrations require tooth isolation by paint on rubber dam material or traditional dam.

157. Which method of bleaching produces the best results?

Split arch comparisons seem to indicate that no discernable differences in lightening are achieved by any properly performed home or energized method and that the affect is a function only of concentration and time.

158. What are the two major complications of vital tooth bleaching?

Tooth sensitivity and gingival irritation may affect up to two-thirds of patients during the course of treatment. Tooth sensitivity is often mild and self-limiting and usually involves increased response to cold. Gingival irritation is often attributed to peroxide contact with tissues or poorly contoured trays that irritate the marginal tissues. There are no structural or functional effects on teeth.

159. What is believed to be the cause of bleach-induced tooth sensitivity?

Pulpal penetration of peroxide, dehydration, and tray-related tooth movements have been implicated. This sensitivity is transient and generally dissipates within a short time.

160. If a patient reports tooth sensitivity during the initial phase of treatment, what strategies may be implemented?

Decreasing the contact intervals may be a start—using one-hour instead of two-hour contact times or even every other day. Decreasing the product concentration chosen, 10% or less carbamide peroxide rather than higher levels, is a second choice. Recently it has been reported that not prebrushing the teeth decreases sensitivity without undue impairment in bleaching result. Dentifrices contain detergents (sodium lauryl sulfate) that may readily denature proteins on contact, which allows greater penetration of peroxide into the tooth and increases transient irritation. A prescription-strength fluoride dentifrice such as Prevident 5000 Plus (Colgate) can be used to resolve persistent cases.Soft tissue irritation can occur with in-office methods unless proper isolation is used. Home bleaching trays must be well adapted and properly contoured to prevent prolonged soft tissue contact. Patients should be instructed not to overfill their trays to avoid swallowing excessive bleach material upon insertion.

161. What contributes to the safety of peroxide as an oral bleaching agent?

Natural tissue peroxidases available on tooth and tissue surfaces limit the penetration of peroxide and degrade it readily. These enzymes are thought to play a role in the efficacy and tolerability of vital bleaching.

162. All methods of tooth-whitening improve tooth color to some degree provided there is what?

A sufficient degree of peroxide diffusion into the tooth surface.

163. Is bleaching safe for children?

Studies in 11- to 18-year-old groups have shown no ill effects greater than those seen in the general population. The use of whitening strips is well accepted because of the shortened application intervals required—2 times for 30 minutes each day vs. hours per day with trays.

164. What concentrations of bleaching gel are used for home bleaching?

Available products for home bleaching come in concentrations ranging from 10% to 30%. Higher concentrations allow shorter exposure times within the trays, which may decrease the effects of dehydration and lessen the chances of sensitivity. When using higher concentrations, bleaching trays must be especially well adapted and trimmed to prevent soft tissue exposure.

165. Can tetracycline-stained teeth be successfully treated with home bleaching?

Depending on the nature and severity of the discoloration, significant esthetic improvement of tetracycline-stained teeth can be achieved with home bleaching. Tetracycline stain exists primarily in the dentin of teeth; discoloration in the incisal two-thirds responds more favorably than that in the gingival one-third. Deeper and more pronounced stain is the most resistant to extensive color change.

166. How would you modify the home bleaching regimen for patients with tetracycline-stained teeth?

If only certain teeth exhibit stain, bleaching may be selectively limited. Treatment times often must be extended to between 2 and 6 months. Fee structures for these cases must be modified accordingly

167. When is the optimal time to bleach in the treatment-planning sequence?

In general, the optimal time is before beginning the final restorative phase. Bleaching lightens tooth color. Subsequent shades of crowns and composites need to be matched to the final tooth color. This is necessary because composite and porcelain restorations do not change color and will be mismatched if subsequent bleaching is performed.

168. Describe the technique of enamel microabrasion.

Microabrasion is the controlled removal of discolored enamel using a rubber cup and a paste composed of medium pumice and an acid, usually 20% hydrochloric acid. This technique is effective for treating superficial enamel discolorations (white or brown spots) often seen post-orthodontically and in cases of fluorosis.

169. How can microabrasion be used as an adjunct to vital bleaching procedures?

Although vital bleaching is extremely effective in many esthetic cases, it tends to make areas of decalcification, (white spots) even whiter in contrast to the surrounding tooth. Additionally, stains common with fluorosis are usually minimally affected by bleaching. Microabrasion is an effective technique for removing such lesions if they are superficial in nature.

170. What are the limitations of the microabrasion technique?

Microabrasion is useful only for the removal of enamel lesions in the outer few hundred microns of the tooth. Lesions that penetrate deeper into enamel or into dentin must be restored with restorative materials. Teeth with deeper intrinsic staining, such as that due to tetracycline, cannot be treated effectively with microabrasion.

171. Should you wait to do bonded restorations on recently bleached teeth?

Alterations in the surface microstructure from peroxide treatments can reduce bond strength. It is advised that one wait 3 or more weeks before doing bonded restorations.

172. Describe a logical sequence for whitening an anterior dentition with older class 3 and 4 composite restorations.

Most often older restorations are replaced after whitening because they will not match the new enamel shade. Before gel application, these older restorations should be carefully disked back to uncover all facial enamel. This process allows full bleach coverage of exposed enamel and leaves a more uniformly colored surface to replace and match the composite restorations.

173. Are reservoirs necessary in prefabricated bleaching trays.

It has been thought that leaving a space on the facial surface of models before making a custom tray allows more of the gel to stay in contact with the teeth. There is generally no difference reported with or without tray reservoirs; they may not be necessary.

174. How effective are whitening toothpastes?

Generally, given their low concentration of bleaching agent and short tooth contact time, whitening toothpastes have a minimal effect on actual tooth color but may prolong the effect of direct bleaching.

175. How are endodontically treated teeth bleached?

Most discoloration of pulpal degeneration is internal and/or from remnants of endodontic paste fillers. Such teeth generally require bleaching from the access cavity. The sooner the bleaching is started after the endodontic event, the more successful the lightening. Often the pulp chamber is packed with a mixture of hydrogen peroxide and sodium perborate, the so-called "walking bleach." This mixture is changed as needed until the result is satisfactory. Care must be taken not to allow the bleach mixture to leach into the pulp canal, especially if there is any doubt about the integrity of the pulpal seal.

176. What is the BriteSmile tooth-whitening system?

BriteSmile is a franchised whitening system that uses a proprietary 15% hydrogen peroxide gel in conjunction with a gas plasma light source to provide a one-hour in-office bleaching treatment. The unique marketing and distribution network has shown rapid growth and patient acceptance (www.britesmile.com).

At-Home Bleaching Products

COMPANY NAME	PRODUCT NAME	WHITENING COMPONENT	CONCEN-TRATION	MAXIMAL RECOM-MENDED WEAR TIME	NO. OF SESSIONS TO COMPLETE TREATMENT	SHELF LIFE
Den-Mat Corp	Rembrandt Xtra-Comfort	Carbamide peroxide	10%, 22%, 30%	Overnight if tolerated	Twice daily for 14 days	3 years
Dentsply Professional	Nupro Gold Whitening	Carbamide peroxide	10%, 15%	4–6 hours	7–14 days	1.5 years
Discus Dental	Day White 2Z	Hydrogen peroxide	7.5%, 9.5%	30 min twice/ day	7–10 days	3 years
Ivoclar Vivadent	Viva Style	Carbamide peroxide	10%, 16%	2 hours	10–12 treatments	2 years
Temrex Corp.	StarWhite	Carbamide peroxide	16%	1 hour	7–10 treatments	3 years
3M Espe	Zaris Tooth Whitening	Carbamide peroxide	10%, 16%	4 hours or overnight	Variable	2 years
Ultradent Products Inc.	Opalescence PF	Carbamide peroxide	10%, 15%, 20%	8–10 hours	5–7 overnight sessions	2 years refrigerated

In-Office Bleaching Products

COMPANY NAME	PRODUCT NAME	WHITENING COMPONENT	CONCEN-TRATION	HEAT OR LIGHT SOURCE	TREATMENT TIME	ISOLATION REQUIRED
Biolase Technology, Inc	LaserSmile	Proprietary	Proprietary	Laser	15–20 min.	Paint-on dam
BriteSmile, Inc.	BriteSmile	Hydrogen peroxide	15%	Gas plasma/ LED	3 treatments, 20 min. each	Paint-on gel
DenMat Corp.	One-Hour Smile	Hydrogen peroxide	35%	Xenon light	1–2 treatments, 45 min. each	Paint-on dam
Discus Dental	Zoom!	Hydrogen peroxide	25%	Metal halide light	3 treatments, 20 min. each	Paint-on dam
LumaLite, Inc.	LumaArch	Hydrogen peroxide	35%	Xenon-halogen light	Less than 1 hour	Paint-on dam
Ultradent Products	Xtra Boost	Hydrogen peroxide	38%	Neither	20–60 min.	Paint-on gel

DENTAL LASERS

177. List the categories of application of dental lasers.

Dental lasers are used primarily in four categories of application: soft tissue, hard tissue, curing, and caries detection.

178. What is the purpose of the lasing medium in dental lasers? Give examples.

The lasing medium is the material within the laser system that is electrically stimulated to produce energy. Lasing materials can be solid, liquid, or gas, and the laser is generally named after the medium. Examples include carbon dioxide, argon, ND:YAG, and erbium:YAG. The erbium:YAG lasers are currently those most often considered for hard tissue use.

179. What are the current uses and limitations of hard tissue lasers in restorative dentistry?

Currently, hard tissue lasers allow the trained practitioner to perform many aspects of restorative dentistry including class I–V cavity preparations and the removal of carious tooth structure, in many cases without the use of local anesthesia. However, more complex procedures requiring more refined tooth preparation, such as crown preparation, onlays, and veneers, still require the use of high-speed handpieces.

180. Describe the mechanism by which hard tissue lasers remove tooth structure and caries.

Highly energetic, short-pulsed laser light causes a rapid heating of dental tissue in a small area. An explosive shock wave is created when the energy causes a volumetric expansion of the water in the hard tissue. In other words, the water molecules in the tissue are superheated, explode, and, in turn, ablate tooth structure and caries. Additionally, the increased water content of caries allows the laser to interact preferentially with the carious tissue, helping to preserve sound tooth structure.

181. How does the laser preparation of enamel, dentin, and caries differ?

The laser parameters required for ablation of enamel, dentin, and caries differ because these structures have different water contents. Because erbium wavelength has an affinity for the water content of hard tissue, less laser energy is required to ablate caries than either enamel or dentin.

182. Should hard tissue lasers be used to remove amalgam fillings?

Laser ablation of dental amalgam is strictly contraindicated because of the potential release of mercury vapor. Lasers currently do not have FDA clearance for this procedure.

Hard Tissue Laser Manufacturers

COMPANY NAME	PRODUCT NAME	PROCEDURES PERFORMED	LASING MEDIUM	LIFETIME OF LASING MEDIUM
American Dental Technologies	PulseMaster 600 IQ	Hard and soft tissue procedures	Solid state Nd: YAG crystal	No limit
Biolase Technologies	Millennium II	Hard and soft Tissue procedures	Er, Cr:YSGG	Depends on usage
Continuum Biomedical	DELight Dental Laser System	Hard and soft Tissue procedures	Erbium:YAG	N/A—solid state

NA = not applicable.

AMALGAM

183. What is the difference between an alloy and an amalgam?

An **alloy** is a mixture of metals; an **amalgam** is an alloy containing mercury.

184. What is the composition of dental amalgam?

Dental amalgam is an alloy composed of silver, tin, copper, and mercury. The basic setting reaction involves the mixing of the alloy complex of silver (Ag) and tin (Sn) with mercury (Hg) to form the so-called gamma phase alloy (original silver/tin) surrounded by secondary phases called gamma-1 (silver/mercury) and gamma-2 (tin/mercury). The weakest component is the gamma-2 phase, which is less resistant to corrosion.

$$Ag_2Sn + Hg \rightarrow Ag_3Sn \quad + \quad Ag_2Hg_3 \quad + \quad Sn_3Hg$$
$$\text{Gamma} \qquad \text{Gamma-1} \qquad \text{Gamma-2}$$

Alloys are manufactured as either filings or spherical particles; dispersed alloys are mixtures of both. Smaller particle size results in higher strength, lower flow, and better carvability. Spherical, high amalgams high in copper usually have the best tensile and compressive characteristics.

185. What is the function of each component?

- Silver increases strength, hardness, and reactivity while decreasing creep.
- Tin increases reactivity and corrosion but decreases strength and hardness.
- Copper increases strength, expansion and hardness while decresing creep.
- Zinc increases plasticity, strength, and the Hg:alloy ratio; it also decreases creep and causes secondary expansion.
- Mercury wets alloy particles, but decreases strength in excessive amounts.

186. How can one tell when an amalgam is properly triturated?

A properly triturated amalgam mix appears smooth and homogeneous. No granular appearance or porosity should be evident. An overtriturated mix is preferable to an undermixed preparation.

187. What types of amalgam alloys are commonly used today?

Alloys are supplied in different particle shapes and sizes to influence the handling and setting properties. The blended alloy is a mixture of fine-cut and spherical particles, whereas all-spherical alloys are composed of spherical particles. Because spherical alloys are very fast setting, they are particularly suitable for core build-ups and impression taking in one visit.

Current Amalgam Products

SPHERICAL	SPHEROIDAL	ADMIXED
Tytin	Tytin FC	Contour
Valiant		Valiant PhD
Unison, Megalloy		Dispersalloy

188. What are the indications for the various amalgam product types?

- All class I preparations: spherical or spheroidal
- Class II preparations: admix or spheroidal
- Around pins and for internal retention: spherical

It is not advisable to combine spherical and admixed types.

189. List current principles for amalgam tooth preparations.

Basically a conservative preparation that salvages the maximal amount of tooth structure while removing carious material is advocated:

- Use of the 333 and 245 burs allows slot and tunnel preparations.
- Prepare rounded internal line angles, 90° cavosurface margins with removal of unsupported enamel during excavation of all caries past the DEJ.
- Use a caries detector solution when necessary.
- Create mechanical retention by undercuts, channels and grooves or bonding.
- Properly wedge, and create tight interproximal contacts.
- Seal dentine tubules with adhesive liners.
- Provide enough amalgam bulk for strength.

190. List six common causes of amalgam failure.

1. Inadequate retention.
2. Insufficient bulk for strength; amalgam should be in peripheral contact with tooth structure to avoid a "trampoline effect" of a stiff structure bouncing on a too flexible base.
3. Nonremoval of unsupported enamel.
4. Incomplete caries removal.
5. Inadequate condensation.
6. Recurrent caries due to microleakage.

191. Should all amalgams be bonded?

State-of-the-art practice says yes, however, this practice has not been confirmed over time. A better view is that amalgam bonding effectively seals dentin tubules, eliminating postoperative sensitivity with the added benefits of retention of the restorative and a stronger total cohesive mass to support all remaining cuspal segments of the tooth.

192. What is the mechanism of bonding amalgams?

The use of a self-curing resin liner (Amalgambond, Parkell, or All Bond 2, BISCO) provides a bond to tooth substrate and to amalgam. As the amalgam is condensed into the unpolymerized resin, a micromechanical bond is formed.

193. What is the purpose of finishing and polishing amalgam restorations?

Amalgram restorations should be finished and polished for three main reasons: (1) to reduce marginal discrepancies and to create a more hygienic restoration; (2) to reduce marginal breakdown and recurrent decay; and (3) to prevent tarnishing and increase the quality of appearance of the restoration. Polishing is often a neglected part of treatment, either for lack of opportunity for recall visits or from the feeling of not being compensatedfor the added service. However, polishing a restoration or two at each recall may allow this quality service to define state-of-the-art dental practice.

194. Describe the sequence for polishing amalgams.

Begin gross contouring with multifluted finishing burs usually at least 1 day after insertion. Burs come in a variety of round, pear, flame, and bullet-nosed shapes and allow anatomic contouring. Shofu-type brownie and greenie points can be used to create a high luster. Final pumicing with rubber cups can complete the finishing.

195. What additional means may be used to retain alloy restorations?

Optimal retention warrants the use of pins, grooves, channels, or holes placed in sound tooth areas. While bonding has replaced much of pin usage, it arguably still provides the best possible retention.

196. List guidelines for the use of pins to retain dental restorative material.

1. Pins should extend 2 mm into tooth structure and then backed off one-half turn to reduce stress.

2. Pins should be placed fully in dentin. If they are too close to the DEJ, the enamel may fracture from the tooth. In general, they should be placed at the line angles where the root mass is the greatest and at least 0.5 mm from the DEJ.

3. Pins should extend 2 mm into amalgam; further extension only weakens the tensile and shear strength of the amalgam.

4. Pins should be aligned parallel to the radicular emergence profile or parallel to the nearest external enamel wall. Additional angulations may be used when there is no danger of pulpal or periodontal ligament perforation.

5. If the tooth structure is flat, the use of small retentive channels cut into the tooth structure prevents potential torsional and lateral stress.

197. What are the major complications to the use of pins to retain restorations?

Pin placement can result in pulpal exposure, perforation through the periodontal ligament and fracture of a tooth. Additionally, pins may weaken an amalgam if they extend more than 2 mm into the mass. The use of a dentin-bonded resin liner can help to seal any potential fracture lines, but placement requires skill and expert technique

198. What should be done if accidental exposure of the pulp or perforation of the periodontal ligament occurs during pin placement?

If the pulp is exposed by the pinhole, allow the bleeding to stop, dry with a sterile paper point, and place calcium hydroxide in the hole. Bond over with an adhesive glass ionomers resin. Do not place a pin in the hole. Usually the pulp will heal. If a penetration of the gingival sulcus or periodontal ligament space occurs, clean , dry, and place the pin to the measured depth of the external tooth surface to seal the opening.

199. What alternatives to pins are available for increasing retention and resistance in large amalgam restorations?

Practitioners use bonding resin along with boxes, slots, grooves, dovetails, parallel walls, and divergent amalgapins to increase resistance and retention substantially without the inherent disadvantages of pins.The amalgapin concept uses 245 burs to create 2-mm points into dentin, which are the packed with amalgam. The resistance is comparable to pins, but the retention is less.

200. Discuss current concepts of pulpal protection.

Former concepts advocated a thermal liner or base under amalgam restorations. If 1–3 mm of dentin remains under the cavity preparation, sufficient thermal protection is present. Sealing dentin tubules is considered important to minimize postoperative pulpal sensitivity and prevent bacterial contamination by microleakage. It is known that microleakage can wash out such liners as calcium hydroxide. Sealing dentin tubules by bonding protects the pulp from postoperative sensitivity and offers long-term protection against bacterial contamination from microleakage.

201. Discuss the classic role of calcium hydroxide.

Calcium hydroxide compounds have a long tradition of providing pulpal protection as a "liner" under restorative materials. Calcium hydroxide is known to serve as an insulator, stimulator of repair dentin via bridge formation, and bactericidal agent due to its high pH. However, it does not bond to dentin, does not seal tubules, and is prone to wash out if microleakage occurs. If calcium hydroxide is used, it should be sealed by the use of some type of bonded resin system.

202. What compounds stimulate dentin bridging?
- Calcium hydroxide
- Zinc phosphate cements
- Resin composite systems

Eugenol and amalgam compounds do *not* show bridge formation

203. Summarize the recommended treatment for a direct vital pulp exposure.
1. Control hemorrhage using irrigation with saline or sodium hypochlorite.
2. Apply a calcium hydroxide capping agent (Dycal).
3. Cover with a layer of glass ionomer cement.
4. Etch, bond, and restore.
5. Alternatively some advocate direct etching, priming, and bonding after hemorrhage control as a direct cap procedure.

204. What is the purpose of a cavity varnish?

Classically, cavity varnishes, such as Copalite, were used to seal dentin tubules without adding bulk and to protect pulpal tissue from the phosphoric acid in zinc phosphate cements. Current dentin-bonding systems fulfill the concept of a cavity varnish more ideally, and the use of co-pal varnishes is probably obsolete.

205. What is a cavity liner? What are the indications for use?

A cavity liner is a relatively thin coating over exposed dentin. It may be self-hardening or light-cured, and it is usually nonirritating to pulpal tissues. The purpose is to create a barrier between dentin and pulpally irritating agents or to stimulate the formation of reparative, secondary dentin. Calcium hydroxide has traditionally been placed on dentin with a thickness of 0.5 mm as a pulpal protective agent. Contemporary practice uses newer dentin-bonding agents for liner materials. They not only provide a barrier to pulpally toxic agents but also seal the dentin tubules from bacterial microleakage and provide a bondable surface to increase the retention of the restoration. Glass ionomer cements and dentin-bonding systems have become the standard liner materials in restorative dentistry.

206. What is a base? What are the indications for use?

Generally, cements that are thicker than 2–4 mm are termed *bases* and as such function to replace lost dentin structure beneath restorations. A base may be used to provide thermal protection under metallic restorations, to increase the resistance to forces of condensation of amalgam, or to block out undercuts in taking impressions for cast restorations. A base should not be used unnecessarily. Pulpal thermal protection requires a thickness of at least 1 mm, but covering the entire dentin floor with a base is not thought to be necessary. Generally, the following guidelines may be used:
1. For deep caries with frank or near exposures or with < 0.5 mm of dentin, apply calcium hydroxide.
2. Under a metal restoration, a hard base may be applied (over the calcium hydroxide) up to 2.0 mm in thickness to increase resistance to forces of condensation.
3. If > 2 mm of dentin is present, usually no base is needed under amalgam; a liner may be used under the composite.
4. Use of a dentin-bonding agent that seals the dentin tubules and bonds to the restorative material is desirable.

POSTS AND CORES

207. What is the purpose of placing a post in an endodontically treated tooth?
Posts are needed only to retain coronal build-up when the remaining coronal tooth structure to support a build-up by itself. Although the cast post has been the standard for years, it is insufficient requires additional time and expense and is being replaced by alternatives. The use of titanium posts and metal-free fiber reinforced posts for better esthetics in anterior teeth has become a popular trend. Retention of posts is usually by micro (sand blasting) or macro (channel undercuts) mechanical methods. Furthermore, posts are now bonded into place either by self-cured or dual-cured resin cements.

208. Does a post strengthen endodontically treated teeth?
Contrary to former thought, posts do not reinforce teeth and may weaken some root structures. Widening a canal space for a larger post can weaken a root. Long posts are more retentive, but too much length may perforate a root or cause compromise in the apical seal. A good guide is to make the length about one-half of the bone supported root length, allow at least 1 mm of dentin lateral to the apical end of the post, and leave at least 3- 5 mm of apical gutta purcha filling.

209. Which canals are generally chosen for post space?
Generally the largest canal is chosen: in maxillary molars the palatal canal and in mandibular molars the distal canal. Two-rooted bicuspids with minimal tooth structure may require one post in each canal.

210. How may vertical fractures develop in roots?
- Wedged or tight fitting posts may cause fractures.
- Overpreparation of the internal canal space may weaken a root and cause fractures.

211. When are posts indicated? When are they not needed?
Indicated
- If more than one-half of the coronal tooth structure is missing, place a post to attach the core material to the root structure.
- If all of the coronal tooth structure is missing, place a post to attach the core material to the root structure.

Not needed
- If minimal coronal tooth structure is missing, as when an access cavity is made centrally with no caries on proximal walls, no post is required. Placement of a bonded filling material to the level of pulpal floor adequately restores the endodontic access preparation.
- If up to one-half of coronal tooth structure is missing, a post may not be needed except for teeth with high lateral stresses, such as cuspids with cuspid rise occlusion. Place a bonded crown build-up.

212. How are antirotational features created?
1. Cast cores can be placed in anterior teeth with recessed boxes to limit rotation.
2. Small cut boxes or channels 1–1.5 mm deep and about the width of a 330 bur may be placed into remaining tooth structure.
3. Accessory pin (Minim or Minikin) may be placed nonparallel to the posts.

213. When a crown preparation is made, where should the finish line be placed?
The gingival margin should be 1–1.5 mm *apical* to the core build-up material and on the root surface for optimal retention and antirotational resistance. If there is a ferrule post and core, the crown margin may be placed on the core material.

214. List the characteristics of ideal posts.
- The post space must provide adequate retention and support for the core, and the core must provide adequate support for the fixed restoration.
- Passive fitting posts are best.
- Resin-bonded posts transmit less force to the root and increase the structural integrity by bonding the post to the root.

215. What are the indications for a cast post?
For build-up of single rooted teeth with little supragingival structure or thin-walled roots, a cast post/core with an inset lock preparation and ferrule design may strengthen the root and prevent rotation. The casting is air-abraded or microetched and bonded into the root.

216. Of what materials are prefabricated posts constructed?
The most common types are made of stainless steel and titanium alloys. Carbon fiber posts are gaining popularity for anterior esthetic preparations.

217. Outline the clinical steps in resin-bonding cast or prefabricated posts.
1. Prepare the canal space with a hot instrument to remove gutta percha to a depth of one-half of bone-supported root length, or as governed buy root shape.
2. Refine the canal preparation with Parapost drills or diamonds.
3. Cleanse the canal of debris with hydrogen peroxide with a syringe.
4. Treat with etchant 37% for 15 seconds or with 17% EDTA for 1 minute to remove the smear layer.
5. Rinse well with water and lightly dry.
6. Microetch the post with air abrasion.
7. Apply resin cement primers and resins to the post and the canal according to product directions
8. Mix the resin cement and inject into the canal quickly, seating the post.
9. Wipe the excessive cement with a brush dipped in resin while holding the post until cement has set.

218. Summarize the guidelines for fillers, build-ups, and post and cores.
For full-crown preparations, all old restorative material should be removed after preliminary tooth preparation. Small areas or missing tooth can be replaced with a bonded filler (compomer, reinforced glass ionomers, flowable composite); larger sections of missing tooth should be replaced with a build-up (bonded composite); and an endodontically treated tooth with more than one-half of its coronal structure missing should have a titanium alloy post and core with a composite build-up.

219. What materials are used to rebuild tooth core structure?
Gold, amalgam, composites, and resin ionomers.

220. List advantages of using composite materials for core build-ups.
- Composite materials can bond to tooth structure.
- Usually they achieve adequate strength in 5–10 minutes so that preparation of core may be done at the same appointment as placement
- They may be tooth-colored to avoid shade-matching problems with final restoration.
- They may also be shaded to differentiate core structure from tooth when placing finish lines.
- They can be prepared easily and placed in a matrix, core form, or freehand.

221. What current types of core composite materials are available?
Light cure. Traditional large-particle materials that are made to cure deeply. Any hybrid composite also may be used.

Dual cure. These materials have the advantage that the surface may be light-cured immediately, whereas deeper layers can chemically cure, allowing preparation to take place soon after placement.

Self-cure. In areas where light penetration cannot be achieved, such as around posts and in deep recesses, these materials may be the best choice.

Note: Some self-cure or dual-cure materials will not bond to light-cured adhesives. It is important to use a self-cure adhesive system and to read the manufacturer's instructions carefully.

AMALGAM, MERCURY, AND HEALTH ISSUES

222. Summarize the current status of the use of amalgam.

Dental amalgam continues to be the most common material for the restoration of carious teeth worldwide. In the United states 100 million people have amalgam fillings, and 100 million amalgams are placed each year. To date there are no epidemiologic links between its use and ill health. The National Institutes of Health reports that only 50 documented cases of allergy to mercury have been reported since 1906. As newer materials evolve, which are as durable and cost-effective, it is likely that mercury-containing restorations will be phased out. Until that time, it is the opinion of world health agencies, medical and dental societies, and the scientific community at large that amalgam is a safe, durable, and cost-effective restorative material. The choice of using a particular material should be left to an informed patient, with adequate scientific information supplied by a knowledgeable professional. The goal is to separate emotion from science in making decisions.

223. What three forms of mercury are found in the environment and may result in human exposure?

Elemental mercury is a small contributor to the total human body burden. It is very short-lived because of rapid oxidation. It is the common form found in dentistry; it is is lipid-soluble and adsorbed in the lungs. Elemental mercury is the least toxic form.

Inorganic mercury is formed by the oxidation of elemental mercury and has limited solubility. It is sequestered in the kidney and excreted slowly in urine with a half life of about 60 days. It is of moderate toxicity.

Organic mercury is most commonly methyl mercury. It is only found in nondental sources. Organic mercury forms in the gut of fish from the bacterial action on mercury and accumulates in red blood cells; it is sequestered in the central nervous system and liver and has high lipid solubility. It is not found in urine but is secreted in feces. Ninety percent is absorbed in the gut. Organic mercury is the most toxic form.

224. What should a dentist know to be prepared to respond to a patient's inquiry about amalgam restorations and safety?

The clinician must know all of the facts about amalgam, health-related sensitivities, ethics of replacements, and alternative restorative choices.

225. What consideration should be given to a patient's concern about sensitivity to dental alloys?

It is important to differentiate the type of inquiry:

1. A real allergy or hypersensitivity (as differentiated from toxicity or poisoning) to dental alloys and metals is not uncommon. Approximately 3% of the population has some type of metal sensitivity. Health questionnaires should ask questions about skin reactions to jewelry and/or known metal sensitivities. Allergy testing can confirm these sensitivities.

2. Patients who have esthetic concerns and do not wish to have non–tooth-colored restorations.

3. Patients who have phobias about alleged toxicity of various dental materials.

4. Patients who have chronic diseases, such as multiple sclerosis, and are looking for some causative agent and a miracle cure.

Each group of patients requires appropriate information from dental and medical sources to help them make informative choices about dental health.

226. What dental materials are reported the most allergenic? What are the manifestations of these exposures?

Allergic reactions have been reported to chromium, cobalt, copper, nickel (the most common), palladium, tin, zinc, silver, and gold/platinum (least allergenic). The symptoms may range from localized chronic inflammation around restorations and crowns to more generalized oral lichen planus, geographic glossitis, angular chelitis, and plicated tongue.

227. Are certain people hypersensitive to mercury?

Yes. But according to the North American Contact Dermatitis Group, true sensitivity to mercury in subtoxic doses is rare. Studies show that 3% of people respond to a 1% mercury patch test. Of these, $< 0.6\%$ have any clinical manifestations of mercury sensitivity allergy. It is important to note that these testing levels are extreme in relation to the exposure possible from dental amalgam restorations.

228. Are there any known harmful effects from the mercury content of dental amalgam?

As a restorative material, silver amalgam has been used in dentistry for over 150 years. Its safety has been studied through this incredibly long period, and no epidemiologic evidence associates general health problems with this amalgram. Many health groups around the world have reviewed and contributed to this conclusion. The World Health Organization, the Swedish Medical Research Council and the Swedish National Board of Health and Welfare (1994), the British Dental Association (1995), the U.S. Public Health Service (1993), the National Institutes of Health and the Institutes of Dental Research, the Food and Drug Administration (1991), and even Consumer Reports (1991) attest that dental amalgam fillings are safe to use and that no beneficial health benefits will result from the removal of existing restorations. Organizations such as the National Multiple Sclerosis Society characterize claims of recovery after removal of dental amalgams as unsubstantiated, unscientific, and a "cruel hoax." A recent study of aging and Alzheimer's disease found no evidence that amalgams reduced cognitive functions in a group of 129 Roman Catholic nuns between the ages of 75 and 102 years. In conclusion, in nonallergic patients, no scientific evidence implicates dental amalgam as a harm to general health.

In conclusion, repeated studies on humans with and without amalgam restorations show no significant difference in any organ system. Comparisons of immune cells show no difference in function. Furthermore, no recoveries or remissions from any chronic diseases after removal of amalgams has been scientifically demonstrated.

229. Discuss the relative safety of composite resins as restorative materials.

Although they appear safe, health concerns have been raised about the use of composite resins. Composite materials contain many components that are potentially hazardous and possibly carcinogenic. To consider these materials a "nontoxic" alternative to dental amalgam is premature and surely warrants further study.

230. By what physical pathways can mercury enter the body?

Elemental mercury is abundant in the earth's environment. It exists in the soil, the oceans, and the air. The burning of fossil fuels and even volcanic eruptions have contributed to the widespread decimation of this element. The use of mercury in manufacturing through the centuries has led to much of the environmental contamination. Furthermore, in high enough doses, mercury is neurotoxic. The questions of exposure to mercury from dental amalgams require some clinical elucidation.

Dental amalgam fillings contain up to 50% mercury and elements of silver, tin, and copper, bound into a metallic complex from which the mercury is not free. Small amounts of mercury vaporize from the surface with function, pass into the air, and are exhaled. This amount, which is absorbed into the body as a function of the number of surface of amalgam, is largely excreted by the kidneys into the urine. The smaller amount that may accumulate in other organs has raised concern. Mercury accumulates in such organs as the brain, lungs, liver, and GI tract, but this accumulation represents exposures from all environmental sources. The ultimate question is the percentage of the dental amalgam component to *total* mercury exposure from all sources.

The daily intake of mercury attributable to dental amalgams, as measured by urine levels of mercury, is reported to be only one-seventh (14%) of that measured from eating one seafood meal per week. The total daily intake from 8–12 amalgam surfaces is about 1–3 μg. This is again seven times lower than the intake from one seafood meal per weak and only about 10–20% of the average total exposure (9 μg/day) from all environmental sources. Clearly the general environmental exposure is much more of a concern.

By comparison the maximal limit of elemental mercury inhalation exposure for industrial workers yields urine levels of 82 μg/L. People *without* amalgam fillings have urine levels of 5–10 μg/L, and dentists have urine levels of < 10 μg/L. It may be easily seen that the ambient environmental exposure to mercury is the significant exposure.

There should there be an overall effort to lower environmental mercury, and there appears to be no dispute on this issue. It is therefore predicted that as newer substitutes for silver amalgam are developed that prove to be as durable, simple to use, and cost-effective, we may see the gradual phasing out of its use.

231. What has contributed to the "amalgam phobia"?

Because it is well known that elemental mercury is an environmentally toxic waste and because hundreds of millions of people have dental amalgams containing mercury, it is only natural for people to question the safety to human health. In what has become a disservice to many, the media have used sensationalism in reporting stories related to health and dental amalgam in much the same distorted way that fluoride has been reported by some media as as a harmful water additive for caries prevention. Furthermore, as scientific efforts continue to describe the biocompatibility of mercury, various animal models have been extrapolated to humans without scientific validity (e.g., sheep absorb 18–25 times more mercury than humans). Even the dental profession was implicated when analytical mercury vapor detectors were sold to dentists, who then found distortedly high levels of mercury vapor over amalgam restorations because their calibrations were inaccurate. The sampling rate of the intake manifolds of the vapor analyzers was much greater than the rates of human inspiration, and the air intake calculated for humans was in error by as much as 16 times. The use of these detectors left many responsible dental clinicians with erroneous conclusions.

Finally, the reports of many people who experienced a health improvement when their amalgams are replaced or removed must be viewed carefully before coming to any causality links. A few weeks of monitoring the newsgroup AMALGAM@Listserv.gme.de will show hundreds of "cases" of people who *experience* better health after amalgam removal. Many psychodynamic issues can be observed in people who report such changes, and direct links to the amalgam contribution needs scientific scrutiny. After all, some people have genuine allergies to some materials, and it is from the observation of human experience that we as a profession learn to ask the questions that lead to productive clinical research.

232. What are the ethical issues related to removing a patient's amalgams?

According to the ADA's Council on Ethics, Bylaws and Judicial Affairs:

Based on available scientific, the ADA has determined . . . that removal of amalgam restorations from the non-allergic patient for the alleged purpose of removing toxic substances from the body, when such treatment is performed solely at the recommendation or suggestion of the dentist, is improper and unethical."

If a dentist represents that such dental treatment has the capacity to cure or alleviate systemic disease, when there is no scientific evidence or knowledge of such, this action is considered unethical. However, a dentist may remove amalgams at a patient's request, as long as no inference is made to improving the patient's health and the risk/benefits are discussed. A dentist may also ethically decline to remove the amalgam if there is no sound medical reason.

233. How can one maintain mercury hygiene in the dental office?
- Use capsulated amalgam.
- Calibrate amalgam triturators.
- Use rubber dam, high-volume suction, and amalgam traps in office procedures.
- Dispose of amalgam waste by certified collectors.

234. What health groups agree on amalgam safety?
ADA News, July 2001
Food and Drug Administration
National Institute of Dental and Craniofacial Research
Public Health Service
Centers for Disease control
World Health Organization
American Association for Dental Research
Consumers Union (Consumer Reports Magazine)

Other comments

Mackert R: *ADA News,* July 2001: "Unlike organic forms of mercury found in seafood, or free volatile elemental mercury in home thermometers, the mercury in dental amalgam exists as intermetallic compounds and is not 'bioavailable' to cause adverse effects. For that reason, to regard amalgam as half mercury and therefore dangerous is not appropriate".

Dental Board of California, Dental Materials Fact Sheet, October 2001: "There is no research evidence that suggests pregnant women, diabetics and children are at increased health risk from dental amalgam fillings in their mouths."

BIBLIOGRAPHY

Miller MB (ed): Reality 2002, vol.16. Houston, Reality Publishing, 2002 Available at <www.realityesthetics. com>.
Clinical Research Associates News Letter. Provo, Utah, 2002. Available at <www.cranews.com>.
Quintessence International, Quintessence Publishing, Chicago. Available at <www.quintpub.com>.

GENERAL REFERENCES

1. Freedman G, Goldstep F, Seif T: Ultraconservative resin restorations. Dentistry Today 19:66–73, 2000.
2. Garcia-Godoy F (ed): Restorative dentistry. Dent Clin North Am 46(2), 2002.
3. Hedge T, Mason E, Hale T: Selecting the most appropriate milling block for use with the Cerec system. Contemp Esthet Restor Pract 6(3): 24–34, 2002.
4. Huckabee T: Combining microabrasion with tooth whitening to treat enamel defects. Dentistry Today 20(5):98–101, 2001.
5. Kidd EAM, Joyston-Bechal S: Essentials of Dental Caries. London, Oxford Medical Publications, 1998.
6. Kugel G, Garcia-Godoy F. Direct esthetic adhesive restorative materials: A review." Contemp Esthet Restor Pract 4(9):6–10, 2000.
7. Leinfelder K, Kurdziolek S: Indirect resin restorative systems. Contemp Esthet and Restor Pract, 4(9): 14–18, 2000.
8. Lussi A, Imwinkerleid S, Pitts N, et al: Performance and reproducibility of a laser fluorescence system for detection of occlusal caries in vitro. Caries Res 33(4):261–266, 1999.
9. Milicich G. The use of air abrasion and glass ionomer cements in microdentistry. Compend Contin Educ Dentistry 22(11A):1026–1039, 2001.
10. Rainey JT: Understanding the applications of microdentistry. Compend Contin Educ Dentistry 22(11A): 1018–1025, 2001.

11. Ross S: One visit makeovers. Contemp Esthet Restor Pract 5(9):42–53, 2001.
12. Small BW: Direct resin composites for 2002 and beyond. Gen Dentistry 50:30–33, 2002.
13. Small BW: The esthetic use of cast and direct gold in 2001. Contemp Esthet Restor Pract, 5(7):16–24, 2001.
14. Wahl, MJ: Amalgam resurrection and redemption. Part 1: The clinical and legal mythology of anti-amalgam. Quint Int: 32:525–535, 2001.
15. Wahl MJ: Amalgam resurrection and redemption. Part 2: The medical mythology of anti-amalgam. Quint Int 32;696–710, 2001.
16. Wefel JS, Donly KJ (eds): Cariology. Dent Clin of North Am 43(4), 1999.

Amalgam safety issues web Resources
www.quackwatch.com/01quackeryRelatedTopics/mercury.html
www.quackwatch.com/01quackeryRelatedTopics/mercurytests.html
www.cda.org/public/factsheet_amalgam.htm

9. PROSTHODONTICS

Ralph B. Sozio, D.M.D.

FIXED PROSTHODONTICS

1. What is the definition of "fit" for a full-crown restoration? What is the clinical acceptance of the fit of a full-crown restoration?

The fit of a full-crown restoration is normally measured in relationship to two reference areas: (1) the occlusal seat and (2) the marginal seal. The two areas are interrelated and affect each other. The ideal fit of a full crown (marginal discrepancy) is related to the film thickness of the cementing medium (normally 10–30 μ). The clinical acceptance of marginal discrepancy is approximately 80 μ.

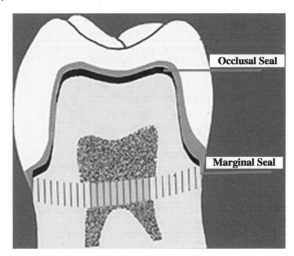

Fit is a relationship between occlusal seal and marginal seal.

2. What is the best marginal tooth preparation?

There is no ideal marginal tooth preparation. The selection of the marginal design depends on many factors, including:

1. The material used in construction of the full crown:
   - All-ceramic restoration — shoulder or deep chamfer
   - Metal-ceramic with porcelain extended to marginal edge — shoulder or deep chamfer
   - Metal-ceramic with metal collars — shoulder with bevel or chamfer
   - Full gold crown — feathered edge, bevel, or chamfer
2. The amount of retention needed: beveled or feathered edge affords the most retention.
3. Seating resistance: shoulder preparation affords the least resistance.
4. Sealing capability: beveled or feathered edge affords the best seal.
5. Pulpal consideration: more tooth reduction is necessary with a shoulder preparation than with a chamfer; the feathered edge requires the least reduction.

3. How does one determine the number of abutments to be used?

There is no rigid rule. Determining factors include:

1. The greater the number of pontics, the greater the increase in loading forces on the abutments.

2. The position of the pontics affects the loading forces of the abutments: the more posterior the pontics, the greater the loading forces on the abutments.

3. The crown-to-root ratio of the abutments (bone support): a periodontally compromised mouth increases the abutment-to-pontic ratio.

4. Roots of the abutments that are parallel to each other distribute the loading forces down the long axis of the teeth. When the loading forces do not fall within the long axis of the tooth, the lateral forces on the abutments are increased. This situation necessitates the use of additional abutments.

4. In periodontally compromised patients, is splinting the entire dental arch with a one-piece, "round-house" fixed bridge the treatment of choice?

Splinting an entire dental arch with a round-house fixed bridge is far from the treatment of choice because it is fraught with potential problems:

1. All tooth preparations must be parallel to each other.

2. Impression taking and die construction are extremely difficult.

3. Accuracy of fit for the one-piece unit is extremely difficult.

4. Premature setting of the cement is a major risk, because total seating of the fixed bridge onto the abutments is made extremely difficult by the mobility of the existing teeth.

5. If one of the abutments fails, it may be necessary to replace the entire prosthesis.

It is better to split up the prosthesis in some fashion than to construct a one-piece unit.

5. Is the cantilever fixed bridge a sound treatment?

A cantilever fixed bridge places more torquing forces on terminal abutments than desirable. Certain guidelines should be followed if a cantilever is used:

1. Cantilever pontics are limited to one per fixed bridge.

2. If the cantilever is replacing a molar, the size of the pontic should be the same as for a bicuspid, and at least one more abutment unit should be incorporated than in a conventional bridge. In addition, there should be no lateral occlusal contact on the pontic, and the bridge should be cemented with a rigid medium.

3. If the cantilever pontic is anterior to the abutments, the mesial aspect of the pontic should be designed to allow some interlocking effect.

6. Can a three-quarter crown be used as an abutment for a fixed bridge?

A three-quarter crown can be used successfully as an abutment for a fixed bridge if certain guidelines are followed:

1. Because there is less tooth reduction than with a full crown, retention may be compromised. Internal modifications, such as grooves or pins, must be used to compensate for potential loss of retention.

2. Proper tooth coverage is necessary for a three-quarter crown abutment:
   • Anterior: linguoincisal
   • Posterior/upper: linguoocclusal
   • Posterior/lower: linguoocclusal plus coverage over the buccal cusp tips

3. A three-quarter crown should be made only of metal; therefore, esthetics may be compromised.

7. Must a post and core be constructed for an endodontically treated tooth that is to be used in a fixed bridge?

An endodontically treated tooth is generally more brittle than a vital tooth. Because of the tooth reduction for the full-crown restoration and preparation of the access cavity for the endodontic procedure, the remaining coronal tooth structure is likely to be small. Therefore, a post and core is more likely to be necessary in the anterior and bicuspid region. If the access cavity is small and sufficient tooth structure remains after tooth preparation in the molar region, a post and core may not be necessary. In this instance, the coronal chamber should be filled, preferably with a bonded material.

8. What is the proper length for the post? Should a post be made for each canal in a multi-rooted tooth?

In general, the length of a post should be such that the fulcrum point, determined from measuring the height of the core to the apex of the tooth, is in bone. This guideline normally places the post approximately two-thirds into the root length. Improper length allows a potential for root fracture. It is not necessary to construct a post for each canal in a multirooted tooth, provided that the dominant root (i.e., palatal root of maxillary molar) is used and proper length has been established. If proper length cannot be obtained, it is necessary to place posts in at least one of the other remaining roots.

9. Can one use the preformed, single-step post and core in place of the two-step cast post and core?

A preformed, single-step post and core can be used in fixed prosthodontics, but the potential for failure is greater with many of the single-step systems than with a cast-gold post and core for the following reasons:

1. The canal preparation must be shaped to the configuration of the preformed post. This requirement may lead to overpreparation of the canal and potential root perforation. In contrast, a cast post is made to fit the existing configuration of the canal.

2. A screw-type post has the greatest retentive value, but it also has the greatest stress forces during insertion.

3. The core build-up of the single-step post and core may not be as stable as a cast-gold core.

4. If the single-step post is metal, the modulus of elasticity is normally much higher than that of the root. This may lead to root fracture during loading. In contrast, a type-three cast-gold post has a modulus of elasticity similar to that of the root.

10. Where should a crown margin be placed in relationship to the gingiva: supragingivally, equigingivally, or subgingivally?

It is better for gingival health to place a crown margin supragingivally, 1–2 mm above the gingival crest, or equigingivally at the gingival crest. Such positioning is quite often not possible because of esthetic or caries considerations. Subsequently, the margin must be placed subgingivally. The question then becomes whether the subgingival margin ends slightly below the gingival crest, in the middle of the sulcular depth, or at the base of the sulcus. In preparing a subgingival margin, the major concern is not to extend the preparation into the attachment apparatus. If the margin of the subsequent crown is extended into the attachment apparatus, a constant gingival irritant has been constructed. Therefore, for clinical simplicity, when a margin is to be placed subgingivally, it is desirable to end the tooth preparation slightly below the gingival crest.

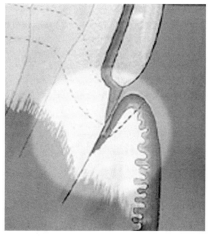

The subgingival margin should not impinge into the attachment apparatus.

MATERIALS

11. What materials are employed in the construction of a full crown?

Gold alloy	Composite resin
Nongold alloy	Composite resin with a metal alloy
Acrylic resin	Ceramic with a metal alloy
Acrylic resin with a metal alloy	All ceramic

12. Are the same materials used in the construction of a fixed bridge?

In general, a fixed bridge needs a metal support for strength. The veneer coating may be acrylic, composite, or ceramic. Newer ceramic materials, including alumina and zirconium, have increased strength that in some cases may eliminate the metal substructure.

13. What are the major advantages and disadvantages of the metal-ceramic crown?

In general, the metal-ceramic crown combines certain favorable properties of metal in its substructure and of ceramic in its veneer coating.

Advantages

1. The metal substructure gives high strength that allows the materials to be used in fixed bridgework and for splinting teeth.

2. The fit of a metal casting can also be achieved with the metal-ceramic crown.

3. Esthetics can be achieved by the proper application of the ceramic veneer.

Disadvantages

1. To allow enough space for the metal-ceramic materials, adequate tooth reduction is necessary (1.5 mm or more). The marginal tooth preparation is critical in relation to the design of the metal with the ceramic.

2. The fabrication technique is complex. The longer the span of bridgework, the greater the potential for metal distortion and/or porcelain problems.

14. What tooth preparation is necessary for the metal-ceramic crown?

The amount of tooth reduction necessary for the metal-ceramic crown depends on the metal and ceramic thickness. The necessary thickness of the metal is 0.5 mm, whereas the minimal ceramic thickness is 1.0–1.5 mm. Therefore, the tooth reduction is approximately 1.5–2.0 mm. With this porcelain-metal sandwich, a shoulder preparation is generally necessary for adequate tooth reduction.

15. What happens if tooth preparation or reduction is inadequate in the marginal area?

If the tooth reduction is < 1.5 mm at the marginal area, only metal can be present in that area. If porcelain is applied on metal that has been reduced in thickness because of lack of space, marginal metal distortion is likely during the firing cycle. If the porcelain thickness is reduced to compensate for the reduced space, the opaque porcelain layer is likely to be exposed or to dominate, leading to an unesthetic result. If both the porcelain and metal have adequate thickness, then the crown is overcontoured.

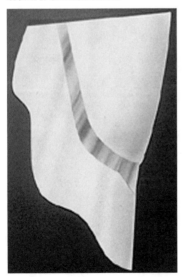

Margin tooth reduction (1.0–1.5 mm) is necessary for acceptance of porcelain to cover metal.

16. Can the marginal area of a metal-ceramic crown be constructed in porcelain without metal?

There are many techniques with which to construct a porcelain margin with optimal esthetics, proper fit, and correct contour (emergence profile).

17. If the tooth preparation is sufficient to accept the porcelain edge of the metal without distortion, why is it necessary to construct a margin in porcelain solely for esthetic reasons?

It is possible to cover the metal correctly with porcelain in the marginal area, but most often the esthetic results fall short of expectation in the most critical area. Incident light that transmits through the porcelain and reflects from the metal often creates a shadowing effect. If porcelain is present only at this marginal area, light transmission and reflection through the porcelain and the tooth create the proper blend between the marginal aspect of the crown and the tooth.

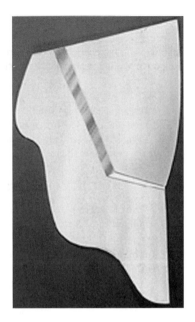

Diagram of porcelain margin.

18. For a successful porcelain marginal construction, how far should the metal extend in relation to the shoulder?

Originally the metal was finished slightly shy of the edge of the shoulder, with porcelain extending to the edge. Another technique finished the metal at the axiocaval line angle of the preparation, creating a porcelain margin that totally covers the horizontal shoulder. With both techniques, however, shadowing was still present. To create proper light transmission and reflection of the porcelain/tooth interface, the metal should be finished to about 1–2 mm above the axiocaval line angle of the shoulder.

19. What are noble alloys?

Noble alloys in general do not oxidize on casting. This feature is important in a metal substrate so that oxidation at the metal-porcelain interface can be controlled by the addition of trace oxidizing elements. If oxidation cannot be controlled on repeated firings, porcelain color may be contaminated and the bond strength may be weakened. Noble alloys are gold, platinum, and palladium. A silver alloy that oxidizes is considered semiprecious.

20. What is a base metal alloy? Can it be used in the construction of a metal-ceramic crown?

The base metal or nonprecious alloys most often used in the construction of a metal-ceramic crown are nickel and chromium. Because such alloys readily oxidize at elevated temperatures, they create porcelain-to-metal interface problems. The oxidation must be controlled by a metal-coating treatment, which is somewhat unpredictable. Casting and fitting are also difficult. Authorities agree that a noble alloy is preferable.

21. What are the criteria for selecting a specific alloy?

1. Compatibility of the coefficient of thermal expansion with the selected porcelains
2. Controllability of oxidation at interface
3. Ease in casting and fabrication
4. Fit potential
5. High yield of strength
6. High modulus of elasticity (stiffness) to avoid stress in the porcelain

22. How does porcelain bond to the alloy?

Ceramic adheres to metal primarily by chemical bond. A covalent bond is established by sharing O_2 in the elements in the porcelain and the metal alloy. These elements include silicon dioxide (SiO_2) in the porcelain and oxidizing elements such as silicon, indium, and iridium in the metal alloy.

23. How is a porcelain selected?

The criteria for selecting a specific porcelain include:

1. Compatibility with the metal used in regard to their respective coefficients of thermal expansion (of prime importance)
2. Stability of controlled shrinkage with multiple firings
3. Color stability with multiple firings
4. Capability of matching shade selection with various thicknesses of porcelain
5. Ease of handling (technique-sensitive)
6. Full range of shades and modifiers

24. How many layers or different porcelains can be applied in the buildup of a metal-ceramic crown?

1. Shoulder
2. Opaque
3. Opacious dentin
4. Body
5. Incisal
6. Translucent
7. Modifiers in every layer
8. External colorants

25. What is the function of the opaque layer?

The elements in the opaque layer create the chemical bond of the porcelain to the metal substrate. The opaque layer masks the color of the metal and is the core color in determining the final shade of the crown.

26. What is opacious dentin?

Opacious dentin is an intermediary modifying porcelain that affords better light transmission than the opaque layer, in part because of its optical properties. Opacious dentin is less opaque than the opaque layer but less translucent than the body (dentin) porcelain. It is also used for color shifts or effect properties.

27. What differentiates shoulder porcelain from dentin (body) porcelain?

The principal difference between shoulder and body porcelain is the firing temperature. Because the shoulder porcelain is established before the general build-up, its color and dimension must remain stable during subsequent firings. Therefore, the shoulder porcelain matures at a higher temperature than the subsequent body porcelain firings.

28. What is segmental build-up in the construction of the metal-ceramic crown?

Segmental build-up refers to the method of applying the porcelain powders in incremental portions horizontally. Each increment differs from the others in either opacity and translucency or hue, value, or chrome. This technique is used to construct a crown that attempts to mimic the optical properties of a natural tooth. (See figure, top of next page.)

29. What is the coefficient of thermal expansion? What is its importance in prosthodontics?

The coefficient of thermal expansion is the exponential expansion of a material as it is subjected to heat. The coefficient is extremely important during joint firing of two dissimilar materials. For example, the coefficient of thermal expansion should be slightly higher (rather than the same) for the metal substrate than for the porcelain coating. This slight difference results in compression of the fired porcelain coating, which gives it greater strength.

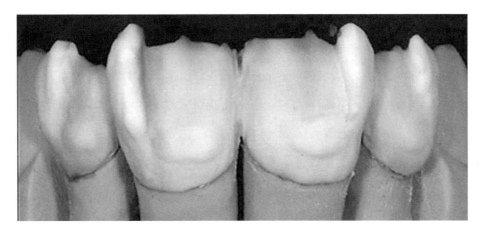

Segmental build-up to construct a porcelain crown.

30. What is the proper coping design for the metal-ceramic restoration?

The purpose of the metal coping is to ensure the fit of the crown and to maximize the strength of the porcelain veneer. The metal must have the proper thickness so as not to distort during the firing. The coping should be reinforced in load-bearing areas, such as the interproximal space, and can be strengthened in areas where metal exists alone, such as the lingual collar. To maximize the strength potential of the porcelain, uniform thickness should be attempted in the final restoration. This thickness can be obtained by designing the wax-up of the framework to accommodate the porcelain layer.

31. How does the marginal tooth preparation affect the design of the metal-ceramic crown?

The marginal tooth preparation determines the marginal configuration of the metal-ceramic crown. The three options are:

1. Beveled or feathered edge: the preparation is covered only in metal.
2. Chamfer: if the depth of the chamfer is at least 1 mm, the porcelain can extend over the metal and a supported porcelain margin can be constructed.
3. Shoulder: the preparation must be 1 mm for the porcelain to cover the metal.

32. Is the design of the metal framework of a fixed bridge different from the design of a single unit?

The design of the metal framework must incorporate four basic interrelationships: strength, esthetics, contour, and occlusion. In fixed bridgework, however, strength of the substrate plays the dominant role. Therefore, greater attention must be paid to reinforcement of the framework than of a single unit.

33. How do design problems of the metal framework influence the function of the metal-ceramic restorations?

1. The color of the porcelain is compromised between abutments and pontics if the thickness of the porcelain varies.
2. If the porcelain veneer is too thick (> 2 mm) because of improper framework design, much of the strength of the interface bond is lost.
3. If the porcelain veneer is too thin (≤ 0.75 mm), the esthetic effect is compromised.
4. The metal framework is designed to resist deformation. If strut-type connector design is not used in the fixed bridgework, the bridge may flex and result in porcelain fracture.

34. What is metamerism? How does it affect the metal-ceramic restoration?

Metamerism is the optical property by which two objects with the same color but different spectral reflectance curves do not match. This property is important in matching the shade of the metal-ceramic restoration to the natural tooth. Even if the colors are the same, different reflectance curves create the "just noticeable" difference.

35. What is the importance of fluorescence in porcelain?

Fluorescence is the optical property by which a material reflects ultraviolet radiation. Fluorescence reflects different hues. Natural teeth can fluoresce yellow-white to blue-white hues. Fluorescence in porcelain is important to minimize metamerism of porcelain to natural teeth in varying light conditions.

36. What are hue, value, and chroma? What is their importance in dentistry?

Color consists of three properties:
1. Hue refers to color families (e.g., red, green).
2. Value refers to lightness or darkness as related to a scale from black to white.
3. Chroma refers to the saturation of a color at any given value level.

The properties have a practical use in ordering color.

37. What is opalescence?

Opalescence is the optical property seen in an opal during light transmission and light reflection. During transmission, the opal takes on an orange-white hue, whereas during reflection it takes on a bluish-white hue. This phenomenon also occurs in the natural tooth as a result of light scattering through the crystalline structure of the opal. The structure size is in the submicron range (0.2–0.5 μ). A porcelain restoration can demonstrate the opal effect by incorporating submicron particles of porcelain into the enamel (incisal) layer.

38. How do you select a shade to match the natural teeth?

There is no truly scientific method to analyze the shade of a natural tooth and to apply this information to the selection of porcelain and fabrication of the crown. Attempts to establish such a technique have met with limited success. At present, shade determination is designed to match natural teeth with a man-made replication (shade guide) that results in a range of acceptability rather than an absolute match.

39. Can you change a shade with external stains?

External stains or colorants are frequently used to minimize the differences between natural and ceramic teeth. They should be used rationally rather than empirically. An understanding of the color phenomenon is necessary in all aspects of shade control and is essential if extrinsic colorants are to be used correctly. Extrinsic colorants follow the physical laws of substractive color.

40. What guidelines derived from the color phenomenon apply to the use of external colorants?

The understanding of hue, value, and chroma and their effect on external staining of a crown are essential. The major guidelines are as follow:

Hue: drastic change of the shade of the ceramic restoration by use of external colorants is quite often impossible. Slight changes in shade may be accomplished (e.g., orange to orange-brown).

Value: external colorants can be used to lower the value of the ceramic. The complementary color of the shade to be altered may have a darkening effect. It is almost impossible to increase the value or shade of the ceramic.

Chroma: chroma can be successfully increased by external colorants, most frequently in the gingival or interproximal areas.

41. What effects can be created with surface stains?
1. Separation and individualization with interproximal staining
2. Coloration of a cervical area to emulate root surface and to produce the illusion of change of form
3. Coloration of hypocalcified areas
4. Coloration of check lines
5. Coloration of stain lines
6. Neutralization of hue for increase of apparent translucency (usually violet)
7. Highlighting and shadowing
8. Incisal edge modifications—emulated opacities, high chrome areas, stain areas
9. Synthetic restorations
10. Aging

42. Are external colorants stable in the oral cavity?
External colorants are metallic oxides that fuse to the ceramic unit during a predetermined firing cycle. Although quite stable in an air environment, they are susceptible to corrosion when subjected to certain oral environments. Depending on the stain and the pH of the oral fluids, external colorants may be lost from the ceramic unit over a long period of time.

43. What is the most important factor in determining the strength of a ceramic?
The most important factor in the strength of a ceramic material is control of small flaws or microcracks, which often are present both at the surface and internally. In most cases, the strength of the ceramic depends on surface flaws rather than porosity within the normal range.

44. Should porcelain be used on the occlusal surface of a metal-ceramic crown?
In general, the surface hardness of dental porcelains is greater than that of tooth structure, metal alloys, and all other restorative materials. This may lead to excessive wear of the opposing dentition if certain occlusal guidelines are not followed. In the best scenario, the opposing material is porcelain, but results are good if the occlusal loads have good force distribution. Porcelain is contraindicated in patients who indulge in bruxism or parafunctional activities in which occlusal overloading may occur.

45. Can a porcelain fracture of a metal ceramic restoration be repaired?
It is now possible to bond composite or ceramic materials to a fractured restoration. The bond, which may occur on porcelain or on the metal substrate, is sufficiently strong to be resistant in a non– or low stress-bearing area. However, if the fracture occurs in a stress-bearing area, the probability of a successful repair is low.

46. On what basis do you choose between an all-ceramic or a metal-ceramic crown?
In recent times all-ceramic crowns have been frequently used. As with their predecessor, the porcelain jacket crown, which was introduced at the turn of the century, the main reason for their use is superior esthetics. Unlike the metal-ceramic crown, which is hindered by the metal substrate, the all-ceramic crown has the capability to mimic the optical properties of the natural tooth. However, all other factors—including strength, fit, ease of fabrication, and tooth selection and preparation—may inhibit its use.

47. Is tooth preparation the same for an all-ceramic crown and a metal-ceramic restoration?
The same amount of overall tooth reduction is needed for a metal-ceramic restoration as for an all-ceramic crown (1.0–1.5 mm labially, lingually, and interproximally). However, unlike the metal-ceramic restoration, which will accept any marginal design, marginal tooth preparation for the all-ceramic crown must be a shoulder or deep chamfer (minimum of 1.0 mm tooth reduction). (See figure, top of next page.)

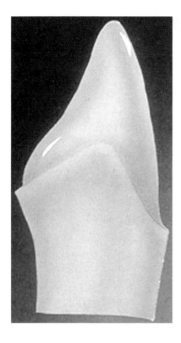

Tooth preparation for an all-ceramic crown.

48. Can the newer all-ceramic materials with high strength values be used in place of metal-ceramic restorations?

Some manufacturers claim that the newer ceramic materials with high theoretical strength values can be used in place of metal-ceramic restorations for any tooth and for small-unit, anterior fixed bridges. However, the guidelines for usage, such as tooth preparation, are more critical and in general more complicated than for metal-ceramic restorations. It is advisable, therefore, to use the all-ceramic crown in the anterior segment, where esthetics is the dominant factor.

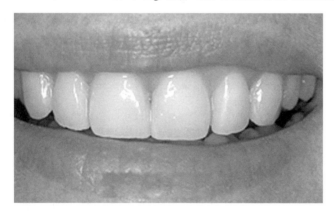

All-ceramic crowns on maxillary anterior segment (teeth 6–11).

49. What are the different types of all-ceramic crowns?

All-ceramic crowns may be categorized by composition and method of fabrication:

Composition
1. Feldspathic porcelain, such as a conventional porcelain jacket crown.
2. Aluminous porcelain: Vitadur, Hyceram, Cerestore, Procera, Inceram

3. Mica glass: Dicor, Cerapearl
4. Crystalline-reinforced glass; Optec, Empress

Method of fabrication

1. Refractory die technique: Optec, Mirage, Hyceram, Inceram
2. Casting: Dicor
3. Press technique: Cerestore, Procera, Empress

50. What is crystalline-reinforced glass?

A crystalline-reinforced glass is a glass in which a crystalline substance such as leucite is dispersed. This composition is used in the Optec or Empress systems. Strength is derived from the crystalline microstructure within the glass matrix. The higher concentration of leucite crystals in the matrix limits the progress of microcracks within the ceramic.

51. What is the importance of alumina in an all-ceramic restoration?

Alumina (Al_2O_3) is a truly crystalline ceramic, the hardest and probably the strongest oxide known. Alumina is used to reinforce glass (as in Hyceram). The strength is determined by the amount of alumina reinforcement. Alumina is also used in total crystalline compositions (Cerestore, Procera, Inceram), which may serve as the substructure much like metal coping. With this technique, the ceramic has high strength.

52. Is the cementing of an all-ceramic crown different from the cementing of a metal-ceramic crown?

The major difference is that a trial cement is not recommended for the all-ceramic crown, which obtains much of its strength from the underlying support of the tooth. If the cement washes out, the unsupported crown is susceptible to fracture. In general, all rigid cements can be used, but a bonded resin cement is highly recommended to maximize the underlying support.

53. Can all of the all-ceramic materials be bonded to the tooth preparation?

It is important that the ceramic material be chemically etched for bonding to a tooth. If the ceramic material cannot be properly etched, alumina is used in the substrate.

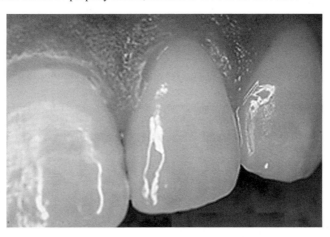

Ceramic veneer (tooth 10) bonded to tooth.

54. What is the significance of the refractory die?

A refractory die is used in many techniques for the construction of different types of all-ceramic crowns and veneers. Basically it is a secondary die obtained by duplicating the master die. The ceramic material is applied on the refractory die for the firing cycles. Once the cycles have

been completed, the refractory die is removed, and the ceramic piece is returned to the master die. Refractory die material must have the following properties:
1. Compatibility with impression materials
2. Dimensional stability for measurements
3. Tolerance of high-heat firing cycles
4. Compatible coefficient of thermal expansion with the ceramic material used
5. Easy removal from the ceramic piece

55. What determines the design of the pontic?

The design of the pontic is dictated by the special boundaries of (1) edentulous ridge, (2) opposing occlusal surface, and (3) musculature of tongue, cheeks, or lips. The task is to design within these boundaries a tooth substitute that favorably compares in form, function, and appearance with the tooth it replaces. The tooth substitute must provide comfort and support to the adjacent musculature, conformity to the food-flow pattern, convenient contours for hygiene, and cosmetic value, if indicated.

56. How should the contact area of the pontic on the edentulous ridge be designed?

Three concepts in pontic design are currently popular:
1. The sanitary pontic design leaves space between poetic and ridge.
2. The saddle pontic design covers the ridge labiolingually. Total coronal width is usually concave.
3. The modified ridge design uses a ridge lap for minimal ridge contact. Labial contact is usually to height of the ridge contour (straight emergence profile).

The selection of the design depends on the following factors:
1. Spatial boundaries
2. Shape of edentulous ridge (normal, blunted, or excessive resorption)
3. Maxillary or mandibular posterior arch (in contrast to the mandibular posterior pontic, the maxillary edentulous ridge is usually broad and blunted and has superior cosmetic effects)
4. Anterior pontic (the overriding cosmetic requirement is that form and shape reproduce the facial characteristics of the natural tooth)

57. What is the emergence profile? What is its importance?

The emergence profile is the shape of the marginal aspect of a tooth or a restoration and relates to the angulation of the tooth or restoration as it emerges from the gingiva. This gingival contour is extremely important for tissue health after placement of a crown.

The most obvious error of the emergence profile of a crown is overcontouring, which creates abnormal pressure of the gingival cuff and leads to inflammation in the presence of bacteria. Overcontouring and poor emergence profile are due primarily to (1) inadequate tooth preparation, (2) improper handling of materials, and/or (3) inadequate communication between the dentist and the technician.

58. After periodontal therapy, when can the dentist complete the marginal tooth preparation?

A certain waiting time is necessary between completion of periodontal therapy and completion of the marginal tooth preparation both to establish and to stabilize the attachment apparatus on the root surface. If this waiting time is not observed, impingement of the restoration into the attachment apparatus quite frequently occurs. The result is an iatrogenic gingival inflammation. The amount of waiting time necessary depends on the aggressiveness of the gingival procedure. A reasonable guideline, however, is to wait at least 6 weeks for tissue resolution.

59. What is a biologically compatible material?

A biologically compatible material elicits no adverse response either in the tissue or systemically. Adverse tissue response may be due to any of the following:

1. Allergic reaction
2. Toxic response
3. Mechanical irritation
4. Promotion of bacterial colonization

In general, highly polished noble alloys and highly glazed porcelains are the most biologically compatible materials.

60. Is any material used to construct crowns suspected of biologic incompatibility?

In general, most materials used in the construction of crowns are biologically compatible. Adverse reactions have occurred to some materials, primarily because of unpolished metal or unglazed porcelain surfaces. However, reports in the literature indicate that nickel-chrome alloys used in castings may be biologically incompatible. An allergic response may occur in 10% of women and 5% of men.

REMOVABLE PARTIAL DENTURES

61. What is the most important factor in determining the success of a bilateral, free-end mandibular removable partial denture (RPD)?

The most important factor in determining success is proper coverage over the residual ridge. Coverage should extend over the retromolar pad to create stability of the RPD and to minimize the torquing forces on the abutment teeth.

62. When clasps are to be used on the abutment teeth, what important factors must be considered?

When clasps are used, it is important to design the prosthesis so that the path of insertion is parallel to the abutment teeth. This factor is important in eliminating torquing forces on the abutment teeth during insertion and removal of the partial denture. If the planes are not parallel, then the abutment teeth must be adjusted. The abutment teeth also must be evaluated for placement of the retentive clasps and the reciprocal bracing arm. The abutment teeth are then shaped to accept the clasps. The proper positioning of occlusal rests on the abutment teeth is extremely important, and the teeth are prepared to optimize positioning.

63. What are the advantages and disadvantages of the cingulum bar as a connector?
   Advantages

1. Space problems for bar placement seldom exist unless anterior teeth have been worn down by attrition.

2. No pressure is exerted on the gingival tissues with movement of the RPD.

3. The major connector forms a single unit with the anterior teeth, thus contributing to comfort of the RPD.

4. Indirect retention is provided.

5. Repair of the RPD is simple when natural anterior teeth are lost.

   Disadvantages

1. The metal bar situated on the lingual surface of the anterior teeth is relatively bulky, especially where crowding is present.

2. Esthetics are compromised if spacing exists.

3. Marked lingual inclination of the anterior teeth precludes use of the bar.

64. What laboratory requirements should be implemented when a cingulum bar is used?

1. For sufficient rigidity, a minimal height of 4 mm and a thickness of 2.5 mm are necessary. These dimensions should be increased when the cingulum bar traverses more natural teeth.

2. No notches should be made in the metal to stimulate tooth contour because they weaken the bar. In the presence of reduced height, the bar is placed more gingivally and made thicker to provide rigidity.

3. The junction of the bar to the denture base must be sufficiently strong. The bar can cover the lingual surfaces of premolars, if present. The contour of the teeth should be adapted to the path of insertion of the RPD.

65. Are indirect retainers necessary in the construction of an RPD? If so, where should they be placed?

The function of an indirect retainer is to prevent dislodgement of the RPD toward the occlusal plane. In a total tooth-bearing RPD, it is unnecessary to include indirect retainers. However, when the RPD has a free-end saddle portion, it is advisable to include indirect retention to prevent vertical dislodgement.

The ideal positioning of the indirect retainer is at the furthest point from the distal border of the free-end saddle. For example, if the free-end saddle is on the lower right quadrant, the indirect retainer is placed on the lower left canine.

66. Is it advantageous to place stress-breaking attachments adjacent to a free-end saddle in an RPD?

The advantage of constructing a stress-breaking attachment next to a free-end saddle is to relieve torquing forces on abutment teeth that have been periodontally compromised. However, further displacement of the free-end saddle toward the underlying ridge may cause an acceleration of resorption of the residual ridge. It is preferable, therefore, to compensate for torquing forces on the abutment teeth by the proper extension of the saddle area.

67. Is it necessary to use clasps around abutment teeth in an RPD?

Clasps may be eliminated around abutment teeth if the teeth are restored with a partial or full crown containing some form of attachment that replaces the functions of the clasps. These functions include:

1. Guide planes for the RPD
2. Prevention of vertical displacement toward the ridge by the occlusal and cingular rest
3. Retentive function from the retentive arm
4. Bracing function from the reciprocal arm

Depending on the type of attachment, all or part of these functions may be replaced. With partial replacement, the remaining functions are incorporated into the RPD.

68. What is the difference between a precision and a semiprecision attachment?

A **precision attachment** is preconstructed with male and female portions that fit together in a precise fashion with little tolerance. Normally, there is no stress, and retention can be adjusted within the attachment. The attachment parts, constructed of a metal that can be placed into the crown and the RPD, normally are joined by solder. In general, no other clasps are necessary.

A **semiprecision attachment** is cast into the crown and the RPD. The female portion is normally made of preformed plastic that is positioned into the wax form and then cast. The male portion is cast with the RPD framework. The female and male parts fit together with much more tolerance than in the precision attachment, resulting in less retention. Secondary retentive clasping is necessary. Less torque is induced on the abutments with a semiprecision than with a precision attachment.

69. Do unlike metals in the male and female portions of the semiprecision attachment pose a problem?

The female portion of the attachment is cast with the crown and is made of the same metal as the crown. The male portion is cast into the RPD. The male portion is made of a harder metal than the female portion, which thus is subjected to greater wear. The wear pattern normally occurs on the vertical walls rather than on the occlusal seat. This creates a loosening of the attachment but no significant vertical displacement of the RPD. The result is the need for an adjustable retentive clasp.

70. What is the difference between an intracoronal and an extracoronal attachment?

An intracoronal attachment is placed within the body of the crown, whereas the extracoronal attachment is attached to the outer portion. The selection of one over the other depends on many factors; if designed properly, both types can be used successfully.

71. What are the advantages and disadvantages of an intracoronal attachment?
Advantages
1. Placement of torquing forces near the long access of the tooth, thus minimizing these forces
2. Elimination of clasps
3. Parallel guide planes for proper RPD insertion
4. Capability to establish proper contour at the abutment-RPD interface
Disadvantages
1. More tooth reduction
2. Need for adequate coronal length
3. Lack of stress-bearing capability
4. Difficulty in performing repairs

72. What are the advantages and disadvantages of an extracoronal attachment?
Advantages
1. Same amount of reduction of the abutment tooth and conventional restoration
2. Elimination of clasps
3. Incorporation of stress-breaking into attachment
4. Ease of replacing parts
5. Improved esthetics
Disadvantages
1. The attachment is positioned away from the long axis of the tooth, creating a potential for torquing forces on the abutment tooth.
2. Adequate vertical space is necessary for placement of the attachment.
3. Interproximal contour at the crown-attachment interface is difficult to establish correctly.

73. Is the unilateral RPD an acceptable treatment modality?

In general, a unilateral RPD is not an ideal treatment modality because cross-arch stabilization is necessary for success. A unilateral RPD may be used, however, when a single tooth is replaced and abutment teeth are on either side of the replacement tooth (Nesbitt appliance).

FULL DENTURES

74. What is the best material for taking a full-denture impression?

In taking a full-denture impression, it is important to understand that the topography of an edentulous arch includes soft, displaceable tissue with undercut areas. An impression material must not distort the tissues. Therefore, the material must be low in viscosity and elastomeric so that it can rebound in the undercut areas.

75. Is border molding necessary for a full lower denture?

Unlike a full upper denture, a lower denture does not rely on a peripheral seal for retention. Thus one may assume that border molding is an unnecessary procedure during impression taking. This assumption is incorrect because inadvertent overextension can greatly reduce denture stability as well as irritate tissue. Underextension of the peripheral border decreases tissue-bearing surfaces, thereby affecting denture stability.

76. What is the importance of the posterior palatal seal? How is its position determined?

The posterior palatal seal is an important component because it completes the entire peripheral sealing aspect of a maxillary denture. Anatomically, the seal is located at the juncture of the hard and the soft palate and joins the right and left hamular notches. If the seal is positioned more posteriorly, then tissue irritation, gagging reflex, and decreased retention can result. If the seal is positioned more anteriorly, tissue irritation and decreased retention can result. Manual palpation and phonetics (the "ah" sound) are the best ways to determine the anatomic position for the palatal seal.

77. What are the critical areas in the border-molding procedure of taking impressions for a maxillary arch?

The most critical area to capture in an impression is the mucogingival fold above the maxillary tuberosity area. Proper three-dimensional extension of the final prosthesis is extremely important for maximal retention. Other critical areas are the labial frena in the midline and the frena in the bicuspid area. Overextension in these areas often leads to decreased retention and tissue irritation.

78. Should an impression be taken under functional load or passively at one static moment?

The answer to this question has been debated for years. Soft tissue constantly changes, and a static impression captures the tissue at one point in time. On the other hand, a functional impression is taken with abnormal masticatory loads. Therefore, there is no absolute method of taking the impression. Denture stability with occlusal forces and periodic tissue evaluation, however, are critical with both methods.

79. What are the critical areas to capture in an impression of a mandibular arch?

Mandibular dentures do not rely on suction from a peripheral seal for retention but rather on denture stability in covering as much basal bone as possible without impinging on the muscle attachments. Movement of the tongue, lips, and cheeks greatly affects the amount of tissue-bearing area. Therefore, apart from identifying and covering the retromolar areas, the active border molding performed by the lip, cheeks, and tongue determines the peripheral areas of a mandibular arch, thus establishing maximal basal bone coverage.

80. How do you determine the peripheral extent of a denture?

For a peripheral border impression, a moldable material should be used around a well-fitting tray. The material should have moderate or low viscosity so as not to displace tissue and should set in a brief period of time. The lips, cheeks, and tongue dictate the extent of the peripheral impression. The impression is captured by exaggerated movements of the anatomic structures made by the patient or manipulated by the dentist.

81. If an impression does not capture everything that is intended, can you realign the existing impression?

One must always bear in mind that an edentulous ridge has soft, displaceable tissue. Thus it is important to relieve the pressure before relining an existing impression. If this is not done, tissue is compressed, and dimensional stability of the final impression is compromised. This inevitability leads to an undersized, ill-fitting denture.

82. How is vertical dimension established in a totally edentulous mouth?

Vertical dimension is established with the aid of bite rims. The most important aspect of vertical dimension is to establish the freeway space. The minimal opening in freeway space, which is determined phonetically (the "s" sound), is normally 1–2 mm.

83. How are overlap and overjet established?

Overlap and overjet are established by the maxillary bite rim, which also establishes the occlusal plane. The bite rim is adjusted by its position relative to the lip and cheek.

84. Is the bite registration taken in the centric relation or centric occlusion position?

This controversy has been argued for years and remains unresolved. However, certain principles are generally accepted:

1. A centric relation position may be duplicated.
2. Centric relation is the same position in various openings of the vertical dimension.
3. Centric relation should be an unstrained position.
4. Centric occlusion may be employed if the bite registration is done without increasing the vertical dimension.

85. Is it necessary to take multiple bite registrations?

It is not necessary to take multiple bite registrations to capture a maxillary/mandibular relationship. However, because tissue displacement makes it difficult to obtain a stable bite with wax rims, a single accurate bite registration is unlikely. It is advisable, therefore, to take multiple bite registrations throughout the fabrication procedure and even after insertion of the final dentures.

86. What does the tooth try-in appointment accomplish?

The most obvious reason for the try-in appointment is to visualize the esthetics of the final teeth in regard to lip line, overbite and overjet, shape, and arrangement. The try-in appointment can also determine the fullness of the labial flanges in relationship to the cheeks and lips. Occlusal relationship can be checked and verified, and a new bit registration can be performed. Above all, the try-in appointment affords both the dentist and the patient a preview of the final completed denture.

87. How is posterior occlusion selected with regard to tooth morphology?

Posterior occlusion can range from monoplane (flat plane) to steep anatomic occlusal cusps. In general, the more anatomic the occlusion, the more efficient its function. However, it is more difficult to establish balanced occlusion with a steep anatomic denture, and lack of balance leads to denture instability. It is, therefore, easier to establish occlusal harmony with monoplane teeth. Overbite and overjet of the anterior teeth also affect selection of the posterior teeth.

88. How do overbite and overjet affect the selection of cuspid inclines of the posterior teeth?

Overbite and overjet of the anterior teeth affect selection of the cuspid inclines of the posterior teeth when balanced occlusion is to be achieved in lateral and protrusive movements:

Steep overbite—steep cuspal incline
Small overbite—monoplane
Wide overjet—monoplane
Narrow overjet—steep cuspal incline

89. Of what materials are denture teeth composed? How are they selected?

Denture teeth are made from basically three materials: porcelain, acrylic, and composite-filled resin. All three materials afford excellent esthetic capabilities.

Porcelain teeth afford the greatest degree of hardness and best withstand wear. However, they are brittle and difficult to change or adjust; they also have a low mechanical bond strength to the resin base.

Acrylic teeth, on the other hand, are the softest of the materials and therefore the least resistant to wear. They are, however, easy to use, they can be easily changed or adjusted, and they have the best bond strength to the denture base.

Composite-filled resin teeth have hardness and strength values between porcelain and acrylic; they bond well to denture base and can be adjusted easily.

90. What procedure should be followed for insertion of a full upper and full lower denture?

During the processing of the denture base, the probability of dimensional change is high. Dimensional change affects the adaptation of the base to the tissue-bearing area and also affects the occlusion. It is advisable, therefore, to verify the adaptation of the dentures to the tissue-bearing areas. This procedure can be accomplished by placing some type of pressure-indicating material inside the denture. The extension of the peripheral borders, especially in the frenum area, should be evaluated. Once the individual bases are adjusted, the occlusal balance should be carefully checked and adjusted. A remount procedure is recommended for this equilibration.

91. When the treatment plan calls for an immediate (transitional) denture, what are the expectations?

If the anterior teeth are to be extracted at the time of denture insertion, the patient should be informed that the denture teeth can be placed in the same position as the existing teeth. However, facial appearance will change because of the presence of the labial flange, which affects the fullness of the lip. The patient also should be made aware of the necessary process of adaptation to the palate and of the increase in salivary flow that over time will become normal. Finally, the patient should be told that most people adapt well to such oral changes.

92. Is the impression procedure the same for a transitional denture as for a conventional denture?

The impression procedure is approximately the same for establishing the peripheral border. The major concern in taking an impression around existing teeth and exaggerated undercut area is to select a material that has the lowest viscosity and is nonrigid after setting. These properties are important to avoid damage of existing teeth during the removal of the impression.

93. How is vertical dimension established in the construction of a transitional denture?

It is important to use the existing teeth to establish the centric occlusal position, regardless of the amount and position of the teeth. At the bite registration phase, a bite rim is constructed in the edentulous space adjacent to the existing teeth, and the teeth with the wax rim are used to capture the occlusal relationship.

94. If the master casts are altered in a transitional denture procedure (e.g., elimination of gross tissue undercuts), how is the surgical procedure altered?

It is necessary during the surgical procedure to know exactly how the master cast has been altered. This knowledge is critical for successful insertion of the transitional denture. It is advisable to construct a second denture base that is transparent. This surgical stent is placed over the ridge after the teeth are extracted. Pressure points and undercuts are readily visible, and surgical ridge correction can be performed.

95. When a transitional denture is inserted, what procedures should be followed?

It is always beneficial to have a surgical stent available to ascertain the fit of the denture base. Because many soft-tissue undercut areas may be present, it is critical to establish a single path of insertion of the denture. Gross removal of areas inside the dentures may lead to poor adaptation of the denture base and instability. In this situation an immediate soft-lining material is indicated.

96. During the healing phase, what procedures should be followed?

The patient should be instructed not to remove the denture and to return after 24 hours. At that time, tissue irritation and occlusion are checked, and the denture is adjusted. Then the patient is instructed about insertion and removal of the denture and told that as the ridges heal, resorption will occur. Each case varies, but in general resorption leads to a loosening of the denture. Therefore, transitional soft-lining procedures should be performed throughout the healing phase, on approximately a monthly basis. The final healing may take from 3–6 months, at which time a permanent lining in the existing denture or a new denture is constructed.

97. Is a face-bow transfer necessary in jaw registration in the full-denture construction?

It is advisable to take a face-bow transfer in the construction of a full denture. The purpose of the registration is to relate the maxillary bite rims to the temperomandibular joint and facial planes. This registration aids in determining not only esthetic factors but also the type of occlusal plane.

98. Is it necessary to take eccentric bite registrations in the construction of full dentures?

Although eccentric bite registrations are not essential, they aid in establishing a balanced occlusion. A stable occlusion is important for the retention and stability of dentures as well as for functional efficiency.

99. What is the neutral zone? How does it relate to the alveolar ridge?

The neutral zone is the potential space between the lips and cheeks on one side and the tongue on the other. Natural or artificial teeth in this zone are subject to equal and opposite forces from the surrounding musculature. The alveolar ridge, which normally dictates the position of the denture teeth, may conflict with the neutral zone. Therefore, the neutral position zone also should be considered when denture teeth are positioned.

100. Are there any advantages to retaining roots under a denture apart from retention properties?

Retention is a critical aspect in root-retained dentures. Of equal importance, however, retained roots help to prevent resorption of the residual ridges. Retained roots also afford the patient some proprioceptive sense of "naturalness" in function of dentures.

101. What is the ideal type of attachment in a root-retained denture?

The ideal type of attachment affords maximal retentive forces for the denture with minimal torquing forces to the roots. Because these ideal properties cannot be totally obtained, a compromise is necessary. Many factors determine how much retention a tooth can withstand without subjection to harmful forces, including:
    1. The amount of supportive bone around the retained roots
    2. The number of existing roots
    3. The type and amount of occlusal forces
    4. The type of attachment (i.e., intra- or extraradicular, rigid or stress-bearing attachments)
    5. Splinting or nonsplinting of roots

102. In a root-retained denture, which is better—intraradicular or extraradicular attachment?

Both attachments can be equally retentive, but the intraradicular attachment places the fulcrum forces more deeply into the bone than an extraradicular attachment and thus helps to withstand deleterious torquing forces. The intraradicular attachments, however, are more difficult to implement because of (1) length of existing root, (2) width of existing root, (3) paralleling to other roots, (4) inability to splint, and (5) difficulty in hygiene.

103. Is splinting a preferred treatment in a root-retained denture?

The main purpose of splinting roots in a tooth-borne denture is to dissipate the forces, thus minimizing the torque on the existing roots. Splinting does not necessarily result in increased denture retention, but it creates a more difficult construction procedure. Splinting should be attempted after certain aspects are evaluated, such as (1) paralleling, (2) amount of freeway space, (3) placement of bar to ridge, and (4) type of bar.

104. What is the difference between a rigid and a stress-breaking attachment?

In **rigid attachment** the male and female components join in a precise fashion, allowing almost no movement between the two parts. This creates a rigid, nonflexible attachment that affords the greatest amount of retention but also produces the greatest amount of torque on the retained roots. A rigid attachment is not recommended on periodontically compromised teeth.

A **stress-bearing attachment** affords movement between the male and female components, thereby relieving torque. In most cases, a stress-bearing attachment is recommended.

105. How many roots must be retained to construct a root-retained denture?

There is no fixed rule. A root-retained denture can be constructed with only one root. The fewer the roots, the less the retentive force that should be applied to them. The ideal distribution of retained roots would be both cuspid regions and bilateral molar regions.

106. Is it necessary to place attachments or to cover the roots of a root-retained denture?

It is not always necessary to cover a root beneath an overdenture. Retention is not the only goal of this treatment modality. Equally important is preservation of the residual ridge by retaining the roots. However, if a root is not covered, the exposed surfaces are highly susceptible to decay. Oral hygiene must be stringently maintained.

107. Are the principles the same for a maxillary as for a mandibular overdenture?

Many of the principles for root-retained dentures are the same for the maxillary arch as for the mandible, including (1) selection of roots to be retained with regard to position and stability, (2) types of attachments, (3) paralleling, and (4) splinting. One aspect that may differ is related to morphologic differences of the residual ridges. The maxillary arch has a greater probability of undercut areas in the anterior region above the roots. This difference is quite apparent in the canine area. It is necessary to design the path of insertion to take the undercuts into consideration. Therefore, attachment selection may have to be altered, and the peripheral border of the denture may have to be reduced or eliminated.

108. Can the palate be eliminated in a root-retained maxillary denture?

If retention is adequate from the retained roots with their attachments, it is possible to eliminate the palate. It must be remembered that the palatal area affords the denture the greatest bearing area and also creates cross-arch stabilization.

109. What are the causes of denture stomatitis? How can it be treated?

Denture stomatitis is caused by trauma from poorly fitting dentures, by poor oral and denture hygiene, and by the oral fungus *Candida albicans*. Denture stomatitis can be treated by using resilient denture liners that stabilize ill-fitting dentures, thereby treating the inflamed tissue. Some liners may also inhibit fungal growth.

IMPLANTS

110. What types of implants are most commonly used for prosthetic replacement of the tooth?

1. **Endosteal implants:** blades, screws, or cylinders are implanted into the maxilla or mandible. These implants support the dental prosthesis.

2. **Subperiosteal implants:** a metal framework is inserted on top of the maxillary or mandibular bone. Vertical posts attached to the framework protrude the soft tissue and support the dental prosthesis.

111. What is an osseointegrated implant?

An osseointegrated implant is a cylinder or screw constructed of a biocompatible material that is precisely imbedded into the ridge of the maxilla or mandible (see figure, top of next page). The fixture is allowed to integrate with the bone without any loading forces for a certain period. Histologically, the bone cells grow tightly around this anchor with no membrane attachment at the interface (unlike natural tooth-bone interface).

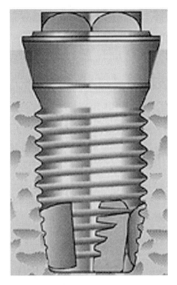

Osseointegrated implant. (Courtesy of NobelBiocare, Westmont, IL.)

112. Describe the components of an implant and the clinical procedures used with each.

The technique and the biocompatible materials used in the osseointegrated implant were developed by Per-Ingvar Branemark, an orthopedic surgeon, more than 50 years ago. Branemark identified the biocompatible material, titanium, and described the following components:

1. **Fixture:** the anchor imbedded into the edentulous ridge. It is constructed of titanium and may be coated with biocompatible, bone-regeneration materal such as hydroxyapatite. The fixture is carefully imbedded into precision-drilled holes and allowed to integrate with the bone undisturbed for 3–6 months.

2. **Abutment:** the transitional piece that connects the fixture to the prosthesis. The abutment is normally attached to the fixture after a second surgical procedure.

3. **Dental prosthesis:** the dental prosthesis can then be constructed and attached to the abutment. This stage may begin a few weeks after the second surgery.

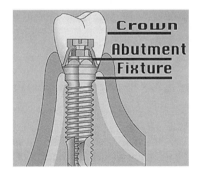

Components of an implant. (Courtesy of NobelBiocare, Westmont, IL.)

113. What is the success rate of an osseointegrated implant prosthesis?

Many factors affect the success rate of an implant prosthesis; however, studies for long-term predictability have demonstrated a success rate of more than 90%.

114. What factors affect the success rate of the implant?
- Careful patient selection
- Exacting diagnostic records
- Integrated treatment planning
- Precise clinical procedures

115. What are the important factors in patient selection?
  1. Patient's general health
     • Medical considerations
     • Medications
     • Psychiatric considerations
  2. Intraoral factors
     • Bone tissue site of fixture installation is free from pathologic conditions (e.g., cysts)
     • Site free from unerupted or impacted teeth, root remnants, or any other foreign bodies
     • No open communication between the bone and oral cavity
     • The mucosa must be healthy and free from ulceration
     • Anatomic factors

116. What type of bone is important to osseointegration?
  Good bone consists of a thick layer of compact bone surrounding a core of dense trabecular bone of favorable strength. Poor bone consists of a thin layer of cortical bone surrounding a core of low-density trabecular bone.

117. What anatomic factors are important to consider for implant replacement?
  • Transverse shape of the jaw bone
  • Degree of resorption
  • Maxilla—location of sinuses, nasal cavity, and incisive canal
  • Mandible—mental foramen, inferior alveolar nerve, and blood vessels

118. How is the intraoral condition evaluated?
  The intraoral condition is determined through radiographic evaluation:
  • Intraoral radiograph of proposed site
  • General view of the jaws (an orthopontomogram reveals any pathologic processes)
  • Lateral cephalometric radiograph (to show relationship between jaws)
  • Tomographic records (valuable information about the width of the alveolar crest and the location of important anatomic structures)

119. How do you plan for the proper treatment modality?
  Planning the actual course of therapy is essential to success. Before the surgery, an evaluation should be made of the desired prosthetic results. This evaluation dictates the following:
  • Type of prosthetic replacement
  • Number of implants
  • Placement of fixtures
  • Models of the jaw mounted on an articulator, if necessary. Set-up of teeth on these models determines the prosthesis and helps the dentist performing the surgery to visualize the proposed prosthesis. The surgeon also may be guided for implant placement by the use of a surgical template.

120. What are radiographic and surgical stents?
  Radiographic and surgical stents are templates constructed on the diagnostic models that aid in the position and placement of the implants. A stent with metal markers over the proposed fixture sites should be used to aid in the evaluation of radiographs. A surgical stent is also useful when the fixtures are implanted. The optimal position from a prosthetic point of view can be visualized.

121. What are the treatment modalities for a totally edentulous jaw?
  • Overdenture supported by implants
  • Fixed "high-water" prosthesis
  • Conventional fixed crown and bridges using implants

122. Describe the concept of implant-supported overdenture.

An implant-supported overdenture is supported both by the implants and the edentulous ridge covered by resilient mucosa. The surgeon must accommodate for this resiliency in the attachments of the implants to permit small rotational movements.

123. What are the indications for the overdenture treatment?

This treatment modality is a comparatively simple procedure with relatively low cost and meets the demands imposed by many patients. The most common indications are:
- Retention of denture
- Compromised hygiene skills (i.e., reduced dexterity, as with elderly people)
- Interarch positions (difficulty in placing proper interdental relationships with fixed restorations)
- Phonetics/esthetics (especially in the maxilla, an overdenture may improve esthetic and/or phonetic results compared with an implant-supported fixed prosthesis).

124. How many implants are necessary to support the overdenture?

The number of implants ranges from a minimum of two fixtures to an ideal of four. It is also important to consider the loading forces on the implant.

125. What is the effect of loading forces on implant-supported overdentures?

The loading forces are important to fixture survival because overloading can lead to implant failure. To reduce improper loading conditions, the following points should be considered:

1. The implants should be positioned as perpendicular to the occlusal plane as possible.

2. Shear loads and bending movements are reduced if leverages are shortened by using short abutments and low attachments.

3. Resilient attachments reduce bending movements. Occlusal forces are shared between fixtures and overdenture-bearing mucosa.

4. Extension bars represent a potential risk of overloading.

126. What is the fixed "high-water" prosthesis on an edentulous arch?

The fixed prosthesis supported by implants on an edentulous arch was first developed and investigated by Branemark in the 1960s:
- Placement of fixtures with transmucosal abutments as parallel as possible to each other
- Cast metal frameworks that fit precisely on the abutments and support the prosthesis
- Denture teeth and processed denture material on the metal framework

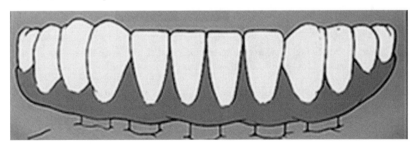

High-water prosthesis. (Courtesy of NobelBiocare, Westmont, IL.)

127. What does "high water" mean?

High water refers to the design of an implant-supported prosthesis. The implants support the prostheses without the aid of the mucosal edentulous ridge, which is utilized in the implant-supported overdenture. Space between the prosthesis and the mucosa is necessary for proper hygiene, thus leading to the descriptive term "high water."

128. What happens when the fixtures are not parallel in a fixed prosthesis?
A precise prosthesis fit is necessary for osseointegrated rigid fixtures; therefore, relative paralleling is required. Lack of parelleling, however, can be compensated with proper abutment selection. The divergence of axial fixtures can differ up to 40°.

129. How many fixtures are necessary to support a high-water fixed prosthesis?
Many factors determine the number of fixtures necessary to support a fixed prosthesis, including quality of bone, placement and length of fixture, and loading of fixtures. In general, however, 4–6 fixtures are sufficient to support a fixed high-water prosthesis.

130. Can conventional fixed bridgework be used over implants to restore a totally edentulous arch?
Conventional fixed bridgework rather than the high-water prosthesis can be used with implants to restore a totally edentulous arch. However, fixture positioning, loading forces, and esthetic and phonetic considerations are more critical. In addition, more fixtures are necessary to support the prosthesis (minimum of 6).

131. Should an implant prosthesis be considered in partially edentulous patients?
The partially fixed implant-supported prosthesis is a viable treatment and should be considered as the treatment of choice when the only alternatives are a removable partial denture or a fixed bridge attached to previously untouched teeth, or if the proposed abutments are periodontally compromised. Conventional bridgework may be the appropriate treatment of choice when the proposed abutment teeth are periodontally sound but need extensive restorative work.

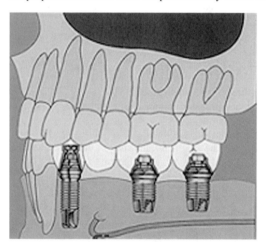

Fixed implant-supported prosthesis. (Courtesy of NobelBiocare, Westmont, IL.)

132. What aspects should be considered in selecting implant treatment for partially edentulous patients?
1. Implant placement is limited and defined by existing edentulous space; therefore, fixture placement may be near sensitive structures such as nerves and blood vessels.
2. Good esthetic results may be difficult to achieve.
3. Greater horizontal loading forces place high demands on the anchorage of the fixture.
4. Topographic conditions of the existing bone and its relationship to the remaining teeth must be considered.
5. Occlusal considerations are essential (i.e., when canines and premolar teeth are replaced in a cuspid-protected articulator with a deep overbite).
6. Periodontal disease on remaining teeth creates a pathologic condition that may contraindicate implantation.

133. What factors influence abutment selection?

The abutment selection is an important prosthodontic phase of treatment because it may determine the final prosthesis design. Factors for abutment selection should include the following:

1. Articulated casts with diagnostic wax-up of the proposed prosthesis aid in size and angulation of the abutment.

2. Type of abutment depends on whether the prosthesis is to be screwed to the implant or cement-retained.

3. Transmucosal space should be determined because it affects the height selection of the abutment.

4. Esthetic/phonetic considerations also affect the selection of abutment.

134. What diagnostic procedure may be used for abutment selection?

To determine the proper abutment angulation height, esthetic factors, and occlusal considerations, it is necessary to know the position of the fixture to the bone in relation to the gingival mucosa and interarch space between the fixture and the opposing dentition. Fixture angulation and transmucosal height can be measured intraorally with diagnostic gauges. However, a more precise method is the following:

1. Obtain an impression of the arch with the fixtures.

2. Construct a cast that contains replicas of the fixtures with its relationship to the mucosa.

3. Articulate this model to the opposing dentition. This method facilitates proper abutment selection and fabrication.

135. What is an angulated abutment?

An angulated abutment is positioned in an angulated direction from the axial position of the fixture. This angulation may vary up to 30°. Angulated abutments are used when the fixtures have been installed with an unfavorable inclination in relation to the desired position of the prosthesis.

136. Is an angulated abutment clinically safe?

In vitro studies have shown that as abutment increases, compressive and tensile strains around the implant also increase. A 3-year clinical evaluation by Balshi et al., however, showed that angulated abutments do not necessarily promote periimplant mucosal problems. The success rate is comparable to that of the standard abutment.

137. What is the UCLA-type abutment?

The UCLA abutment is custom-fabricated on the fixture replica. Normally, the fabrication is done so that the final abutment appears like a full-crown preparation on which the prosthesis is

(Courtesy of NobelBiocare, Westmont, IL.)

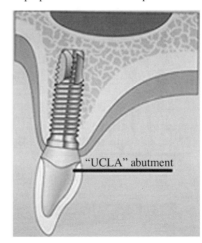

cemented. It also may be screw-retained. This customized fabrication technique allows control of angulation, transmucosal shape and height, esthetic considerations, and interocclusal space.

138. Can an implant be used for single-tooth replacement?
Yes. However, careful patient selection and presurgical analysis are critical so that function and esthetics approximate the natural tooth.

139. Can implants and natural teeth be used together to support a final prostheses?
Natural teeth are suspended in bone by the periodontal membrane. This situation allows tooth movement in relationship to bone. An osseointegrated implant, which is fixed rigidly to the bone, allows no movement at its interface. Joining a movable natural tooth and rigid implant with a fixed prosthesis may cause support problems that lead to failure. It is better to separate the prosthesis if possible (implant with implant, natural tooth with natural tooth). This strategy may not always be possible. If the prosthesis calls for joining natural teeth, provisions should be made in the prosthesis to allow movement of the natural tooth abutment. This goal is quite often accomplished with a nonrigid interlocking attachment.

BIBLIOGRAPHY

1. Balshi I, Ekfeldt A, Stember T, Vrielinck L: Three-year evaluation of Branemark implants connected to angulated abutments. Int J Oral Maxillofac Implants 12:52–58, 1997.
2. Chiche GJ, Pinault A: Esthetics of Anterior Fixed Prosthodontics. Chicago, Quintessence, 1993.
3. Lucia VO: Treatment of the Edentulous Patient. Chicago, Quintessence, 1986.
4. Magnussen S, Nilson H, Lindh T: Branemark Systems: Restorative Dentist's Manual. Gothenburg, Sweden, Nobel Biocare AB, 1992.
5. McLean JW: The Science and Art of Dental Ceramics, vol. I. Chicago, Quintessence, 1979.
6. McLean JW: The Science and Art of Dental Ceramics, vol. II. Chicago, Quintessence, 1980.
7. Morrow RM, Rudd KD, Rhoads JE: Dental Laboratory Procedures: Complete Dentures, vol. I, 2nd ed. St. Louis, Mosby, 1986.
8. Phillips R: Skinner's Science of Dental Materials, 9th ed. Philadelphia, W.B. Saunders, 1991.
9. Rudd KD, Morrow RM, Rhoads JE: Dental Laboratory Procedures: Removable Partial Dentures, vol. 3. St. Louis, Mosby, 1986.
10. Shillingburg HT Jr, et al: Fundamentals of Fixed Prosthodontics, 2nd ed. Chicago, Quintessence, 1981.
11. Smith R, Kournjian J: Understanding Dental Implants. San Bruno, CA, Kramer Communications, 1989.
12. Yamamoto M: Metal Ceramics: Principles and Methods of Makoto Yamamoto. Tokyo, Quintessence, 1990.

10. ORAL AND MAXILLOFACIAL SURGERY

Bonnie L. Padwa, D.M.D., M.D., and Stephen T. Sonis, D.M.D., D.M.Sc.

GENERAL TOPICS

1. Why should a patient be hospitalized for routine oral surgical procedures?

The most common reason for hospitalizing a patient for routine oral surgical procedures is behavioral management. Patients who are severely handicapped, for example, may not be able to tolerate care in an office setting. Patients who are at high medical risk are often best treated in the controlled environment of the operating room, where constant monitoring and quick treatment of a problem are more easily managed. The final reason for treating a patient in the operating room is an inability to tolerate or obtain local anesthesia.

2. List the American Heart Associations' recommendation for antibiotic prophylaxis before dental procedures.
- Amoxicillin, 2 gm 1 hour before procedure, *or*
- Clindamycin, 600 mg 1 hour before procedure, *or*
- Cephalexin, 2 gm 1 hour before procedure, *or*
- Azithromycin or clarithromycin, 500 mg 1 hour before procedure

3. What are the basic technical considerations in performing an incision?
- Use a sharp blade of appropriate size.
- A firm, continuous stroke is preferable to short, soft, repeated strokes.
- Avoid vital structures; incising the lingual artery can ruin your morning.
- Use incisions that are perpendicular to epithelial surfaces.
- Consider the anatomy of the site in placement of the incision.

4. What factors influence the placement of incisions in the mouth?
- Anatomy and location of vital structures
- Convenience and access

5. For making an incision in an epithelial surface, how should the scalpel blade be oriented?

To avoid bias, the incision should be made perpendicular to the epithelial surface.

6. What are the principles of flap design?
- Flap design should ensure adequate blood supply; the base of the flap should be larger than the apex.
- Reflection of the flap should adequately expose the operative field.
- Flap design should permit atraumatic closure of the wound.

7. What are the most frequent causes of the tearing of mucogingival flaps?
1. Flaps are too small to provide adequate exposure.
2. Too much force is used to elevate the flaps.

8. What are the means of obtaining hemostasis?

Pressure	Ligation with sutures
Thermal coagulation	Use of vasoconstrictive substances

9. Describe and discuss the function of Allis forceps in oral surgery.

Allis forceps have a locking handle similar to a needle holder and small beaks at the working end of the instruments. These beaks are useful in grasping tissue for removal.

10. What is an arthrocentesis?

It is irrigation of the superior joint space of the temporomandibular joint. Sterile saline irrigation is used to flush out the inflammatory mediators associated with degenerative arthritis and pain.

11. What is a genioplasty?

Genioplasty is a procedure by which the position of the chin is surgically altered. The most common techniques are osteotomy or augmentation with natural or synthetic materials.

12. Define distraction osteogenesis.

It is the slow application of a force using a distraction device to widen a surgically created bone gap in the mandible or maxilla. The distraction gap fills with a collagen matrix whose fibers are oriented parallel to the force of distraction. Calcification of the collagen fibers occurs from the periphery

13. What is the role of the general dentist in managing oral cancer?

The general dentist has three major roles in managing oral cancer:

1. Perhaps the most important is detection. As the primary provider of oral health care, the dentist is in the position to detect the presence of early lesions. A high degree of suspicion should lead to aggressive evaluation of any abnormality of the oral soft tissues. Biopsy of most areas of the mouth is within the realm of the generalist.

2. Once a diagnosis of oral cancer has been established, the dentist has the responsibility of ensuring that there are no areas of latent oral infection that may predispose to the development of osteoradionecrosis or other complications of therapy.

3. Because xerostomia and subsequent caries are common among patients receiving radiation therapy to the head and neck, the generalist should educate the patient about factors and behavior that increase the risk and should provide the patient with trays for the self application of fluoride gels. An aggressive recall schedule should be established.

14. List the symptoms of obstructive sleep apnea.

- Snoring
- Excessive daytime sleepiness
- Impaired cognition and memory loss
- Hypertension
- Heart failure (cor pulmone)
- Cardiac arrhythmias

15. Explain the concept of guided tissue regeneration in preprosthetic surgery.

Guided tissue regeneration is based on the fact that different cell types grow at various rates. The membrane physically prevents fast growing fibroblasts and epithelium from entering the osseous defect before the slower growing osteoblasts can repopulate the defect.

16. What are the advantages of using allogeneic or alloplastic materials under a barrier membrane?

- They stabilize the blood clot under the membrane.
- They provide a matrix for bone growth.
- They may increase the rate of bone growth.

17. What are the optimal dimensions (ratio) for an elliptical incisional biopsy?

To ensure adequate margins for an incisional biopsy of an elliptical lesion, the length of the ellipse should be 3 times the width.

Golden DP, Hooley JR: Oral mucosal biopsy procedures—Excisional and incisional. Dent Clin North Am 38:279–300, 1994.

18. What are the major oral side effects of radiation to the head and neck?

Xerostomia

Mucositis

Caries

Osteoradionecrosis

SUTURES: TECHNIQUES AND TYPES

19. What is the most common suture method? What are its advantages?

The interrupted suture is the most common method. Because each suture is independent, this procedure offers strength and flexibility in placement. Even if one suture is lost or loosens, the integrity of the remaining sutures is not compromised. The major disadvantage is the time required for placement.

20. What are the advantages of a continuous suture?

- Ease and speed of placement
- Distribution of tension over the whole suture line
- A more watertight closure than interrupted sutures

21. What factors determine the type of suture to be used?

Tissue type

Wound condition

Healing process

Expected postoperative course

22. How are sutures sized?

Size refers to the diameter of the suture material. The smallest size that provides the desired wound tension should be used. The higher the number, the smaller the suture. For example, 3-0 sutures are thicker than 4-0 sutures. The larger the diameter, the stronger the suture. In general, sutures for intraoral wound closure are 3-0 or 4-0.

23. What are the types of resorbable sutures? Nonresorbable sutures?

Resorbable	Nonresorbable
Plain gut	Silk
Chromic gut	Synthetic
Monocryl	Nylon
Vicryl	Mersilene
Dexon	Prolene

24. What is the difference between monofilament and polyfilament sutures?

Monofilament sutures consist of material made from a single strand. They resist infection by not harboring organisms. Plain and chromic gut are examples. Polyfilament sutures are made of multiple fibers that are either braided or twisted. They generally have good handling properties. The most common examples used in oral surgery are silk, Dexon, and Vicryl.

25. What are the principles of suturing technique?

- The suture should be grasped with the needle holder three-fourths of the distance from the tip.
- The needle should be perpendicular when it enters the tissue.
- The needle should be passed through the tissue to coincide with the shape of the needle.
- Sutures should be placed at an equal distance from the wound margin (2–3 mm) and at equal depths.
- Sutures should be placed from mobile tissue to fixed tissue.
- Sutures should be placed from thin tissue to thick tissue.
- Sutures should not be overtightened.
- Tissues should not be closed under tension.
- Sutures should be 2–3 mm apart.
- The suture knot should be on the side of the wound.

26. When should intraoral sutures be removed?
In uncomplicated cases, sutures generally may be removed 5–7 days after placement.

TOOTH EXTRACTION

27. What are the three principles of exodontia according to Shira?
1. Obtain adequate access.
2. Create an unimpeded path of removal.
3. Use controlled force.

28. What forceps are typically used for the removal of maxillary teeth?
Single-rooted teeth are usually removed with a maxillary universal forceps (150) or a no. 1 forceps. Premolars can be extracted with the maxillary universal forceps. To extract maxillary molars, 150 forceps usually can be used. Alternatively, the upper molar cowhorn can be used for fractured or carious teeth if care is applied.

29. What forceps are typically used for the removal of mandibular teeth?
Ashe forceps are generally the most effective for the removal of mandibular incisors, canines, and premolars. A lower universal forceps (151) is an alternative. The 151 also can be used for most molars, although a mandibular cowhorn forceps (no. 23) and no. 17 forceps are alternatives.

30. Name the indications for tooth extraction.
- Severe caries resulting in a nonrestorable tooth
- Pulpal necrosis that is not treatable with endodontic therapy
- Advanced periodontal disease resulting in severe, irreversible mobility
- Malpositioned, nonfunctional teeth
- Cracked or fractured teeth that are not amenable to conservative therapy
- Prosthetic considerations
- Impacted teeth when indicated (not all impacted teeth require extraction)
- Supernumerary teeth (when indicated)
- Teeth associated with a pathologic lesion, such as a tumor, that cannot be eliminated completely without sacrificing the tooth
- Before severe myelosuppressive cancer therapy or radiation therapy, any tooth that has a questionable prognosis or may be a potential source of infection should be extracted.
- Teeth involved in jaw fractures

31. What are the major contraindications for tooth extraction?
Contraindications may be either systemic or local. Systemic contraindications are related to the patient's overall health and may include the presence of a coagulopathy; uncontrolled diabetes mellitus; hematologic malignancy, such as leukemia; uncontrolled cardiac disease; and certain drug therapy. Elective extractions in pregnant patients is contraindicated. Local factors include radiation therapy to the area, active infection, and nonlocalized infection. The presence of a localized, dentoalveolar abscess is not a contraindication for extraction.

32. Give reasons for extracting third molars in a teenaged patient rather than waiting until the patient is in his or her 40s.
Younger patients have a follicle surrounding the crown, whereas this space is occupied by dense bone in older patients. Similarly, the periodontal ligament space is more prominent in younger patients. Finally, whereas the roots are likely to be incompletely formed in younger patients, they are completely formed in older patients and may add to the complexity of extraction.

33. What factors affect the difficulty associated with tooth extraction?

- Position of the tooth in the arch. In general, anterior teeth are more easily extracted than posterior teeth. Maxillary teeth are less difficult than mandibular teeth.
- Condition of the crown. Carious teeth may be easily fractured, thus complicating the extraction.
- Mobility of the tooth. Teeth that are mobile as a consequence of periodontal disease are more easily extracted. Ankylosis or hypercementosis increases the difficulty of tooth removal. In assessing mobility, the operator needs to ensure that the crown is not fractured; fracture may produce a false sense of overall tooth mobility.
- Root shape and length
- Proximity of associated vital structure
- Patient attitude and general health

34. What conditions may influence the difficulty of extraction of an erupted tooth?

- Root form
- Caries
- Hypercementosis
- Prior endodontic therapy
- Internal or external root resorption

35. What are the major forces used for tooth extraction?

Rotation and luxation are the major forces used for tooth extraction.

36. For multiple extractions, what is the appropriate order of tooth removal?

In general, maxillary teeth are removed before mandibular teeth and posterior teeth before anterior teeth.

37. What principles guide the use of elevators in tooth extraction?

- Elevators may be used to assess the level of anesthesia and to release the periodontal ligament.
- The bone, not adjacent teeth, should be used as the fulcrum for elevator assistance in tooth extraction.
- Elevators are most useful in multiple extractions.
- Elevators may assist in the removal of root tips by using a wedge technique.

38. What are the steps in postoperative management of an extraction site?

1. Irrigate the site with sterile saline.
2. Remove tissue tags and granulation tissue from the soft tissue of the site.
3. Aggressive curettage of the socket is contraindicated. Pathologic tissue should be removed by gentle scraping of the socket.
4. Compress the alveolar bone with finger pressure.
5. Suture if necessary at the papillae bordering the extraction site and across the middle of the socket.
6. Review postoperative instructions with the patient.

39. What are the indications for third-molar extraction?

- Pericoronitis
- Nonrestorable caries
- Advanced periodontal disease
- Position that prohibits adequate home care of the third molar or compromises maintenance of the second molar
- Associated pathology (e.g., cyst)
- Malposition
- Chronic pain
- Resorption of adjacent tooth

40. Should all impacted third molars be extracted?

No. Fully impacted third molars that do not communicate with the oral cavity need not be extracted. The teeth should be followed regularly, however, to ensure that no pathologic process develops. No data support the suggestion that impacted third molars contribute to crowding of anterior teeth.

41. What is the most common supernumerary tooth? Summarize the indications for its removal.

Mesiodens is the most common supernumerary tooth, followed by fourth molars and extra premolars. Indications for removal are similar to those for impacted teeth: symptoms of pain/infection, evidence of periodontal bone loss, resorption of adjacent teeth, pathology associated with the supernumerary tooth, midline diastema, and orthodontic treatment.

42. What are the major complications of tooth extraction?

Fracture of the root or alveolar plate	Infection
Displacement of a root tip	Perforation of the maxillary sinus
Bleeding	Lingual paresthesia and idiopathic avascular
Dry socket (localized osteitis)	necrosis
Fracture of the tuberosity	Soft-tissue injury

43. What is the most common complication of tooth extraction? How can it be prevented?

The most common complication of tooth extraction is root fracture. The best method of prevention is to expose the tooth surgically and to remove bone before extraction.

44. Which tooth root is most likely to be displaced into an unfavorable anatomic site during extraction?

The palatal root of the maxillary first molar is most likely to be displaced into the maxillary sinus during extraction.

45. What is the most important factor in successful treatment of an impacted lower second permanent molar?

Impaction of the lower second molars generally is due to inadequate arch length. The impacted second molar is usually associated with an impacted third molar that impedes normal eruption. The second molar impaction should be diagnosed as early as possible and the third molar removed to allow eruption of the second molar. If the molar requires surgical repositioning (uprighting), this procedure should be done before full root formation.

46. Describe the prevention and treatment of postoperative bleeding.

A thorough preoperative medical history helps to identify most patients at systemic risk for postoperative bleeding. On leaving the office, patients should receive both verbal and written instructions for postoperative wound care. Of particular relevance regarding bleeding is the avoidance of rinsing, spitting, and smoking during the first postoperative day. The patient should be specifically instructed to avoid aspirin. Patients should be instructed to bite on a gauze sponge for 30 minutes after the extraction.

A patient with postoperative bleeding should return to the office. The wound should be cleared of residual clot or debris, and the source of the bleeding identified. Local anesthesia should be administered, and existing sutures removed. The wound should be irrigated copiously with saline. Residual granulation tissue should be removed. A hemostatic agent, such as gelatin sponge, oxidized cellulose, or oxidized regenerated cellulose, may be placed into the extraction site. The wound margins should be reapproximated and carefully sutured.

47. What is the differential diagnosis for a radiolucent lesion associated with the crown of an impacted third molar?

- Dentigerous cyst
- Odontogenic keratocyst
- Ameloblastoma

48. What is a dry socket?

Dry socket is a localized osteitis of the extraction site that typically develops between the third and fourth postoperative day. The term applies to the clinical appearance of the socket, which is devoid of a typical clot or granulating wound. Consequently, patients develop moderate-to-severe throbbing pain. The frequency of dry socket after routine tooth extractions is around 2%. However, the condition may occur in as many as 20% of cases after extraction of impacted mandibular third molars.

49. How can dry socket be prevented?

Prevention of dry socket is somewhat controversial. It is generally agreed that careful technique to minimize trauma reduces the likelihood of this complication. In addition, preoperative rinsing with chlorhexidine gluconate 0.12% may be of benefit. Placement of antibiotic-impregnated gelfoam or injection of polylactic acid granules into the socket before suturing may be of value, although these interventions are far from being universally accepted.

50. How is dry socket treated?

Curettage of the extraction site is contraindicated. The extraction site should be gently irrigated with warm saline. A medicated dressing is then placed into the socket. The medication used for this purpose has been the topic of much discussion. One alternative consists of eugenol, benzocaine, and balsam of Peru. Alternatively, a gauze dressing impregnated with equal amounts of zinc oxide, eugenol, tetracycline, and benzocaine may be used.

51. What substances should never be placed into a healing socket?

Petrolatum-based compounds and tetracycline powder.

52. If perforation into the maxillary sinus occurs during extraction of a maxillary tooth, what surgical maneuvers and postoperative instructions help prevent formation of an oro-antral fistula?

- Water tight closure of the extraction site
- Sinus precautions: no nose blowing or using a straw
- Antibiotics to prevent infection in the sinus
- Decongestants to decrease swelling of the nasal mucosa and allow normal drainage through the sinus ostium

53. Describe pain control after extraction.

For most patients, adequate control of postoperative pain is obtained with nonsteroidal antiinflammatory drugs (NSAIDs). Data indicate that postoperative pain can be minimized if the first dose of NSAIDs is administered immediately after the procedure. No evidence indicates that preoperative administration of NSAIDs favorably alters the postoperative course. For patients unable to take NSAIDs because of allergies, ulcer disease, or other contraindications, various narcotic analgesics are available. Patients taking such medications must be cautioned about drowsiness and concurrent use of alcohol or other medication. In no instance is persistent postoperative pain (> 2 days) to be expected, and patients should be instructed to call if they have prolonged discomfort, which may indicate infection or another complication.

54. What percent of patients request pain medication after third-molar removal?

90%.

55. Which teeth are most commonly impacted?

The most commonly impacted teeth are the third molars and the maxillary canines.

INFECTIONS AND ABSCESSES

56. What are the major sources of odontogenic infections?

The two major sources of odontogenic infection are periapical disease, which occurs as a consequence of pulpal necrosis, and periodontal disease.

57. What are the three clinical stages of odontogenic infection?

1. Periapical osteitis occurs when the infection is localized within the alveolar bone. Although the tooth is sensitive to percussion and often slightly extruded, there is no soft tissue swelling.

2. Cellulitis develops as the infection spreads from the bone to the adjacent soft tissue. Subsequently, inflammation and edema occur, and the patient develops a poorly localized swelling. On palpation the area is often sensitive, but the sensitivity is not discrete.

3. Suppuration then occurs and the infection localizes into a discrete, fluctuant abscess.

58. What are the significant complications of untreated odontogenic infection?

- Tooth loss
- Spread to the cavernous sinus and brain
- Spread to the neck with large vein complications
- Spread to potential fascial spaces with compromise of the airway
- Septic shock

59. What are the principles of therapy for odontogenic infections as defined by Peterson?

1. Determine the severity of the infection.
2. Evaluate the state of the host defense mechanisms.
3. Determine whether the patient should be treated by a general dentist or a specialist.
4. Treat the infection surgically.
5. Support the patient medically.
6. Choose and prescribe the appropriate antibiotic.
7. Administer the antibiotic properly.
8. Evaluate the patient frequently.

60. What is the treatment of choice for an odontogenic abscess?

The treatment of choice for an odontogenic abscess is incision and drainage, which may be accomplished in one of three ways: (1) exposure of the pulp chamber with extirpation of the pulp, (2) extraction of the tooth, or (3) incision into the soft-tissue surface of the abscess. Antibiotic therapy is indicated in the presence of fever or lymphadenopathy.

61. How are incision and drainage of soft tissue best performed?

Local anesthesia should be obtained first. Care must be taken not to inject through the infected area and thus spread the infection to noninvolved sites. Once adequate anesthesia has been obtained, an incision should be placed at the most dependent part of the swelling. The incision should be wide enough to facilitate drainage and to allow blunt dissection. After irrigation, a drain (e.g., iodoform gauze or rubber) should be placed to maintain the patency of the wound. Postoperative instructions should include frequent rinses with warm saline, appropriate pain medication, and, when indicated, antibiotic therapy. The patient should be instructed to return for follow-up evaluation in 24 hours and the drain advanced or removed.

62. When infection erodes through the cortical plate, it does so in a predictable manner. What factors determine the location of infection from a specific tooth?
- Thickness of bone overlying the tooth apex; the thinner the bone, the more likely it is to be perforated by spreading infection.
- The relationship of the site of bony perforation to muscle attachments to the maxilla or mandible.

63. State the usual site of bone perforation, the relationship to muscle attachment, the determining muscle, and the site of localization for each tooth for odontogenic infections.

INVOLVED TEETH	USUAL SITE OF PERFORATION OF BONE	RELATION OF PERFORATION TO MUSCLE ATTACHMENT	DETERMINING MUSCLE	SITE OF LOCALIZATION
Maxilla				
Central incisor	Labial	Below	Orbicularis oris	Labial vestibule
Lateral incisor	Labial	Below	Orbicularis oris	Labial vestibule
	(palatal)*	—	—	(palatal)
Canine	Labial	Below	Levator anguli oris	Oral vestibule
	Labial	(above)	Levator anguli oris	(canine space)
Premolars	Buccal	Below	Buccinator	Buccal vestibule
Molars	Buccal	Below	Buccinator	Buccal vestibule
	Buccal	Above	Buccinator	Buccal space
	(palatal)	—	—	(palatal)
Mandible				
Incisors	Labial	Above	Mentalis	Labial vestibule
Canine	Labial	Above	Depressor anguli oris	Labial vestibule
Premolars	Buccal	Above	Buccinator	Buccal vestibule
First molar	Buccal	Above	Buccinator	Buccal vestibule
	Buccal	Below	Buccinator	Buccal space
	Lingual	Above	Mylohyoid	Sublingual space
Second molar	Buccal	Above	Buccinator	Buccal vestibule
	Buccal	Below	Buccinator	Buccal space
	Lingual	Above	Mylohyoid	Sublingual space
	Lingual	Below	Mylohyoid	Submandibular space
Third molar	Lingual	Below	Mylohyoid	Submandibular space

*Parentheses indicate rare occurrences.
Modified from Laskin DM: Anatomic considerations in diagnosis and treatment of odontogenic infections. J Am Dent Assoc 69:308, 1964.

64. What is osteoradionecrosis?
Osteoradionecrosis occurs after radiation therapy. It is most commonly noted in the mandible of patients who receive treatment for head and neck cancer and have preexisting dental infection. Thus, the frequency is higher in dentulous patients compared with edentulous patients. Prevention of osteoradionecrosis involves the elimination of infected teeth before initiation of radiation therapy. The patient who receives radiation to the head and neck remains at risk for osteoradionecrosis.

65. What are the indications for hospitalization of patients with infection?
Fever > 101°F
Dehydration
Trismus
Marked pain
Significant and/or spreading swelling
Elevation of the tongue
Bilateral submandibular swelling
Neurologic changes
Difficulty with breathing or swallowing
Leukocytosis (WBC > 10,000)
Shift of WBC to the left (increased immature neutrophils)
Systemic disease known to modify the patient's ability to fight infection
Need for parenteral antibiotics
Inability of patient to comply with traditional treatment
Need for drainage

66. What are the indications for antibiotic therapy in orofacial infection?
- Evidence of systemic involvement, such as fever, leukocytosis, malaise, fatigue, weakness, lymphadenopathy, or increased pulse
- Infection that is not localized but extending or progressing
- No response to standard surgical intervention
- Increased risk for endocarditis or systemic infection because of cardiac status, immune status, or systemic disease

67. What are fascial space infections?
Fascial spaces potentially exist between fascial layers and may become filled with purulent material from spreading orofacial infections. Spaces that become directly involved are termed spaces of primary involvement. Infections may spread to additional spaces, which are termed secondary.

68. What are the primary maxillary fascial spaces?
Canine, buccal, and infratemporal.

69. What are the primary mandibular fascial spaces?
Submental, submandibular, buccal, and sublingual.

70. What are the secondary fascial spaces?

Masseteric	Lateral pharyngeal
Pterygomandibular	Retropharyngeal
Superficial and deep temporal	Prevertebral

71. What is Ludwig's angina?
Ludwig's angina is bilateral cellulitis affecting the submandibular and sublingual spaces. Patients develop marked brawny edema with elevation of the floor of the mouth and tongue that results in airway compromise.

72. What is cavernous sinus thrombosis?
Cavernous sinus thrombosis may occur as a consequence of the hematogenous spread of maxillary odontogenic infection via the venous drainage of the maxilla. The lack of valves in the facial veins permits organisms to flow to and contaminate the cavernous sinus, thus resulting in thrombosis. Patients present with proptosis, orbital swelling, neurologic signs, and fever. The infection is life-threatening and requires prompt and aggressive treatment, consisting of elimination of the source of infection, drainage, parenteral antibiotic therapy, and neurosurgical consultation.

73. What is the antibiotic of choice for odontogenic infection?
Penicillin is the drug of choice; 95% of bacteria causing odontogenic infections respond to penicillin. For most infections, a dose of penicillin VK, 500 mg every 6 hours for 7–10 days, is adequate; 5–7% of the population, however, is allergic to penicillin.

74. What are alternative antibiotics for patients who are allergic to penicillin?
Clarithromycin, clindamycin, and azithromycin.

75. Despite the advent of numerous new antibiotics, penicillin remains the drug of choice for odontogenic infections. Why?
- It is bactericidal with a narrow spectrum of activity that includes the most common pathogens associated with odontogenic infection.
- It is safe; the toxicity associated with penicillin is low.
- It is cheap. A 10-day supply of penicillin cost under $5, compared, for example, with Augmentin, which costs the patient approximately $70.

76. List the major side effects associated with clindamycin
- Diarrhea and abdominal pain
- Nausea and vomiting
- Rash
- Pseudomembranous colitis

77. What factors govern the selection of a particular antibiotic?

Specificity

Toxicity

Cost

Ease of administration

78. When should cultures be used for odontogenic infection?
- Infection in immunocompromised patients (e.g., cancer chemotherapy, diabetes mellitus, or immunosuppressive drugs)
- Before changing antibiotics in a patient who has failed to respond to empirical therapy
- Before initiating antibiotic therapy in a patient who demonstrates signs of systemic infection

79. Why may antibiotic therapy fail?
- Lack of patient compliance
- Failure to treat the infection locally
- Inadequate dose or length of therapy
- Selection of wrong antibiotic
- Presence of resistant organisms
- Nonbacterial infection
- Failure of antibiotic to reach infected site
- Inadequate absorption of antibiotic, as when tetracycline is taken with milk products

80. Does the initiation of antibiotic therapy obviate the need for surgical intervention in a patient with an infection?

No. Failure to eliminate the source of infection through surgical intervention ultimately results in the failure of other forms of therapy.

DENTAL TRAUMA

81. What are the most important questions to ask in evaluating a patient with acute trauma?
1. How did the injury occur?
2. Where did the injury occur?
3. When did the injury occur?
4. Was the patient unconscious, or did the patient have nausea, vomiting, or headache after the accident?
5. Was there prior injury to the teeth?
6. Is there any change in the occlusion?
7. Is there any thermal sensitivity of the teeth?
8. Review of the medical history

Andreasen JO, Andreasen FM: Essentials of Traumatic Injuries to the Teeth. Copenhagen, Munksgaard, 1990.

82. Discuss the primary assessment and management of the patient with trauma.

The initial assessment and management of the traumatized patient are centered on identification of life-threatening problems. The three most significant aspects are (1) establishing and maintaining an airway, (2) adequate ventilation, (3) evaluation and support of the cardiopulmonary system, and (4) control of external hemorrhage. The patient should be assessed and treated for shock.

83. What are the methods of choice for evaluation of the pediatric patient with trauma?

History and physical examination are the mainstays in evaluating the pediatric patient with trauma. The clinician should determine the cause of the trauma, the type of injury and the direction from which it occurred. In the case of a younger child, it is helpful if an adult witnessed the traumatic event. Physical examination should determine the child's mental state, facial asymmetry, trismus, occlusion, and vision. The radiographic evaluation of choice is computed tomography.

Kaban L: Diagnosis and treatment of fractures of facial bones in children. J Oral Maxillofac Surg 51: 722–729, 1993.

84. What are the four best ways for a patient to preserve a recently avulsed tooth until he or she is seen by a dentist?

The four best ways for a patient to preserve a recently avulsed tooth are (1) to replace it immediately into the socket from which it was avulsed; (2) to place it in the mouth, under the tongue; (3) to place the tooth in milk; or (4) to place the tooth in Hank's medium.

85. How should an avulsed tooth be managed?

1. Whenever possible, avulsed teeth should be replaced into the socket within 30 minutes of avulsion. After 2 hours, associated complications such as root resorption increase significantly.

2. The tooth should not be scraped or extensively cleaned or sterilized because such procedures will damage the periodontal tissues and cementum. The tooth should be gently rinsed with saliva only.

3. The tooth should be placed in the socket with a semirigid splint for 7–14 days.

86. What should be included in the clinical evaluation of the traumatized dentition?

Mobility testing   Electric pulp testing
Percussion sensitivity   Soft-tissue evaluation

Andreasen JO, Andreasen FM: Essentials of Traumatic Injuries to the Teeth. Copenhagen, Munksgaard, 1990.

87. Describe the injuries involving the supporting structures of the dentition.

Concussion: injury to the tooth that may result in hemorrhage and edema of the periodontal ligament, but the tooth remains firm in its socket. Treatment: occlusal adjustment and soft diet.

Subluxation: loosening of the involved tooth without displacement. Treatment: same as for concussion.

Intrusion: tooth is displaced apically into the alveolar process. Treatment: if root formation is incomplete, allow the tooth to reerupt over several months; if root formation is complete, then the tooth should be repositioned orthodontically. Pulpal status must be monitored, because pulpal necrosis is frequent in the tooth with an incomplete root and close to 100% in the tooth with complete root formation.

Extrusion: tooth is partially displaced out of the socket. Treatment: manually reposition tooth into socket, and splint in position for 2–3 weeks. A radiographic examination should be performed after 2–3 weeks to rule out marginal breakdown or initiation of root resorption.

Lateral luxation: tooth is displaced horizontally, therefore resulting in fracture of the alveolar bone. Treatment: gentle repositioning of tooth into socket followed by splinting for 3 weeks. A radiographic examination should be performed after 2–3 weeks to rule out marginal breakdown or initiation of root resorption.

Avulsion: total displacement of the tooth out of the socket. Treatment: rapid reimplantation is the ideal. The tooth should be held by the clinical crown and not by the root. Rinse the tooth in saline, and flush the socket with saline. Replant the tooth, and splint in place with semirigid splint for 1 week. Place the patient on antibiotic therapy. Assess the patient's tetanus prophylaxis status and treat appropriately. If the apex is closed, a calcium hydroxide pulpectomy should be initiated at the time the splint is removed. If the tooth cannot be replanted immediately, placing it in Hank's medium, milk, or saliva aids in maintaining the vitality of the periodontal and pulpal tissues. Follow-up radiographic examinations should be performed at 3 and 6 weeks and at 3 and 6 months.

88. What are the types and characteristics of the resorption phenomenon that may follow a traumatic injury?

Inflammatory external and internal resorption occurs when necrotic pulp has become infected, leading to resorption of the external surface of the root or the pulp chamber and/or canal. Immediate treatment with a calcium pulpectomy is indicated to arrest the process. **Replacement resorption** occurs after damage to the periodontal ligament results in contact of cementum with bone. As the root cementum is resorbed, it is replaced by bone, resulting in ankylosis of the involved tooth.

89. When can the above forms of resorption be detected radiographically?

It is possible to detect periapical radiolucencies that indicate internal and external resorption after 3 weeks. Replacement resorption may be detected after 6 weeks.

90. Why should radiographs of the soft tissue be included in evaluation of a patient with dental trauma?

It is not uncommon for fragments of fractured teeth to puncture and imbed themselves into the oral soft tissue. Clinical examination is often inadequate to detect these foreign bodies.

91. When a lip laceration is encountered, what part of the lip is the most important landmark and the first area to be reapproximated?

The vermilion border, the area of transition of mucosal tissue to skin, is evaluated and approximated first. An irregular vermilion margin is unesthetic and difficult to correct secondarily.

92. How should a small avulsion of the lip be managed?

Avulsions can be treated with primary closure if no more than one-fourth of the lip is lost. The tissue margins should be excised so that the wound has smooth, regular margins.

93. How should a full-thickness, mucosa-to-skin laceration of the lip be closed? Which layers should be sutured?

A layer closure ensures an optimal cosmetic and functional results. First a 5-0 nylon suture is placed at the vermilion border. The muscle layer, the subcutaneous layer, and the mucosa layer are closed with 4-0 resorbable sutures; then the skin layer is closed with a 5-0 or 6-0 nylon suture.

94. How should a facial laceration that extends into dermis or fat be closed?

Wounds that extend into dermis or fat should be closed in layers. The dermis should be closed with 4-0 absorbable sutures, the skin with 5-0 or 6-0 nonabsorbable sutures.

95. Why is a layered closure important?

A layered wound closure reestablishes anatomic alignment and avoids dead space, thus reducing the risk of infection and scar formation. Closure of the muscle and subcutaneous tissue layers minimizes tension in the skin layer and thus allows eversion of the skin edges, which results in the most esthetic scar.

96. What structures are at risk when a facial laceration occurs posterior to the anterior margin of the masseter muscle and inferior to the level of the zygomatic arch?

The buccal branch of the facial nerve and the parotid gland duct are at risk with lacerations in this position. When such a laceration is encountered, facial nerve function must be tested, along with salivary flow from the parotid duct.

97. What is a dentoalveolar fracture? How is it treated?

A dentoalveolar fracture is a fracture of a segment of the alveolus and the tooth within that segment. This fracture usually occurs in anterior regions. Treatment consists of reduction of the segment to its original position or best position relative to the opposing dentition, because it may not be possible to determine the exact position before injury. The segment is then stabilized with a rigid splint for 4–6 weeks.

98. What is the Le Fort classification of fractures?

Le Fort I	Horizontal segmented fracture of the alveolar process of the maxilla (also called Guérin's fracture and low maxillary fracture)
Le Fort II	Unilateral or bilateral fracture of the maxilla, in which the body of the maxilla is separated from the facial skeleton and the separated portion is pyramidal in shape; the fracture may extend through the body of the maxilla down the midline of the hard palate, through the floor of the orbit, and into the nasal cavity (also called pyramidal fracture)
Le Fort III	Fracture in which the entire maxilla and one or more facial bones are completely separated from the craniofacial skeleton (also called craniofacial dysjunction)

99. Describe the Ellis classification of dental fractures.

Class I	Enamel only
Class II	Dentin and enamel
Class III	Dentin, enamel, and pulp
Class IV	Whole crown

100. Describe the management of each of the above fractures.

Class I	Enameloplasty and/or bonding
Class II	Dentin coverage with calcium hydroxide and bonded restoration or reattachment of fractured segment
Class III	Pulp therapy via pulp capping or partial pulpotomy
Class IV	If the fracture is supragingival, remove the coronal segment and perform appropriate pulp therapy, then restore. If the fracture is subgingival, remove the coronal segment and perform appropriate pulp therapy, then reposition the remaining tooth structure coronally either orthodontically or surgically. The surgical approach results in loss of pulpal vitality and therefore requires a pulpectomy.

101. What are the most likely signs and symptoms of a mandibular body or angle fracture?

Alteration in occlusion	Mobility at the fracture site
A step or change in the mandibular occlusal plane	Pain at the fracture site
Lower lip numbness	Bleeding at the fracture site or submucosal hemorrhage

102. How is a displaced fracture of the mandibular body or angle treated?

A displaced mandibular fracture is treated by open reduction and rigid internal fixation. Arch bars are placed on the teeth and used with either intermaxillary wires or elastics to establish the preoperative occlusion. This procedure involves exposing the mandible through an incision, reducing the fracture, and fixing the fracture segments with rigid plates and screws. In many cases, rigid internal fixation can be used to avoid intermaxillary fixation. These cases are treated by exposing the fracture area and applying a rigid fixation plate that provides absolute interosseous stability of the fracture. Intermaxillary fixation usually is not required.

103. What are the two causes of mandibular fracture displacement?

Mandible fractures are displaced by the force that causes the fractures and by the muscles of mastication. Depending on the orientation of the fracture line, the attached muscles may cause significant displacement of the segments.

104. Are most fractures of the mandibular condyle treated by closed or open reduction?

Most fractures of the mandibular condyle are treated by closed reduction. Treatment usually consists of 1–3 weeks of intermaxillary fixation followed by mobilization and close follow-up.

105. What radiographs are used to diagnose mandibular fractures?

- CT scan
- Panoramic radiograph
- Occlusal radiograph
- Mandibular series
  Lateral oblique views
  Posteroanterior view
  Towne's view

106. What are the likely signs and symptoms of a zygomatic fracture?

Pain over zygomatic region	Submucosal hemorrhage or ecchymosis
Numbness in the infraorbital nerve distribution	Subconjunctival hemorrhage or ecchymosis
Swelling in the zygomatic region	Submucosal or subconjunctival air
Depression or flatness of the zygomatic prominence	Palpable step at the infraorbital rim (emphysema) Exophthalmos
Nasal bleeding	Diplopia
	Unequal pupil level

107. Which radiographs are used to evaluate and diagnose zygomatic fractures?

1. CT scan
2. Plain film
   Waters' view (posteroanterior obliques)
   Submental vertex

108. Which bones articulate with the zygoma?

- Frontal bone
- Sphenoid bone
- Maxillary bone
- Temporal bone

109. How may mandibular function be affected by a fracture of the zygoma or zygomatic arch?

A depressed zygoma or zygomatic arch fracture can impinge on the coronoid process or temporalis muscle, causing various degrees of hypomobility.

110. Define neurapraxia.

Neurapraxia is the mildest form of nerve injury and denotes a localized conduction block along a nerve. Axonal continuity is maintained, and nerve conduction proximal and distal to the lesion is preserved. No treatment other than documentation of the area of injury is required. Recovery is generally rapid, and impulse conduction is complete within weeks.

111. Define axonotmesis.

Axonotmesis denotes sufficient damage to disrupt the continuity of axons within the connective tissue of the peripheral nerve. Conduction block is complete and distal axon degeneration follows the injury. Prognosis is good because of the continuity of the supportive connective tissue and basement membrane.

112. What is neurotomesis?

The most severe type of injury is neurotemesis. Complete anatomic severance of the peripheral nerve occurs, and no recovery is expected without surgical cooptation of the ends of the fibers. Proximal and distal degeneration is present.

LOCAL ANESTHESIA

113. What are the major classifications of local anesthetics used in dentistry?

Classification of local anesthetics is based on the molecular linkage between hydrophilic and lipophilic groups of the molecule. The amides, such as xylocaine and mepivacaine, are the most commonly used class of local anesthetics and for the most part have replaced esters, such as procaine.

114. Do all local anesthetics used in dentistry have the same duration of action?

No. Long-lasting local anesthetics, such as marcaine, provide surgical grade anesthesia about three times longer than generally used anesthetics, such as lidocaine.

115. What is the role of pH in determining the effectiveness of a local anesthetic?

Anesthetic solutions are acid salts of weak bases and have a pH in the range of 3.3–5.5. For the molecule to be active, the uncharged base must be available. If the tissue into which the solution is placed has a pH lower than the anesthetic solution, dissociation does not occur, and the amount of active base available is not adequate for a substantial anesthetic effect. A clinical example of this phenomenon is the injection of local anesthesia into an area of infection.

116. What are the advantages of including epinephrine in a local anesthetic solution?

There are two major advantages of including epinephrine in local anesthesia: (1) because epinephrine is a vasoconstrictor, it helps to maintain an optimal level of local anesthesia at the site of injection and thus reduces permeation of the drug into adjacent tissue, and (2) the vasoconstrictive properties of epinephrine also result in reduced intraoperative bleeding.

117. How significant is the concentration of epinephrine in local anesthetic solutions in affecting their hemostatic properties?

No difference in the degree or duration of hemostasis has been noted when solutions containing epinephrine of 1:100,000, 1:400,000 or 1:800,000 were compared. Five minutes should be allowed for epinephrine to achieve its maximal effect.

118. Which nerves are anesthetized using the Gow-Gates technique?

1. Inferior alveolar nerve
2. Lingual nerve
3. Mylohyoid nerve
4. Auriculotemporal nerve
5. Buccal nerve

119. Describe the best type of injections of local anesthesia for extractions of the following teeth:

Maxillary lateral incisor	Infiltration at apex
	Infiltration of buccal soft tissue
	Nasopalatine block
Maxillary first molar	Infiltration at apex
	Infiltration over mesial root and over apex of maxillary second molar
	Anterior palatine block
Mandibular canine	Inferior alveolar block
	Lingual nerve block
Mandibular second molar	Inferior alveolar block
	Lingual nerve block
	Buccal block

Peterson LJ, Ellis E, Hupp JR, Tucker MR: Contemporary Oral and Maxillofacial Surgery. St. Louis, Mosby, 1988.

120. What are the symptoms and treatment for inadvertent injection of the facial nerve during the administration of local anesthesia?

The muscles of facial expression are paralyzed. The condition is temporary and self-limiting. However, the patient's eye should be protected, because closure of the eye on blinking may be limited.

121. How does a hematoma form after the administration of a local anesthetic? How is it treated?

Hematoma may occur when the needle passes through a blood vessel and results in bleeding into the surrounding tissue. Posterosuperior alveolar nerve blocks are most often associated with hematoma formation, although injection into any area, particularly a foramen, may have a similar result. Treatment of hematoma includes direct pressure and immediate application of ice. The patient should be informed of the hematoma and reassured. In healthy patients, the area should resolve in about 2 weeks. In patients at risk for infection, hematomas may act as a focus of bacterial growth. Consequently, such patients should be placed on an appropriate antibiotic.

122. What are the reasons for postinjection pain after the administration of a local anesthetic?

The most common causes of postinjection pain are related to injury of the periosteum, which results either from tearing of the tissue or from deposition of solution beneath the tissue.

123. What causes blanching of the skin after the injection of local anesthesia?

Arterial spasms caused by needle trauma to the vessel may result in sudden blanching of the overlying skin. No treatment is required. Epinephrine causes vasoconstriction.

124. What is the toxic dose of most local anesthetics used in dentistry? What is the maximal volume of a 2% solution of local anesthetic that can be administered?

The toxic dose for most local anesthetics used in dentistry is 300–500 mg. The standard carpule of local anesthetic contains 1.8 cc of solution. Thus, a 2% solution of lidocaine contains 36 mg of drug (2% solution = 20 mg/ml × 1.8 ml = 36 mg). Ten carpules or more are in the toxic range.

125. What is the most common adverse reaction to local anesthesia? How is it treated?

Syncope is the most common adverse reaction associated with administration of local anesthesia. Almost half of the medical emergencies that occur in dental practice fall into this category. Syncope typically is the consequence of a vasovagal reaction. Treatment is based on early recognition of a problem; the patient often feels uneasy, queasy, sweaty, or lightheaded. The patient should be reassured and positioned so that the feet are higher than the head (Trendelenburg position); oxygen is administered. Tight clothing should be loosened and a cold compress placed on the forehead. Vital signs should be monitored and recorded. Ammonia inhalants are helpful in stimulating the patient.

POSTOPERATIVE MANAGEMENT AND WOUND HEALING

126. What are the principal components of postoperative orders?
- Diagnosis and surgical procedure
- Patient's condition
- Allergies
- Instructions for monitoring of vital signs
- Instructions for activity and positioning
- Diet
- Medications
- Intravenous fluids
- Wound care
- Parameters for notification of dentist
- Special instructions

Peterson LJ, Ellis E, Hupp JR, Tucker MR: Contemporary Oral and Maxillofacial Surgery. St. Louis, Mosby, 1988.

127. What is "dead space"?

Dead space is the area in a wound that is free of tissue after closure. An example is a cyst cavity after enucleation of the cyst. Because dead space often fills with blood and fibrin, it has the potential to become a site of infection.

128. What are the four ways that dead space can be eliminated?

1. Loosely suture the tissue planes together so that the formation of a postoperative void is minimized.

2. Place pressure on the wound to obliterate the space.

3. Place packing into the void until bleeding has stopped.

4. Place a drain into the space.

129. What is postoperative ecchymosis? How does it occur? How is it managed?

Ecchymosis is a black and blue area that develops as blood seeps submucosally after surgical manipulation. It is a self-limiting condition that looks more dangerous than it actually is. Patients should be warned that it may occur. Although no specific treatment is indicated, moist heat often speeds resolution.

130. What are the causes of postoperative swelling after an oral surgical procedure?

Swelling due to edema usually reaches its maximum 48–72 hours after the procedure and then resolves spontaneously. It can be minimized by application of cold compress to the surgical site for 20-minute intervals on the day of surgery. Beginning on the third postoperative day, moist heat may be applied to swollen areas. Patients should be informed of the possibility of swelling. Swelling after the third postoperative day, especially if it is new, may be a sign of infection, for which patients need appropriate assessment and management.

131. What is primary hemorrhage? How should it be treated?

Primary hemorrhage is postoperative bleeding that occurs immediately after an extraction. In essence, the wound does not stop bleeding. To permit clear visualization and localization of the site of bleeding, the mouth should be irrigated thoroughly with saline. The patient's overall condition should be assessed. Once the general site of bleeding is identified, pressure should be applied for 20–30 minutes. Extraneous granulation tissue or tissue fragments should be carefully debrided. If the source of the bleeding is soft tissue (e.g., gingiva), sutures should be applied. If the source is bone, bone wax can be applied. Placement of a hemostatic agent, such as a surgical gel, in the socket may be followed by the placement of interrupted sutures. The patient should be instructed to bite on gauze for 30 minutes. At the end of that time, coagulation should be confirmed before the patient is dismissed.

A clot may fail to form because of a quantitative or functional platelet deficiency. The former is most readily assessed by obtaining a platelet count. The normal platelet count is 200,000–500,000 cells/mm³. Prolonged bleeding may occur if platelets fall below 100,000 cells/mm³. Treatment of severe thrombocytopenia may require platelet transfusion. Qualitative platelet dysfunction most often results from aspirin ingestion and is most commonly measured by determining the bleeding time. Prolonged bleeding time requires consultation with a hematologist.

132. What is secondary hemorrhage? How is it treated?

Secondary hemorrhage occurs several days after extraction and may be due to clot breakdown, infection, or irritation to the wound. The mouth first should be thoroughly irrigated and the source of the bleeding identified. The wound should be debrided. Sources of local irritation should be eliminated. The placement of sutures or a hemostatic agent may be necessary. Patients with infection should be placed on an antibiotic. If local measures fail to stem the bleeding, additional studies, especially relative to fibrin formation, are indicated.

133. Describe the stages of wound healing.

The **inflammatory stage** begins immediately after tissue injury and consists of a vascular phase and a cellular phase. In the vascular phase initial vasoconstriction is followed by vasodilatation, which is mediated by histamine and prostaglandins. The cellular phase is initiated by the complement system, which acts to attract neutrophils to the wound site. Lymphocytic infiltration follows. Epithelial migration begins at the wound margins.

During the **fibroplastic stage**, wound repair is mediated by fibroblasts. New blood vessels form, and collagen is produced in excessive amounts. Foreign and necrotic material is removed. Epithelial migration continues.

In the **remodeling stage**, the final stage of wound healing, collagen fibers are arranged in an orderly fashion to increase tissue strength. Epithelial healing is completed.

134. What is the difference between healing by primary and secondary intention?

In healing by primary intention, the edges of the wound are approximated as they were before injury, with no tissue loss. An example is the healing of a surgical incision. In contrast, wounds that heal by secondary intention involve tissue loss, such as an extraction site.

135. What are the five phases of healing of extraction wounds?

1. Hemorrhage and clot formation
2. Organization of the clot by granulation tissue
3. Replacement of granulation tissue by connective tissue and epithelialization of the wound
4. Replacement of the connective tissue by woven bone
5. Recontouring of the alveolar bone and bone maturation

IMPLANTOLOGY

136. What are dental implants?

Dental implants are devices that are placed into bone to act as abutments or supports for prostheses.

137. Describe the bone-implant interface found in osseointegrated implants.

Osseointegrated (osteointegrated) implants interface directly with the bone, resulting in a relationship that mimics ankylosis of a tooth to bone. Osseointegrated implants are made of titanium.

138. What are the requirements for successful implant placement?

- Biocompatibility
- Mucosal seal
- Adequate transfer of force

139. The surgical placement of most osseointegrated implants can require two steps. What are they? How long between them?

The first step is the actual placement of the implant. Implants can be covered with soft tissue during the time that they integrate with bone. This process takes between 3–6 months. After this period, a second surgical procedure is performed, during which the implant is exposed. Some brands of implants are not "buried" during the period of osseointegration, and therefore do not require a second surgical procedure.

140. Describe the major indications for the consideration of implants as a treatment alternative.

- Resorption of alveolar ridge or other anatomic consideration does not allow for adequate retention of conventional removable prostheses
- Patient is psychologically unable to deal with removable prostheses
- Medical condition for which removable prostheses may create a risk, i.e., seizure disorder
- Patient has a pronounced gag reflex that does not permit the placement of a removable prosthesis
- Loss of posterior teeth, particularly unilaterally
- Adjacent teeth are without decay or extensive restoration

141. What are the major contraindications for the placement of implants?
- Pathology within the bone
- Limiting anatomic structures such as the inferior alveolar nerve or maxillary sinus
- Unrealistic outcome expectations from patient
- Poor oral health and hygiene
- Patient inability to tolerate implant procedures because of a medical or psychological condition
- Inadequate quantity/quality of bone

142. What is the prognosis of osseointegrated implants placed in an edentulous mandible? Maxilla?

According to studies with implants developed by Branemark, the stability of implant-supported continuous bridges for a 5- to 12-year period was 100% in the mandible and 90% in the maxilla.

143. What are the steps in the assessment of patients prior to implant placement?
- Medical and dental history
- Clinical examination
- Radiographic examination

144. Which radiographic studies are used for patient assessment before implant placement?

For many implant cases, panoramic and periapical radiographs provide adequate information relative to bone volume and the location of limiting anatomic structures. In some instances, CT may be especially useful in providing information relative to multiplanar jaw configuration.

145. During preparation of the implant recipient site, what is the maximal temperature that should develop at the drill-bone interface?

To prevent necrosis of bone, a maximal temperature of 40° C has been recommended. This goal is achieved through the use of copious external or internal saline irrigation and low-speed, high-torque drills. In the final step of implant site preparation, the drill rotates at a speed of only 10–15 rpm.

146. What is the best way to ensure proper implant placement and orientation?

Careful pretreatment evaluation and preparation by *both* surgeon and restoring dentist are critical. A surgical stent fabricated to the specifications of the restoring dentist is an extremely helpful technique. Lack of pretreatment communication and planning may result in implants that are successfully integrated but impossible to restore.

147. Do any data suggest that osseointegration of implants may occur when implants are placed into an extraction site?

Some data suggest that placement of an implant into an extraction site may be successful, especially if the implant extends apically beyond the depth of the extraction site. Conventional treatment, however, consists of a period of 3 months from extraction to implant placement.

148. What anatomic feature of the anterior maxilla must be evaluated before placement of an implant in the central incisor region?

The incisor foramen must be carefully evaluated radiographically and clinically. Variations in size, shape, and position determine the position of maxillary anterior implants. Fixtures should not be placed directly into the foramen.

149. Which anatomic site is the most likely to yield failed implants?

Implants placed in the maxillary anterior region are the most likely to fail. Because short implants are more likely to fail than longer implants, the longest implant that is compatible with the supporting bone and adjacent anatomy should be used.

150. Do definitive data support the contention that implanted supported teeth should not be splinted to natural teeth?

This issue is controversial, but available data refute the claim that bridges with both implant and natural tooth abutments do more poorly than bridges supported only by implants.

Gunne J, Astrand P, Ahlen K, et al: Implants in partially edentulous patients: A longitudinal study of bridges supported by both implants and natural teeth. Clin Oral Implant Res 3:49–56, 1992.

151. Is there any reason to avoid the use of fluorides in implant recipients?

Yes. Acidulated fluoride preparations may corrode the surface of titanium implants.

152. Do implants need periodic maintenance once they are placed?

Like natural teeth, poorly maintained implants may demonstrate progressive loss of supporting bone, which may result in implant failure. Aggressive home care is necessary to ensure implant success. Plastic-tipped instruments are available for professional cleaning.

153. What is the most common sign that an implant is failing?

Mobility of the implant is regarded as an unequivocal sign of implant failure.

PAIN SYNDROMES AND TEMPOROMANDIBULAR JOINT DISORDERS

154. What is trigeminal neuralgia?

Trigeminal neuralgia, or tic douloureux, results in severe, lancinating pain in a predictable anatomic location innervated by the fifth cranial nerve. The pain typically is of short duration but extremely intense. Stimulation of a trigger point initiates the onset of pain. Possible etiologies include multiple sclerosis, vascular compression of the trigeminal nerve roots as they emerge from the brain, demyelination of the gasserian ganglia, trauma, and infection.

155. Discuss the treatment of trigeminal neuralgia.

Drug therapy is the primary treatment for most forms of trigeminal neuralgia. Carbamazepine and antiepileptic drugs are used most often. If drug therapy fails, surgical intervention may be necessary. Surgical options include rhizotomy and nerve decompression.

156. What symptoms are associated with temporomandibular (TMJ) disorders?

TMJ disorders are characterized by the presence of one or more of the following:
- Preauricular pain and tenderness
- Limitation of mandibular motion
- Noise in the joint during condylar movement
- Pain and spasm of the muscles of mastication

157. What are the two most common joint sounds associated with TMJ disorders? How do they differ?

Clicking and crepitus are the two most common joint sounds associated with TMJ disorders. Clicking is a distinct popping or snapping sound; crepitus is a scraping, continuous sound. Sounds are best distinguished by use of a stethoscope.

158. What are the components of evaluation of the patient with TMJ symptoms?

Evaluation of the patient with TMJ symptoms should include a detailed history of the problem, a thorough physical examination, and appropriate radiographic and imaging studies.

159. What should be included in the physical examination of the patient with TMJ symptoms?

- Gross observation of the face to determine asymmetry
- Palpation of the muscles of mastication

- Observation of mandibular motion
- Palpation of the joint
- Auscultation of the joint
- Intraoral examination of the dentition and occlusion

160. What are the parameters for normal mandibular motion?

The normal vertical motion of the mandible results in 50 mm of intraincisor distance. Lateral and protrusive movement should range to approximately 10 mm.

161. What radiographic and imaging studies are of value in evaluating the TMJ?

Panoramic radiograph is a baseline screening radiograph. However, to identify bony disease of the joint and surrounding structures computed tomographic studies provide the most definitive information. Magnetic resonance imaging (MRI) is the technique of choice to evaluate soft-tissue changes (disc displacement) within the joint.

162. What is the likelihood that a patient with TMJ symptoms will demonstrate identifiable pathology of the joint?

Only 5–7% of patients presenting with TMJ symptoms have identifiable pathology of the joint. Based on this frequency, it clearly makes sense to proceed initially with conservative, reversible treatment.

163. What is the most common disorder associated with the TMJ?

Myofascial pain dysfunction (MPD) is the most common clinical problem associated with the TMJ.

164. What is the cause of MPD?

The cause of MPD is multifactorial. Functional, occlusal, and psychological factors have been associated with its onset. Fortunately, most cases are self-limited.

165. What occlusal factors may contribute to MPD?

Clenching and bruxing may be associated with MPD, because they may result in muscle spasm. Lack of posterior occlusion, which results in changes in the relationship of the jaws, also is a potential cause. The placement of restorations or prostheses that alter the occlusion may cause MPD directly or indirectly through the patient's attempt to accommodate changes in vertical dimension.

166. What patient group is at highest risk for MPD?

Of patients with MPD, 70–90% are women between the ages of 20 and 40 years.

167. What are the diagnostic criteria for myofascial pain syndrome?

1. Tender areas in the firm bands of the muscles, tendons, or ligaments that elicit pain on palpation
2. Regional pain referred from the point of pain initiation
3. Slightly diminished range of motion

Sturdivant J, Fricton JR: Physical therapy for temporomandibular disorders and orofacial pain. Curr Opin Dent 1:485–496, 1991.

168. What signs and symptoms are associated with MPD?

Patients with MPD may have some or all of the following:

- Pain on palpation of the muscles of mastication
- Pain on palpation of the joint
- Pain on movement of the joint

- Altered TMJ function, including trismus, reduced opening, and mandibular deviation on opening
- Joint popping, clicking or crepitus
- Stiffness of the jaws
- Facial pain

169. What radiographic findings are associated with MPD?

None. Radiographic studies of the joint of patients with MPD fail to demonstrate the presence of pathology.

170. Describe the treatment approach to MPD.

Because most cases of MPD are self-limiting, a conservative, reversible approach to intervention is recommended. Patients should be informed of the condition and its frequency in the overall population (patients always feel better knowing that they have something that is "going around" rather than some rare, exotic disease), then reassured. Mobility of the joint should be minimized. A soft diet, limited talking, and elimination of gum chewing should be recommended. Moist heat, applied to the face, is often helpful in relieving muscle spasms. Muscle relaxants (flexeril) and benzodiazepores can be prescribed. Pain symptoms generally respond to nonsteroidal antiinflammatory agents. For patients with evidence of occlusal trauma or abnormal function, fabrication of an occlusal appliance may be helpful.

171. What are the indications for superficial heat in the treatment of facial muscle and TMJ pain?

1. To reduce muscle spasm and myofascial pain
2. To stimulate removal of inflammatory byproducts
3. To induce relaxation and sedation
4. To increase cutaneous blood flow

Sturdivant J, Fricton JR: Physical therapy for temporomandibular disorders and orofacial pain. Curr Opin Dent 1:485–496, 1991.

172. What are the contraindications for using superficial heat to treat facial pain?

1. Acute infection
2. Impaired sensation or circulation
3. Noninflammatory edema
4. Multiple sclerosis

Sturdivant J, Fricton JR: Physical therapy for temporomandibular disorders and orofacial pain. Curr Opin Dent 1:485–496, 1991.

173. What is the function of ultrasound in the therapy of myofascial pain?

Ultrasound provides deep heat to musculoskeletal tissues through the use of sound waves. It is indicated for treatment of muscle spasm or contracture, inflammation of the TMJ, and increased sensitivity of the joint ligament or capsule. It is contraindicated in areas of acute inflammation, infection, cancer, impaired sensation, or noninflammatory edema. Ultrasound is typically administered by a physical therapist.

174. What is internal derangement of the TMJ?

Although internal derangement refers to disturbances among the articulating components within the TMJ, it is generally applied to denote changes in the relationship of the disc and the condyle.

175. What are the main categories of internal derangement?

- Anterior displacement of the disc with reduction, in which the meniscus is displaced anteriorly when the patient is in a closed-mouth position but reduces to its normal position on opening. Patients experience a click on both opening and closing.

- Anterior displacement of the disc without reduction (also called a closed lock)
- Disc displacement with perforation

176. What are the common symptoms of internal derangement?
- Pain, usually in the preauricular area and usually constant, increasing with function
- Earache
- Tinnitus
- Headache
- Joint noise
- Deviation of the mandible on opening

177. What imaging techniques are useful in the diagnosis of internal derangement?
MRI is the imaging techniques of choice for evaluating soft-tissue changes of the joint.

178. What is the treatment of internal derangement?
Initial treatment should be similar to MPD and is successful in a reasonable number of cases, particularly in patients with anterior disc displacement with reduction. Surgical intervention may be required in patients who do not respond to conservative therapy.

179. What are the most common causes of ankylosis of the TMJ?
Infection and trauma are the most common causes of ankylosis caused by pathologic changes of joint structures. Severe limitation of TMJ function also may be caused by non-TMJ factors, such as contracture of the masticatory muscles, tetanus, psychogenic factors, bone disease, tumor, or surgery.

180. Are tumors of the TMJ common?
No. Tumors of the joint itself are rare. However, benign connective tumors are common, including osteomas, chondromas, and osteochondromas. Both benign and malignant tumors also may affect structures adjacent to the joint and thereby affect TMJ function.

181. What is the effect of radiation therapy on the TMJ?
Patients receiving radiation therapy for the treatment of head and neck cancer may experience fibrotic changes of the joint. Consequently, they have difficulty with opening. Exercise may help to minimize such functional changes.

182. What is the effect of orthodontic therapy on the development of temporomandibular dysfunction?
The results of many well-controlled scientific studies have revealed no causal relationship between orthodontics and temporomandibular dysfunction.

183. What about extraction therapy?
Again, the results of several well-controlled studies offer no support to the contention that extraction therapy may precipitate TMJ disorders.

184. What degenerative diseases can affect the TMJ?
Osteoarthritis, rheumatoid arthritis, and psoriatic arthritis may affect the TMJ. Over time, radiographs may demonstrate degenerative changes of joint structures. Often patients have a history of one of these conditions elsewhere in the body.

ACKNOWLEDGMENT

The authors thank Willie L. Stephens, D.D.S., for his contribution to compiling the questions for this chapter.

BIBLIOGRAPHY

1. Andreasen JO, Andreasen FM: Essentials of Traumatic Injuries to the Teeth. Copenhagen, Munksgaard, 1990.
2. Branemark P, Zarb G, Alberktsson T (eds): Tissue-integrated Prostheses. Chicago, Quintessence Books, 1985.
3. Donoff RB (ed): Manual of Oral and Maxillofacial Surgery. St. Louis, Mosby, 1987.
4. Kwon PH, Kaskin DM (eds): Clinician's Manual of Oral and Maxillofacial Surgery. Chicago, Quintessence Publishing, 1991.
5. Laskin DM (ed): Oral and Maxillofacial Surgery. St. Louis, Mosby, 1980.
6. Peterson LJ, Ellis E, Hupp JR, Tucker MR: Contemporary Oral and Maxillofacial Surgery. St. Louis, Mosby, 1988.
7. Smith RA: New developments and advances in dental implantology. Curr Opin Dent 2:42, 1992.
8. Tarnow DP: Dental implants in periodontal care. Curr Opin Periodontol 157, 1993.

11. PEDIATRIC DENTISTRY AND ORTHODONTICS

Andrew L. Sonis, D.M.D.

1. What is the difference between natal and neonatal teeth?

Natal teeth are present at birth, whereas neonatal teeth emerge through the gingiva during the first month of life.

2. How common are natal teeth?

There is a large range in the reported incidence of natal teeth. The study by Kates et al., which used two methods of determining incidence, reported the following results: 1 in 3667 birth and 1 in 716 births, respectively. In previous studies, the incidence ranged from 1 in 1000 births to 1 in 30,000 births.

3. Summarize the characteristics of natal teeth.

- 95% are the actual primary teeth; 5% are supernumerary teeth.
- All natal teeth observed in the study by Kates et al. were mandibular central incisors.
- A family history of natal teeth has been established in previous studies; the incidence of a positive family history ranges from 8% to 46%.
- When natal teeth erupt, the enamel is at the normal histologic age for the child. Because the teeth erupt prematurely, the enamel matrix is not fully calcified and wears off quickly. Once the gingival covering is lost, the enamel cannot continue to mature.

4. How are natal teeth managed?

In general, natal teeth are left alone unless they cause difficulty for the infant or mother. Clinical complications include ulceration of the tongue, lingual frenum, or mother's nipple during breast-feeding. Because natal teeth are usually quite mobile, some people worry about aspiration; however, no cases of aspiration have been reported. Treatment includes grinding to smoothen the incisal surface or extraction of the tooth. In three reports, a breast-feeding splint was fabricated. In one study, half of the natal teeth were removed or lost before 4 months of age. If the teeth survive past 4 months of age, the prognosis for continued survival is good; most natal teeth, however, are not esthetically pleasing because of enamel dysplasia.

Kates GA, Needleman HL, Holmes LB: Natal and neonatal teeth: A clinical study. J Am Dent Assoc 109:441–443, 1984.

5. What should be included in an infant dental health program?

1. Prenatal oral health counseling for parents
   - Counsel parents about their own oral health habits and their effect as role models.
   - Discuss pregnancy-related gingivitis.
   - Review **infant dental care:** (1) clean gums daily before eruption of the first primary tooth to help establish healthy oral flora and (2) do not use dentifrice to avoid fluoride ingestion.
   - Review **oral care for toddlers** (1–3 years of age): (1) introduce soft toothbrush, (2) use pea-sized amount of dentifrice at age 2 years, (3) allow child to begin brushing with supervision (parents should remain primary oral caregiver), and (4) discuss timing of eruption of primary teeth and teething.
   - Review of **preschool oral care** (3–6 years of age): (1) parents should continue to supervise and help with oral hygiene, (2) continue with pea-sized amount of dentifrice, and (3) start flossing if teeth are in contact with each other.

2. Discussion of **baby-bottle tooth decay** and how it can be prevented.
   - Avoid putting child to sleep with a bottle.
   - Avoid nocturnal breast-feeding after the first primary tooth begins to erupt.
   - Always avoid juice by bottle.
   - Encourage drinking from a cup around the first birthday.
3. Discussion of timing of first dental visit (see question 7)
Edelstein B: Pediatr Ann 27:569, 1998.

6. What is meant by anticipatory guidance?
Anticipatory guidance is the deliberate and systematic distribution of information to parents as a tool to help them know what to expect, how to prevent unwanted conditions or events, and what to do when an anticipated or unexpected event occurs. Information should include dental and oral development, fluoride status, nonnutritive oral habits (see questions 8–10), injury prevention, oral hygiene, and the effects of diet on the dentition.
Sanchez DM, Childers NK: Anticipatory Guidance in Oral Health: Rationale and Recommendations. American Academy of Family Physicians, 2001.

7. When should children have their first visit to the dentist?
Currently, the American Academy of Pediatric Dentistry (AAPD) and the American Dental Association (ADA) recommend an initial oral evaluation within 6 months of the eruption of the first primary tooth and no later than the child's first birthday. At this visit, the dentist should complete thorough medical and dental histories (covering prenatal, perinatal, and postnatal periods) as well as an oral examination. After completing these tasks, the dentist can best formulate a tailored prevention care plan based on the patient's risk of developing oral and dental disease. In addition, the dentist can use this appointment to provide anticipatory guidance (see question 6).
AAPD Reference Manual: Clinical Guidelines on Infant Oral Health Care. American Academy of Pediatric Dentistry, 2001–2002.
ADA News Release: Baby's First Dental Visit. American Dental Association, 2001.

8. What are nonnutritional sucking habits?
Nonnutritional sucking habits are learned patterns of muscular contraction. The most common types are as follows:
   - Finger habit
   - Lip wetting or sucking
   - Abnormal swallowing or tongue thrusting
   - Abnormal muscular habits

Sucking is the best-developed avenue of sensation for an infant. Deprivation may cause an infant to suck on the thumb or finger for additional gratification.

9. Are nonnutritional sucking habits harmful to the dentoalveolar structures?
If a child stops nonnutritional sucking habits within 3 years of life, the damage usually is limited to the maxillary anterior segment and presents as an open bite. If the habit continues past 3 years, the damage may be long-lasting and detrimental to the developing dentoalveolar structures. After 4 years of age, a finger habit can become well established and is much harder to stop. Oral structures can become further deformed by palatal constriction and posterior crossbite.

Tongue and lip habits are often associated with a finger habit and produce added compensatory forces that can lead to full-blown malocclusion. Thumb and finger habits can cause an anterior open bite, facial movement of the upper incisors, lingual movement of the lower incisors, and constriction of the maxillary arch. Lip sucking and lip biting can procline the maxillary incisors, retrocline the mandibular incisors, and increase the amount of overjet.

Tongue thrusting and mouth breathing also may play a part in the creation of a malocclusion. An anterior open bite is the most common dental problem associated with the anomalies.

10. Describe intervention therapy for nonnutritional sucking habits.

1. Ideally the patient should understand the problem and want to correct it.

2. The timing of intervention is controversial. Some authors suggest that therapy should begin around age 4 years to prevent irreversible changes, whereas others suggest waiting until the patient is about 6–7 years old to ensure that he or she can understand the intent of therapy.

3. Patients who decide to accept appliance therapy should have support and encouragement from their parents to help them during treatment.

4. The dentist should know the patient well in order to provide intervention and advice at the correct time.

5. The dentist should be able to evaluate the deformity and the extent of its effects so that it can be treated in the best possible manner.

11. What is the current schedule of systemic fluoride supplementation?

Fluoride Supplementation

AGE	FLUORIDE CONCENTRATION IN LOCAL WATER SUPPLY (ppm)		
	< 0.3	0.3–0.6	> 0.6
6 months to 3 yr	0.25 mg/day	0	0
3–6 yr	0.50 mg/day	0.25 mg/day	0
6–16 yr	1.00 mg/day	0.50 mg/day	0

12. Summarize the scientific basis for the use of fluoride varnishes in caries management.

1. When used appropriately, varnishes offer a 40–65% reduction in the incidence of caries, with a 36% reduction in fissured caries and a 66% reduction in nonfissured surfaces.

2. Varnishes result in a 51% reversal of decalcified tooth structure and a reduction in enamel demineralization of 21–35%.

3. Varnish application is effective in arresting and reversing active enamel lesions, reducing the need for restorative treatment.

4. Varnishes are as effective as APL gels in controlling approximal caries.

5. In primary teeth of preschool children, varnishes cause a 44% reduction in caries.

Vaikuntam J: Fluoride varnishes: Should we be using them? Pediatr Dent 22:513–516, 2000.

13. Is prenatal fluoride supplementation effective in decreasing caries rates in the primary dentition?

No. No studies to date support the administration of prenatal fluorides to protect the primary dentition against caries.

14. Do home water filtration units have any effect on fluoride content?

Absolutely. For example, reverse-osmosis home filtration systems remove 84%, distillation units remove 99%, and carbon filtration systems remove 81% of the fluoride from water.

Brown MD, Aaron G: The effect of point-of-use water conditioning systems on community fluoridated water. Pediatr Dent 13:35–38, 1991.

15. Why has the prevalence of fluorosis increased in the United States?

The increased prevalence is likely due to three factors: (1) inappropriate fluoride supplementation; (2) ingestion of fluoridated toothpaste (most children under age of 5 years ingest all of the toothpaste placed on the toothbrush); and (3) high fluoride content of bottled juices. For example, white grape juice may have fluoride concentrations greater than 2 ppm.

16. What are the common signs of acute fluoride toxicity?

Acute fluoride toxicity may result in nausea, vomiting, hypersalivation, abdominal pain, and diarrhea.

17. What is the first step in treating a child who has ingested an amount of fluoride greater than the safely tolerated dose?

In acute toxicity, the goal is to minimize the amount of fluoride absorbed. Therefore, syrup of ipecac is administered to induce vomiting. Calcium-binding products, such as milk or milk of magnesia, decrease the acidity of the stomach, forming insoluble complexes with the fluoride and thereby decrease its absorption.

18. Are children born with *Streptococcus mutans*?

Children are not born with *Streptococcus mutans*. Instead, they acquire this caries-causing organism between the ages of about 1 and 3 years. Mothers tend to be the major source of infection. The well-delineated age range of acquisition is referred to as the "window of infectivity."

Caufield PW, Cutter GR, et al: Initial acquisition of *mutans* streptococci by infants: Evidence for a discrete window of infectivity. J Dent Res 72:37–45, 1993.

19. What variable is the best predictor of caries risk in children?

Past caries rates are the single best predictor in assessing a child's future risk.

Disney JA, Graves RC, et al: The University of North Carolina Caries Risk Assessment Study: Further developments in caries risk prediction. Community Dent Oral Epidemiol 20:64–75, 1992.

20. Is milk a contributing factor to early childhood caries?

Several animal and in vitro studies suggest that milk and milk components are not cariogenic. Likewise, human breast milk on its own does not cause demineralization. However, when mixed with a sucrose-containing substance, both cow's milk and human breast milk promote caries.

21. What food components reduce the caries-inducing effects of carbohydrates?

Phosphates, fats, and cheese decrease caries susceptibility. Phosphates apparently have a topical effect that aids in remineralization and improves the structural integrity of the enamel surface. Although the mechanism is not entirely clear, fats may form a protective barrier on the teeth or coat the carbohydrate. Cheese may contribute through a number of mechanisms, including its fat, phosphorus, and calcium content.

22. Is there any dental health benefit to chewing gum?

A recent study found that children of mothers who chewed sugar-free gum sweetened with xylitol (in addition to normal oral hygiene measures) had 70% less dental decay than children of mothers who did not chew the gum.

Isokangas P, et al: J Dent Res 79:1885–1889, 2000.

23. Summarize the mechanisms of xylitol's effect.

- Xylitol has a 5-carbon chemical structure not recognized by oral bacteria.
- Because it is not fermented, no acid production results and pH levels in the mouth do not drop (see question 25).
- Chewing xylitol-sweetened gum promotes stimulation of salivary flow, which in turn helps to rinse away excessive sucrose residues and to neutralize acids from other foods. In addition, saliva contains calcium and phosphate, which promote remineralization of early caries.
- Xylitol is a polyol that inhibits the growth of S. mutans, thereby reducing caries susceptibility. Continued use helps to reduce the number of virulent bacteria in the plaque, although xylitol is not bactericidal.
- Xylitol reduces plaque in the oral cavity and enhances the proportion of soluble to insoluble polysaccharides.
- Xylitol complements fluoride in the oral cavity.

24. Who throws a meaner curve, Ryan or Stephan?

Undoubtedly Stephan! The Stephan curve describes the drop in pH that occurs following a cariogenic challenge. Nolan Ryan, on the other hand, is best remembered for his fastball.

Stephan RM: Changes in the hydrogen ion concentration on tooth surfaces in carious lesions. J Am Dent Assoc 27:718, 1940.

25. What is meant by critical pH?

Critical pH is the pH (around 5.5) at which enamel is demineralized.

26. What is the Vipeholm Study? What did it demonstrate?

In the Vipeholm Study, adult institutionalized patients were followed for several years on a variety of controlled diets. The following results were reported:

- Caries increased significantly when sucrose-containing foods were ingested between meals.
- Sucrose in a retentive form produced greater caries than forms that were rapidly cleared from the mouth.
- Sucrose consumed with meals was the least detrimental form.
- Caries activity differs among people with the same diet.

Gustafson BE, Quensel CE, Lanke LS, et al: The Vipeholm Dental Caries Study: The effect of different levels of carbohydrate intake on caries activity in 436 individuals observed for five years. Acta Odontol Scand 11:232–364, 1954.

27. Why are children with asthma at higher risk of developing dental caries?

The two major classes of medications used to treat asthma are anti-inflammatory agents (corticosteroids and cromolyn sodium) and bronchodilators (beta-adrenergic agonists such as ventolin and albuterol). Over the years, numerous studies have shown that all of these medications can impair salivary function, causing xerostomia (dry mouth) and thus increasing susceptibility to caries. For this reason, it is important to implement appropriate preventive measures in asthmatic patients, such as routine fluoride application and extra attention to oral hygiene.

American Dental Association: Guide to Dental Therapeutics, 2nd ed. Chicago, ADA Publishing, 2000, pp 341 and 523.

Ryburg M, Moller C, Ericson T: Saliva composition and caries development in asthmatic patients treated with beta$_2$-adrenergic agonists: A 4-year follow-up study. Scand J Dent Res 99:212–218, 1991.

28. What is the earliest macroscopic evidence of dental caries on a smooth enamel surface?

A white-spot lesion results from acid dissolution of the enamel surface, giving it a chalky white appearance. Optimal exposure to topical fluorides may result in remineralization of such lesions.

29. Which teeth are often spared in nursing caries?

The mandibular incisors often remain caries-free as a result of protection by the tongue.

30. Does an explorer stick necessarily indicate the presence of caries?

Several studies have demonstrated that an explorer stick more often than not is due to to the anatomy of the pit and fissure and not the presence of caries. It has been suggested that "sharp eyes" are more important than "sharp explorers" in detecting pit and fissure caries.

31. What are the indications for an indirect pulp cap in the primary dentition?

Because of the low success rate, most pediatric dentists believe that indirect pulp caps are contraindicated in the primary dentition.

32. Which branchial arch gives rise to the maxilla and mandible?

The first branchial or mandibular arch gives rise to the maxilla, mandible, Meckel's cartilage, incus, malleus, muscles of mastication, and the anterior belly of the digastric muscle.

33. How does the palate form?

The paired palatal shelves arise from the intraoral maxillary processes. These shelves, originally in a vertical position, reorient to a horizontal position as the tongue assumes a more inferior position. The shelves then fuse anteriorly with the primary palate, which arises from the median nasal process posteriorly and with one another. Failure of fusion results in a cleft palate.

34. When do the primary teeth develop?

At approximately 28 days in utero, a continuous plate of epithelium arises in the maxilla and mandible. By 37 days in utero, a well-defined, thickened layer of epithelium overlying the cell-derived mesenchyme of the neural crest delineates the dental lamina. Ten areas in each jaw become identifiable at the location of each of the primary teeth.

35. After the eruption of a tooth, when is root development completed?

In the primary dentition, root development is complete approximately 18 months after eruption; in the permanent dentition, the period of development is approximately 3 years.

36. Define ankylosis. How is it diagnosed?

Ankylosis is the fusion of cementum with alveolar bone and may occur at any time during the course of eruption. Because affected teeth have retarded vertical growth, they appear to submerge below the occlusal plane. Diagnosis involves visual determination that a tooth may be 1 mm or more below the height of the occlusal plane, radiographic evidence of lack of a periodontal ligament, or lack of physiologic mobility. The ankylosed tooth emits an atypical, sharp sound on percussion. In addition, children with affected siblings are twice as likely to have submerged teeth compared with the general population. Ankylosis often occurs bilaterally; 67% of affected people have two or more submerged teeth.

37. What causes ankylosis? Which teeth are most often affected?

The definitive cause of ankylosis is unknown. Contributing factors cited in the literature include local mechanical trauma, disturbed local metabolism, localized infection, chemical or thermal irritation, and gaps in the periodontal membrane.

Mandibular first primary molars are most often affected, followed by second mandibular molars, first maxillary molars, and, finally, second maxillary molars. The prevalence of infraclusion peaks between 8 and 9 years of age, with a suspected range of 1.3–8.9%.

Douglass J, Tinanoff N: The etiology, prevalence and sequelae of infraclusion of primary molars. J Dent Child Nov–Dec:381–483, 1991.

38. How is ankylosis treated?

The severity of submergence dictates the treatment protocol. Therefore, constant vigilance at recall appointments is crucial. The age at which ankylosis begins determines the rate of submergence. The younger the child at onset of ankylosis, the more quickly the tooth submerges because of the increased rate of growth of alveolar bone height. In minor cases, in which the occlusal surface is within 1 mm of the occlusal plane, the tooth needs only monitoring for exfoliation. In rare cases, the ankylosis is severe enough that the occlusal surface meets the interproximal gingival tissue. In such cases, the affected tooth must be extracted with subsequent space maintenance. For moderate cases, stainless steel crowns or build-up restorations can be used to prevent space loss or supraeruption. With mismanagement or misdiagnosis, the sequelae of infraclussion include space loss, molar tipping, supraeruption of antagnoist teeth, and periodontal defects with decreased height of bone.

Messer LB, Cline JT: Ankylosed primary molars: Results and treatment recommendations from an eight-year longitudinal study. Pediatr Dent 2(1):34–47, 1990.

39. What is the relationship between overjet and dental trauma?

Because of the high prevalence of dental trauma involving maxillary incisors, it is important to determine whether any interceptive treatment can lower a patient's risk for trauma. Children with class II malocclusions face a greater risk of maxillary incisor trauma. A tendency to skeletal open bite with negative overbite and excessive overjet predispose patients to dental trauma. Children with overjets greater than 3 mm are twice as likely to injure the anterior teeth as children with overjets less than 3 mm. The risk of trauma increases with increasing overjet measurements.

Although definitive guidelines are not available, high-risk children with a large overjet, excessive maxillary incisor proclination, and high facial angle types may benefit from an evaluation for early orthodontic intervention. Certainly it is the dentist's role to provide anticipatory guidance about injury prevention and the use of a mouthguard.

Baccetti T, Antonini A: Dentofacial characteristics associated with trauma to maxillary incisors in the mixed dentition. J Clin Pediatr Dent 22(4):281–284, 1998.

Ngyuyen QV, Bezemer PD, Habets L, Prahl-Anderson B: A systematic review of the relationship between overjet size and traumatic dental injuries. Eur J Orthodont 21:503–515, 1999.

40. How should dosages of local anesthetic be calculated for a pediatric patient?

Because children's weights vary dramatically for their chronologic age, dosages of local anesthetic should be calculated according to a child's weight. A dosage of 4 mg/kg of lidocaine should *not* be exceeded in pediatric patients.

41. Should the parent be allowed in the operatory with the pediatric patient?

The debate continues. However, recent studies indicate that many pediatric dentists allow the parent to be present in the operatory.

Marcum BK, Turner C, et al: Pediatric dentists' attitudes regarding parental presence during dental procedures. Pediatr Dent 17:432–436, 1995.

42. What is the treatment for a traumatically intruded primary incisor?

In general, the treatment of choice is to allow the primary tooth to reerupt. Reeruption usually occurs in 2–4 months. If the primary tooth is displaced into the follicle of the developing permanent incisor, the primary tooth should be extracted.

43. What are the potential sequelae of trauma to a primary tooth?

1. Pulpal necrosis usually manifests as a gray or gray-black color change in the crown of the involved primary tooth at any time after the injury (weeks, months, years). No treatment is indicated unless other pathologic changes occur (e.g., periapical radiolucency, fistulation, swelling, or pain).

2. Damage to the succedaneous permanent tooth, including hypoplastic defects, dilaceration of the root, or arrest of tooth development, also has been reported.

44. What are the advantages of fixed vs. removable orthodontic appliances?

Fixed orthodontic appliances offer controlled tooth movement in all planes of space. Removable appliances are generally restricted to tipping teeth.

45. What is the straightwire appliance?

The straightwire appliance is a version of the edgewise appliance with several features that allow placement of an ideal rectangular archwire without bends (a so-called straightwire). These features include (1) variations in bracket thickness to compensate for differences in the labiolingual position and thickness of individual teeth; (2) variations in angulation of the bracket slot relative to the long axis of the tooth to allow mesiodistal differences in root angulation of individual teeth; and (3) variations in torque of the bracket slot to compensate for buccal-lingual differences in root angulation of individual teeth.

46. What are so-called functional appliances? Do they work?

Functional appliances are a group of both fixed and removable appliances generally used to promote mandibular growth in patients with class II malocclusions. Although these appliances have been shown to be effective in correcting class II malocclusions, most studies indicate that their effects are mainly dental, with little if any effect on the growth of the mandible.

47. What are the indications for a lingual frenectomy?

Tongue-tie, or ankyloglossia, is relatively rare and usually requires no treatment. Occasionally, however, a short lingual frenum may result in lingual stripping of the periodontium from the lower incisors, which is an indication for frenectomy. A second indication is speech problems secondary to tongue position as diagnosed by a speech pathologist. Nursing problems have been reported in infants who were "cured" after frenectomy.

48. When should orthodontic therapy be initiated?

There is no one optimal time to initiate treatment for every orthodontic problem. For example, a patient in primary dentition with a bilateral posterior crossbite may benefit from palatal expansion at age 4 years. Conversely, the same-aged patient with a severe class III malocclusion due to mandibular prognathism may best be treated by waiting until all craniofacial growth is completed.

49. What is the difference between a skeletal and dental malocclusion?

Skeletal malocclusion refers to a disharmony between the jaws in a transverse, sagittal, or vertical dimension or any combination thereof. Examples of skeletal malocclusions include retrognathism, prognathism, open bites, and bilateral posterior crossbites. Dental malocclusion refers to malpositioned teeth, generally the result of a discrepancy between tooth size and arch length. This discrepancy often results in crowding, rotations, or spacing of the teeth. Most malocclusions are neither purely skeletal nor purely dental but rather a combination of the two.

50. If a child reports a numb lip, can you be certain that the child has a profoundly anesthetized mandibular nerve?

Children, especially young ones, often do not understand what it means to be numb. The mandibular nerve is the only source of sensory innervation to the labial-attached gingiva between the lateral incisor and canine. If probing of this tissue with an explorer evokes no reaction from the patient, a profound mandibular block is assured. No other sign can be used to diagnose profound anesthesia of the mandibular nerve.

51. Does slight contact with a healthy approximal surface during preparation of a class II cavity have any significant consequences?

Even slight nicking of the mesial or distal surface of a tooth greatly increases the possibility for future caries. Placement of an interproximal wedge before preparation significantly decreases the likelihood of tooth damage and future pathology.

52. Why bother with restoring posterior primary teeth?

Caries is an infectious disease. As at any location in the body, treatment consists of controlling and eliminating the infection. With teeth, caries infection can be eliminated by removing the caries and restoring or extracting the tooth. However, extraction of primary molars in children may result in loss of space needed for permanent teeth. To ensure arch integrity, decayed primary teeth should be treated with well-placed restorations.

53. What is the most durable restoration for a primary molar with multisurface caries?

Stainless steel crowns have the greatest longevity and durability. Their 4.5-year survival rate is over twice that of amalgam (90% vs. 40%).

Einwag J, Dunninger P: Stainless steel crowns versus multisurface amalgam restorations: An 8-year longitudinal clinical study. Quintessence Int 27:321–323, 1996.

54. How should a primary tooth be extracted if it is next to a newly placed class II amalgam?

Two steps can be taken to eliminate the possibility of fracturing the newly placed amalgam:
1. The primary tooth to be extracted can be disked to remove bulk from the proximal surface. Care still must be taken to avoid contacting the new restoration.
2. Placing a matrix band (teeband) around the newly restored tooth offers additional protection.

55. Can composites be used to restore primary teeth?

If good technique is followed, composite material is not contraindicated. Interproximally, however, it may be quite difficult to get the kind of isolation required for optimal bonding. There is no scientific advantage to using composite instead of amalgam for such restorations, and one has to evaluate whether esthetic effects justify the additional time required for the composite technique in primary teeth.

56. List the indications and contraindications for pulpectomy in a primary tooth.

Indications
- Teeth with chronic inflammation or necrosis of the radicular pulp
- Often attempted on the primary second molar before eruption of the first permanent molar

Contraindications
- Teeth with advanced resorption (internal or external), loss of root structure, or evidence of periapical infection involving the crypt of the succedaneous tooth
- Primary root canals that are difficult to prepare because of variable and complex morphology
- Proximity of succedaneous tooth bud (unwanted damage may result from instrumentation, medication, or filling materials)

Fuks AB: Pulp therapy for the primary and young permanent dentitions. Dent Clin North Am 44: 571–596, 2000.

57. How successful is pulpectomy in a primary tooth?

In primary teeth with zinc oxide-eugenol (ZOE) pulpectomies, the success rate is 77.7%. The most important preoperative predictor of success is amount of tooth root absorption (more than 23% resorption reduces the success rate to only 23%). If correctly done, pulpectomy does not cause adverse effects on succedaneous tooth formation, but it does involve a 20% chance of altering the eruption path of the permanent tooth.

Coll JA, Sadrian R: Predicting pulpectomy success and its relationship to exfoliation and succedaneous dentition. Pediatr Dent 18:57–63, 1996.

58. What filling materials may be used for pulpectomy in a primary tooth?

The ideal properties of the filling material for pulpectomy in a primary tooth include resorption rate similar to that of primary root, no damage or irritation of periapical tissues or the permanent tooth bud, antiseptic nature, and no discoloring of teeth. The two most commonly used materials are as follows:
- ZOE paste (different rate of resorption, potential underfilling, mild foreign body reaction with overfilling)
- Iodoform paste (rapid resorption, no deleterious effects on succedaneous tooth)

59. Which syndromes or conditions are associated with supernumerary teeth?

Apert's syndrome	Gardner's syndrome
Cleidocranial dysplasia	Hallermann-Streiff syndrome
Cleft lip and palate	Oral-facial-digital syndrome type 1
Crouzon's syndrome	Sturge-Weber syndrome
Down syndrome	

60. Which syndromes or conditions are associated with congenitally missing teeth?

Achondroplasia	Ectodermal dysplasia
Cleft lip and palate	Hallermann-Streiff syndrome
Crouzon's syndrome	Incontinentia pigmenti
Chondroectodermal dysplasia	Oral-facial-digital syndrome type 1
Down syndrome	Rieger's syndrome

61. What are the differences among fusion, gemination, and concrescence?

Fusion is the union of two teeth, resulting in a double tooth, usually with two separate pulp chambers. Fusion is observed most commonly in the primary dentition.

Gemination is the attempt of a single tooth bud to give rise to two teeth. The condition usually presents as a bifid crown with a single pulp chamber in the primary dentition.

Concrescence is the cemental union of two teeth, usually the result of trauma.

62. What is the incidence of inclusion cysts in the infant?

Approximately 75%.

63. What are the three most common types of inclusion cysts and their etiology?

1. **Epstein's pearls** are due to entrapped epithelium along the palatal rapine.
2. **Bohn's nodules** are ectopic mucous glands on the labial and lingual surfaces of the alveolus.
3. **Dental lamina cysts** are remnants of the dental lamina along the crest of the alveolus.

64. What are the most common systemic causes of delayed exfoliation of the primary teeth and delayed eruption of the permanent dentition?

Cleidocranial dysplasia	Gardner's syndrome	Vitamin D-resistant rickets
Chondroectodermal dysplasia	Down syndrome	Hypothyroidism
Achondroplasia	De Lange syndrome	Hypopituitarism
Osteogenesis imperfecta	Apert's syndrome	Ichthyosis

65. What are the most common systemic causes of premature exfoliation of the primary dentition?

Fibrous dysplasia	Cyclic neutropenia	Acatalasia
Vitamin D-resistant rickets	Histiocytosis	Gaucher's disease
Prepubertal periodontitis	Juvenile diabetes	Dentin dysplasia
Papillon-Lefèvre syndrome	Scurvy	Odontodysplasia
Hypophosphatasia	Chediak-Higashi disease	

66. What are Murphy's laws of dentistry?

1. The easier a tooth looks on radiograph for extraction, the more likely you are to fracture a root tip.
2. The shorter a denture patient, the more adjustments he or she will require.
3. The closer it is to 5:00 PM on Friday, the more likely someone will call with a dental emergency.
4. The cuter the child, the more difficult the dental patient.
5. Parents who type their child's medical histories are trouble.
6. The more you need specialists, the less likely they are to be in their office.
7. When a patient localizes pain to one of two teeth, you will open the wrong one.
8. The less a patient needs a procedure for dental health, the more the patient will want it (e.g., anterior veneer vs. posterior crown).

67. Give the appropriate splinting times for the following traumatic dental injuries: luxation, avulsion, root fracture, and alveolar fracture.

Luxation: 3 weeks

Avulsion: Most sources recommend 7–10 days for teeth with both open and closed apices; however, some sources recommend splinting teeth with open apices for 3 weeks. In either case, caution should be used because of the high risk of ankylosis associated with excessive splinting times.

Root fracture and alveolar fracture: 3 weeks. Splinting times for root and alveolar fractures used to be 2–4 months, but recent studies have shown that splinting for 3 weeks is sufficient.

In all cases, a flexible splint should be used to allow physiologic movement of the teeth. In addition, sound clinical judgment should be exercised to help decide whether longer splinting times are necessary. For example, an avulsed tooth with a closed apex that is still +3 mobile after 1 week may need to be splinted for 2 weeks.

Andreason JO, Bakland LK, Flores MT: Guidelines for the evaluation and management of traumatic dental injuries. Dent Traumatol 17:1–4, 145–148, 193–196, 2001.

Peterson LJ, et al: Contemporary Oral and Maxillofacial Surgery, 3rd ed. St. Louis, Mosby, 1998.

68. What can be done to prevent impaction of permanent maxillary canines?

Within 1 year after the total eruption of the maxillary lateral incisors, either a panoramic radiograph or intraoral radiographs should be taken to determine the axial inclination of the developing permanent canine. If mesial angulation is noted, extraction of the maxillary primary canine and maxillary first primary molars may often eliminate the impaction of the maxillary canine.

69. What is the most important technique of behavioral management in pediatric dentistry?

Tell the child what is going to happen, show the child what is going to happen, and then perform the actual procedure intraorally. The major fear in pediatric dental patients is the unknown. The tell, show, and do technique eliminates fear and enhances the patient's behavioral capabilities.

70. What pharmacologic agents are indicated for behavioral control of the pediatric dental patient in an office setting?

There are no absolutely predictable pharmacologic agents for controlling the behavior of pediatric dental patients. Unless the operator has received specific training in sedation techniques for children, patients with behavioral problems are best referred to a specialist in pediatric dentistry.

71. If a primary first molar is lost, is a space maintainer necessary?

Before eruption of the six-year molar and its establishment of intercuspation, mesial migration of the second primary molar will occur, and a space maintainer is indicated to prevent space loss.

72. Do hypertrophic adenoids and tonsils affect dental occlusion?

The incidence of posterior crossbites is increased in children with significant tonsillar and adenoid obstruction. Eighty percent of children with a grade 3 obstruction have posterior crossbites.

Oulis CJ, Vadiakas GP, et al: The effect of hypertrophic adenoids and tonsils on the development of posterior crossbites and oral habits. J Clin Pediatr Dent 18:197–201, 1994.

73. When should crossbites be corrected?

Whenever a crossbite is noted and the patient is amenable to intraoral therapy, correction is indicated. Although a crossbite can be corrected at a later date, optimal time for correction is as soon as possible after diagnosis.

74. What technique may be used if a pediatric patient refuses to cooperate for conventional bitewing radiographs?

A buccal bitewing is taken. The tab of the film is placed on the occlusal surfaces of the molar teeth, and the film itself is positioned between the buccal surfaces of the teeth and cheek. The cone is directed from 1 inch behind and below the mandible upward to the area of the second primary molar on the contralateral side. The setting is three times that which is normally used for a conventional bitewing exposure.

75. What are the morphologic differences between primary and secondary teeth? How does each difference affect amalgam preparation?

1. Occlusal anatomy of primary teeth is generally not as defined as that of secondary teeth, and supplemental grooves are less common. The amalgam preparation therefore can be more conservative.

2. Enamel in primary teeth is thinner than in secondary teeth (usually 1 mm thick); therefore, the amalgam preparation is more shallow in primary teeth.

3. Pulp horns in primary teeth extend higher into the crown of the tooth than pulp horns in secondary teeth; therefore, the amalgam preparation must be conservative to avoid a pulp exposure.

4. Primary molar teeth have an exaggerated cervical bulge that makes matrix adaptation more difficult.

5. The generally broad interproximal contacts in primary molar teeth require wider proximal amalgam preparation than those in secondary teeth.

6. Enamel rods in the gingival third of the primary teeth extend occlusally from the dentinoenamel junction, eliminating the need in class II preparations for the gingival bevel that is required in secondary teeth.

76. What is the purpose of the pulpotomy procedure in primary teeth?
The pulpotomy procedure preserves the radicular vital pulp tissue when the *entire* coronal pulp is amputated. The remaining radicular pulp tissue is treated with a medicament such as formocresol.

77. What is the advantage of the pulpotomy procedure on primary teeth?
The pulpotomy procedure allows resorption and exfoliation of the primary tooth but preserves its role as a natural space maintainer.

78. What are the indications for the pulpotomy procedure in primary teeth?
1. Primary tooth that is restorable with carious or iatrogenic pulp exposure
2. Deep carious lesions without spontaneous pulpal pain
3. Absence of pathologic internal or external resorption but intact lamina aura
4. No radiographic evidence of furcal or periapical pathology
5. Clinical signs of a normal pulp during treatment (e.g., controlled hemorrhage after coronal amputation)

79. What are the contraindications for pulpotomy in primary teeth?
1. Interradicular (molar) or periapical (caries and incisor) radiolucency
2. Internal or external resorption
3. Advanced root resorption, indicating imminent exfoliation
4. Uncontrolled hemorrhage after coronal pulp extirpation
5. Necrotic dry pulp tissue or purulent exudate in pulp canals
6. Fistulous tracks or abscess formation
7. Contraindication to pulpotomy procedure

80. How does rubber-dam isolation of the tooth improve management of pediatric patients?
1. The rubber dam seems to calm the child as it acts as both physical and psychological barrier, separating the child from the procedure being performed.
2. Gagging from the water spray or suction is alleviated.
3. Access is improved because of tongue, lip, and cheek retraction.
4. The rubber dam reminds the child to open.
5. The rubber dam ensures a dry field that otherwise would be impossible in many children.

81. When do the primary and permanent teeth begin to develop?
The primary dentition begins to develop during the sixth week in utero; formation of hard tissue begins during the fourteenth week in utero. Permanent teeth begin to develop during the twelfth week in utero. Formation of hard tissue begins about the time of birth for the permanent first molars and during the first year of life for the permanent incisors.

82. Summarize the chronology of development and eruption of the primary and permanent teeth.
See table on following page.

Chronology of Development and Eruption of Teeth

TOOTH	TOOTH GERM COMPLETED	CALCIFICATION COMMENCES	CROWN COMPLETED	ERUPTION IN MOUTH	ROOT COMPLETED
Primary					
Incisor	3–4 mth i.u.	2–4 mth	6–8 mth	1/2–2 yr	
Canines	5 mth i.u.	9 mth	16–20 mth	21/2–3 yr	
1st molars	12–16 weeks i.u.	5 mth i.u.	6 mth	12–15 mth	2–21/2 yr
2nd molars	6–7 mth i.u.	11–12 mth	20–30 mth	3 yr	
Permanent					
Central incisors	30 weeks i.u.	3–4 mth	4–5 yr	Max: 7–9 yr Mand: 6–8 yr	9–10 yr
Lateral incisors	32 weeks i.u.	Max.: 10–12 mth Mand.: 3–4 mth	4–5 yr	7–9 yrs	10–11 yr
Canines	30 weeks i.u.	4–5 mth	6–7 yr	Max.: 11–12 yr Mand.: 9–10 yr	12–15 yr
1st premolars	30 weeks i.u.	11/2–2 yr	5–6 yr	10–12 yr	12–14 yr
2nd premolars	31 weeks i.u.	2–21/2 yr	6–7 yr	10–12 yr	12–14 yr
1st molars	24 weeks i.u.	Birth	3–5 yr	6–7 yr	9–10 yr
2nd molars	6 months	21/2–3 yr	7–8 yr	12–13 yr	14–16 yr
3rd molars	6 years	7–10 yr	12–16 yr	17–21 yr	18–25 yr

All dates postnatal, except where designated intrauterine (i.u.).
From Bishara SE: Textbook of Orthodontics. Philadelphia, W.B. Saunders, 2001, with permission.

83. What is leeway space?

Leeway space is the difference in the total of the mesiodistal widths between the primary canine, first molar, and second molar and the permanent canine, first premolar, and second premolar. In the mandible, leeway space averages 1.7 mm (unilaterally); it is usually about 0.9–1.1 mm (unilaterally) in the maxilla.

84. What changes occur in the size of the dental arch during growth?

From birth until about 2 years of age, the incisor region widens and growth occurs in the posterior region of both arches. During the period of the full primary dentition, arch length and width remain constant. Arch length does not increase once the second primary molars have erupted; any growth in length occurs distal to the second primary molars and not in the alveolar portion of the maxilla or mandible. There is a slight decrease in arch length with the eruption of the first permanent molars, but a slight increase in intercanine width (and some forward extension of the anterior segment of the maxilla) with the eruption of the incisors. A further decrease in arch length may occur with molar adjustments and the loss of leeway space when the second primary molar exfoliates.

85. What is ectopic eruption? How is it treated?

Ectopic eruption occurs when the erupting first permanent molar begins to resorb the distal root of the second primary molar. Its occurrence is much more common in the maxilla, and it is often associated with a developing skeletal class II pattern. It is seen in about 2–6% of the population and spontaneously corrects itself in about 60% of cases. If the path of eruption of the first permanent molar does not self-correct, a brass wire or an orthodontic separating elastic can be placed between the first permanent molar and the second primary molar, if possible. In severe cases, the second primary molar may exfoliate or require extraction, necessitating the need for space maintenance or space regaining.

86. When is the proper time to consider diastema treatment?

A thick maxillary frenum with a high attachment (sometimes extending to the palate) is common in the primary dentition and does not require treatment. However, a large midline diastema in the primary dentition may indicate the presence of an unerupted midline supernumerary tooth (mesiodens) and often warrants an appropriate radiograph.

The permanent maxillary central incisors erupt labial to the primary incisors and often exhibit a slight distal inclination that results in a midline diastema. This midline space is normal and decreases with the eruption of the lateral incisors. Complete closure of the midline diastema, however, does not occur until the permanent canines erupt. Treatment of residual midline space is addressed orthodontically at this time.

87. What is the effect of early extraction of a primary tooth on the eruption of the succedaneous tooth?

If a primary tooth must be extracted prematurely and 50% of the root of the permanent successor has developed, eruption of the permanent tooth is usually delayed. If > 50% of the root of the permanent tooth has formed at the time of extraction of the primary tooth, eruption is accelerated.

88. Where are the primate spaces located?

In the maxilla, primate spaces are located distal to the primary lateral incisors. In the mandible, primate spacing is found distal to the primary canines.

89. What is the normal molar relationship in the primary dentition?

Historically both the flush terminal plane and mesial step have been considered normal. More recent studies demonstrate that this may not be the case, because about 45% of children with a flush terminal plane go on to develop a class II molar relationship in the permanent dentition.

90. What is meant by the term "pseudo class III"?

This term refers to the condition in which the maxillary incisors are in crossbite with the mandibular incisors. Although the patient appears to have a prognathic mandible, it is due not to a skeletal disharmony but rather to the anterior positioning of the jaw as a result of occlusion. The ability of the patient to retrude the mandible to the edge-to-edge incisal relationship is often considered diagnostic.

91. What is the space maintainer of choice for a 7-year-old child who has lost a lower primary second molar to caries?

The lower lingual arch (LLA) is the maintainer of choice. The 6-year-old molars are banded. The connecting wire lies lingual to the permanent lower incisors in the gingival third and prevents mesial migration of the banded molars. Unlike the band and loop space maintainer, the LLA is independent of eruption sequence. (The band and loop serve no purpose after the primary first molar exfoliates.)

92. What is the space maintainer of choice for a 5-year-old child who has lost an upper primary second molar to caries?

The distal shoe is the appliance of choice. This appliance extends backward from a crown on the primary first molar and subgingivally to the mesial line of the unerupted first permanent molar, thus preventing mesial migration.

93. A 4-year-old child with generalized spacing loses three primary upper incisors to trauma. What space maintainer is needed?

No space maintainer is necessary.

94. What is the best space maintainer for any pulpally involved primary tooth?

Restoring the tooth with pulpal therapy is the best way to preserve arch length and integrity.

95. If a primary tooth is lost to caries but has no successor, is it necessary to maintain space?

Sometimes it is necessary to maintain the space, sometimes it is not. The decision is based on the patient's skeletal and dental development. Either way orthodontic evaluation is of utmost importance to formulate the future plan for this space.

96. When do you remove a space maintainer once it is inserted?

The space maintainer can be removed as soon as the succedaneous tooth begins to erupt through the gingiva. Space maintainers that are left in place too long make it more difficult for patients to clean. Furthermore, it may be necessary to replace a distal shoe with another form of space maintainer once the 6-year molar has erupted to prevent rotation of the molar around the bar arm.

97. What are the various types of headgear and their indications?

There are four basic types of headgear. Each type of headgear has two major components: intraoral and extraoral. The extraoral component is what generally categorizes the type of headgear.

1. **Cervical-pull headgear.** The intraoral component of cervical-pull headgear is composed of a heavy bow that engages the maxillary molars through some variation on a male-female connector. The anterior part of the bow is welded to an extraoral portion that is connected to an elasticized neck strap, which provides the force system for the appliance. The force application is in a down and backward direction. This headgear is generally used in class II, division 1 malocclusions, in which distalization of the maxillary molars and/or restriction of maxillary growth as well as anterior bite opening is desired.

2. **Straight-pull headgear.** The intraoral component is similar to the cervical-pull headgear. However, the force application is in a straight backward direction from the maxillary molar,

parallel to the occlusal plane. Like cervical-pull headgear, this appliance is also used for the class II, division 1 malocclusions. Because of the direction of force application, this appliance may be chosen when excessive bite opening is undesirable.

3. **High-pull headgear.** The intraoral components of high-pull headgear are similar to those described above. However, the force application is in a back and upward direction. Consequently, it is usually chosen for the class II, division 1 malocclusions where bite opening is contraindicated (i.e., class II malocclusion with an open bite).

4. **Reverse-pull headgear.** Unlike the other headgears, the extraoral component of reverse-pull headgear is supported by the chin, cheeks, forehead, or a combination of these structures. The intraoral component usually attaches to a fixed appliance in the maxillary appliance via elastics. Reverse-pull headgear is most often used for class III malocclusions, in which protraction of the maxilla is desirable.

98. What is the basic sequence of orthodontic treatment?

1. **Level and align.** This phase establishes preliminary bracket alignment generally with a light round wire, braided archwire, or a nickel-titanium archwire.

2. **Working archwires.** This phase corrects vertical discrepancies (i.e., bite opening) and sagittal position of the teeth. A heavy round or rectangular archwire is usually employed.

3. **Finishing archwires.** This phase idealizes the position of the teeth. Generally, light round archwires are used.

4. **Retention.** Retention of teeth in their final position may be accomplished with either fixed or removable retainers.

99. What is a tooth positioner?

A tooth positioner is a removable appliance composed of rubber, silicone, or a polyvinyl material. Its appearance is not unlike that of a heavy mouthguard, except it engages both the maxillary and mandibular dentition. It is generally used to idealize final tooth position at or near the completion of orthodontic therapy. The appliance is usually custom fabricated by taking models of the teeth and then repositioning them to their ideal position. The positioner is then fabricated to this ideal setup. The elasticity of the appliance provides for minor positional changes of the patient's teeth. After completion of treatment, the positioner may be used as a retainer.

100. What is "pink tooth of Mummary"?

Pink appearance of tooth due to internal resorption.

101. What intervention is indicated when permanent maxillary canines are observed radiographically to be erupting palatally?

Extraction of the primary maxillary canine. About 75% of ectopic canines show normalization of eruption at 12 months.

Ericson S, Kurol J: Early treatment of palatally erupting maxillary canines by extraction of the primary canines. Eur J Orthod 10:282–295, 1988.

102. Does teething cause systemic manifestations?

Although teething may be associated with drooling, gum rubbing, or changes in dietary intake, no evidence indicates that it causes systemic illness (e.g., diarrhea, fever, rashes, seizures, or bronchitis). Fever associated with teething in fact may be a manifestation of undiagnosed primary herpes gingivostomatitis.

King DL, Steinhauer W, Garcia-Godoy F, Elkins CJ: Herpetic gingivostomatis and teething difficulty in infants. Pediatr Dent 14:82–85, 1992.

103. Should dental implants be placed in the growing child?

Generally implants should be deferred until growth is completed. In a growing child the implant may become submerged or embedded. In addition, an implant that crosses the midline may limit transverse growth.

104. Should an avulsed primary tooth be reimplanted?
No. The prognosis of reimplanted primary teeth is poor and may adversely affect the developing succedaneous tooth.

105. How should an avulsed primary tooth be managed?
Rinse the tooth with water, and place it under the child's pillow.

106. What variable is most important in the prognosis of an avulsed permanent tooth?
Time out of the mouth is most critical, according to Andreasen. With an extra-alveolar time less than 1 hour, partial PDL healing is possible; an extra-alveolar time longer than 1 hour results in total PDL death and progressive root resorption.

107. What other factors affect prognosis?
Extra-alveolar storage medium and stage of root development.

108. If an avulsed tooth cannot be reimplanted immediately, what transport medium is best?
In order of preference: Hank's balanced salt medium, milk, saliva, and water.

109. How do closed vs. open apices affect prognosis?
Closed apices
- Revascularization is not likely
- Pulp extirpation in 7–10 days
- Pulpal necrosis (radiolucency) noted usually as early as 3–4 weeks (usually apical one-third and within 1 year)

Open apices
- Revascularization is possible
- Pulp necrosis is evident after 2–4 weeks and presents with periapical pathology, sometimes with signs of IRR

110. What are the most common complications after reimplantation of an avulsed tooth?
- Pulpal necrosis, ankylosis
- Inflammatory resorption, replacement resorption
- Internal calcification with pulpal obliteration (common in non-endodontically treated reimplants)

111. Describe the occurrence of ankylosis after reimplantation of an avulsed tooth.
- Irreversible and progressive
- More rapid progression with younger age
- Mobility and dull percussion noted as early as 5 weeks (on radiographs at 8 weeks)
- Small areas of ankylosis are reversible with functional mobility

112. Why must care be taken not to "nick" the adjacent interproximal surface in preparing a class II restoration?
Damaged noncarious primary tooth surfaces are 3.5 times more likely to develop a carious lesion and to require future restoration than undamaged surfaces, and damaged noncarious permanent tooth surfaces are 2.5 times more likely to develop a carious lesion and to require future restoration than undamaged surfaces.

113. Do all discolored primary incisors require treatment?
The gray discoloration of primary teeth is usually the result of a traumatic episode. This discoloration is due to either (1) hemorrhage into the dentinal tubules or (2) a necrotic pulp. In the case of hemorrhage into the dentinal tubules, the discoloration usually appears within 1

month of the injury. Often the teeth return to their original color as the blood breakdown products are removed from the site. Discoloration due to a necrotic pulp may take days, weeks, months, or years to develop. It does not improve with time and in fact may worsen. A tooth that is light gray may progress to dark gray. A yellow opaque discoloration is usually indicative of calcific degeneration of the pulp. Discolored teeth do not require treatment unless there is radiographic and/or clinical evidence of pathology of the periodontium (soft and/or hard tissues).

114. How stable is the orthodontic correction of crowding?

Approximately two-thirds of all patients treated for crowding experience significant relapse without some form of permanent retention. This relapse rate is about the same whether the patient is treated with a nonextraction or extraction approach; whether third molars are present, congenitally missing, or extracted; and whether treatment is started in mixed dentition or permanent dentition. Unfortunately, no variables that correlate with relapse potential have been identified. And to add further insult, relapse potential continues throughout life.

115. Does eruption of third molars cause crowding of the incisors?

No. The eruption of third molars with real or perceived increase in crowding of the incisors is coincidental. Studies have revealed that patients who are congenitally missing third molars experience the same crowding phenomenon.

116. What is the ideal molar relationship in the primary dentition?

Mesial step. Although many pediatric dentistry and orthodontic texts suggest that both the mesial step relationship and the flush terminal plane are considered normal, a longitudinal study by Bishara et al. revealed that almost 50% of flush terminal plane relationships in the primary dentition later develop into class II malocclusions.

Bishara SE, Hoppens BJ, Jakobsen JR, Kohout FJ: Changes in the molar relationship between the deciduous and permanent dentitions: A longitudinal study. Am J Orthod Dentofac Orthop 93:19–28, 1988.

117. Which two dentists have appeared on the cover of *Time* magazine?

Dr. Harold Kane Addelson, the originator of the tell-show-do technique, and Dr. Barney Clark, the first human recipient of a mechanical heart.

BIBLIOGRAPHY

 1. AAPD Reference Manual: Clinical Guidelines on Infant Oral Health Care. American Academy of Pediatric Dentistry, 2001–2002.
 2. American Dental Association: Guide to Dental Therapeutics, 2nd ed. Chicago, ADA Publishing, 2000.
 3. Andreasen JO, Andreasen FM: Essentials of Traumatic Injuries to the Teeth. Copenhagen, Munksgaard, 1990.
 4. Andreasen JO, Bakland LK, Flores MT: Guidelines for the evaluation and management of traumatic dental injuries. Dent Traumatol 17:1–4, 145–148, 193–196, 2001.
 5. Baccetti T, Antonini A: Dentofacial characteristics associated with trauma to maxillary incisors in the mixed dentition. J Clin Pediatr dent 22(4):281–284, 1998.
 6. Bishara SE: Textbook of Orthodontics. Philadelphia, W.B. Saunders, 2001.
 7. Brown MD, Aaron G: The effect of point-of-use water conditioning systems on community fluoridated water. Pediatr Dent 13:35–38, 1991.
 8. Caulfield PW, Cutter GR, et al: Initial acquisitions of *mutans* streptococci by infants: Evidence for a discrete window of infectivity. J Dent Res 72:37–45, 1993.
 9. Coll JA, Sadrian R: Predicting pulpectomy success and its relationship to exfoliation and succedaneous dentition. Pediatr Dent 18:57–63, 1996.
10. Douglas J, Tinanoff N: The etiology, prevalence and sequelae of infraclusion of primary molars. J Dent Child Nov–Dec:381–483, 1991.
11. Einwag J, Dunninger F: Stainless steel crowns versus multisurface amalgam restorations: An 8-year longitudinal clinical study. Quintessence Int 27:321–323, 1996.
12. Enlow DH: Facial Growth, 3rd ed. Philadelphia, W.B. Saunders, 1990.
13. Fuks AB: Pulp therapy for the primary and young permanent dentitions. Dent Clin North Am 44:571–596, 2000.

14. Gorlin RJ, Cohen MM Jr, Levin LS: Syndromes of the Head and Neck. New York, Oxford University Press, 1990.
15. Disney JA, Graves RC, et al: The University of North Carolina Caries Risk Assessment: Further developments i caries risk prediction. Community Dent Oral Epidemiol 20:64–75, 1992.
16. Kaban LB: Pediatric Oral and Maxillofacial Surgery. Philadelphia, W.B. Saunders, 1990.
17. Marcum BK, Turner C, et al: Pediatric dentists' attitudes regarding parental presence during dental procedures. Pediatr Dent 17:432–436, 1995.
18. McDonald RE, Avery DR: Dentistry for the Child and Adolescent. St. Louis, Mosby, 1994.
19. Moyers R: Handbook of Orthodontics. Chicago, Year Book, 1986
20. Nguyen QV, Bezemer PD, Habets L, Prahl-Anderson B: A systematic review of the relationship between overjet size and traumatic dental injuries. Eur J. Orthodont 21:502–515, 1999.
21. Peterson LJ, et al: Contemporary Oral and Maxillofacial Surgery, 3rd ed. St. Louis, Mosby, 1998.
22. Pinkham JR, Casamassimo PS, Fields HW, et al: Pediatric Dentistry: Infancy through Adolescence, 2nd ed. Philadelphia, W.B. Saunders, 1994.
23. Proffit W, Fields HW: Contemporary Orthodontics. St. Louis, Mosby, 1993.
24. Ryburg M, Moller C, Ericson T: Saliva composition and caries development in asthmatic patients treated with beta$_2$-adrenergic agonists: A 4-year follow-up study. Scand J Dent Res 99:212–219, 1991.
25. Sanchez DM, Childers NK: Anticipatory Guidance in Oral Health: Rationale and Recommendations. American Academy of Family Physicians, 2001.
26. Scully C, Welbury R: Color Atlas of Oral Diseases in Children and Adolescents. London, Mosby-Year Book Europe Limited, 1994.
27. Vaikuntam J: Fluoride varnishes: Should we be using them? Pediatr Dent 22:513–516, 2000.

12. INFECTION AND HAZARD CONTROL

Helene Bednarsh, R.D.H., B.S., M.P.H., *Kathy J. Eklund*, R.D.H., B.S., M.H.P.,
John A. Molinari, *Ph.D.*, *and Walter W. Bond*, M.S.

1. What is the difference between infection control and exposure control?

Infection control encompasses all policies and procedures to prevent the spread of infection and/or the potential transmission of disease. A newer term, exposure control, refers to procedures for preventing exposures to potentially infective microbial agents.

2. What are the major mechanisms by which diseases are transmitted?

Disease may be transmitted by direct contact with the source of microorganisms (e.g, percutaneous injury, contact with mucous membrane, nonintact skin, or infective fluids, excretions, or secretions) and by indirect contact with contaminated environmental surfaces or medical instruments and aerosols.

3. What is aerosolization?

Aerosolization is a process whereby mechanically generated particles (droplet nuclei) remain suspended in the air for prolonged periods and may be capable of contributing to **airborne transmission** of disease, even considerable distances from the source. Aerosols are airborne particles in the range of 5–10 μm in diameter and are capable of being inhaled and penetrating the bronchial tree to the alveoli of the lungs. In contrast, larger particles may be "airborne" in the sense they travel through the air, but only for short times and distances; they are too large to be inhaled. They do not play a role in airborne transmission of disease per se, but they may contribute to **direct transmission** (e.g., if they are from an infected source and hit a susceptible host in the mucous membranes of the eyes, nose, or mouth) or **indirect transmission** of disease (e.g., when they "fall out" onto horizontal surfaces and are subsequently transferred to the proper portal of entry into a susceptible host by hand/finger contamination). It is important to recognize the actual meaning of "true aerosol," because effective strategies for protecting against aerosol transmission of disease versus diseases transmitted by splash, spatter, and perhaps contaminated surfaces are significantly different.

4. What barriers may be used to block the above routes?

A surgical mask or an appropriate face shield provides some degree of protection from contact with larger airborne particles such as splash and spatter. Surgical masks were neither designed nor intended to protect the worker from true aerosols (see question 3). Surgical masks and protective eyewear, in fact, help prevent mucous membrane exposures. Clinic attire and gloves offer skin contact protection. The basic idea is to put a barrier between exposed areas of the body and microbially laden materials. In regard to tuberculosis, a surgical mask is not the appropriate barrier for the prevention of transmission of airborne organisms such as *Mycobacterium tuberculosis* found in droplet nuclei. The National Institute for Occupational Safety and Health (NIOSH) recommends the use of a personal respirator.

5. What does the Occupational Safety and Health Administration (OSHA) require in a written exposure control plan?

OSHA requires at least the following elements:

1. The employer's "exposure determination," which identifies at-risk employees
2. An implementation schedule and discussion of specific methods of implementing requirements of the OSHA Bloodborne Pathogens Standard.
3. The method for evaluating and documenting exposure incidents
4. That consideration was given to the use of safety devices as evidenced by staff evaluation and determination whether they were or were not feasible for use in the practice.

6. How often must a written exposure control plan be reviewed?

OSHA's Bloodborne Pathogens Standard requires an annual review of a written exposure control plan. The plan must be reviewed and updated after any changes in knowledge, practice, personnel, guidelines, or regulations that may affect occupational exposure.

7. Are there any revisions to the exposure control plan (ECP)?

OSHA revised some of the requirements for the ECP in the Needlestick Safety and Prevention Act of 2000. There has always been a requirement to review and update the ECP annually. This update and review must now include the changes in technology that eliminate or reduce exposure to bloodborne pathogens. Therefore, the plan should document consideration and implementation of appropriate safer devices that are designed to eliminate or minimize occupational exposure. This documentation must include evidence that employees who use the devices have had input into the identification, evaluation, and selection of the devices.

8. What is an exposure incident?

According to OSHA, an exposure incident is any reasonably anticipated eye, skin, mucous membrane, or parenteral contact with blood or other potentially infectious fluids during the course of one's duties. In more general terms, an exposure incident is an occurrence that puts one at risk of a biomedical or chemical contact/injury on the job.

9. What should be included in the procedure for evaluating an exposure incident?

At least the following factors should be considered in evaluating an exposure incident:

1. Where the incident occurred in terms of physical space in the facility
2. Under what circumstances the exposure occurred
3. Engineering controls and work practices in place at the time of the exposure, including the use of a safety device
4. Policies in place at the time of the incident
5. Type of exposure and severity of the injury
6. Any information available about the source patient
7. The presence of visible blood on the device

10. How does OSHA define a "source individual" in the context of an exposure incident?

The standard defines "source individual" as any individual, living or dead, whose blood or other potentially infectious materials may be a source of occupational exposure.

11. Are students covered by OSHA standards?

In accordance with the Occupational Safety and Health Act of 1970, OSHA jurisdiction extends only to employees and does not cover students if they are not considered to be employees of the institution. If, however, the student is paid by the institution, he or she becomes an employee. Regardless of employee status, most aspects of the OSHA Bloodborne Pathogens Standard are considered to be standards of practice for all health care workers and are designed to prevent the potential transmission of disease. Therefore, the safe practices and procedures outlined in the standard should be followed by all health care workers.

12. How do you determine who is at risk for a bloodborne exposure?

The first step is to conduct a risk assessment, which begins by evaluating the tasks that are always done, sometimes done, and never done by an employee. If any one task carries with it an opportunity for contact with any potentially infective (blood or blood-derived) fluid or if a person may, even once, be asked to do a task that carries such an exposure risk, that employee is at risk and must be trained to abate or eliminate risk.

13. Can the receptionist help out in the clinic?

Only if he or she has been trained to work in a manner that reduces risk of an exposure incident, understands the risk, and has received (unless otherwise waived) the hepatitis B vaccine or demonstrates immunity from past infection.

14. What is an engineering control?

The term refers to industrial hygiene and is used by OSHA for technologically derived devices that isolate or remove hazards from the work environment. The use of engineering controls may reduce the risk of an exposure incident. Examples include ventilation systems, ergonomic design of equipment and furnishings, and safety devices.

15. Give examples of engineering controls used in dentistry.

A needle-recapping device is an engineering control, as is a sharps container. These items are designed to isolate sharps, wires, and glass. A rubber dam, which serves as a barrier between the operator and potentially infective patient fluids, is also an engineering control because it reduces aerosols and splashing and spattering of large droplets during dental procedures. A newer engineering control in the dental setting is safety devices.

16. What is an SESIP?

SESIP is a **s**harps with **e**ngineered **s**harps **i**njury **p**rotection. It refers to a nonneedle sharp or a needle device with a built-in safety feature or mechanism that effectively reduces the risk of an exposure incident.

17. Where is the most reasonable location for a sharps container?

To be most effective in reducing the hazard associated with nonreusable sharps, the container should be placed in a site near where the sharps are used and not in a separate area that requires transport or additional handling.

18. What needle-recapping devices are acceptable?

First, any recapping must be done with a mechanical device or a technique that uses only one hand ("scoop technique"). Such techniques ensure that needles are never pointed at or moved toward the practicing health care worker or other workers, either on purpose or accidentally. Newer, self-sheathing anesthetic syringes and needle devices do not require any movements associated with recapping.

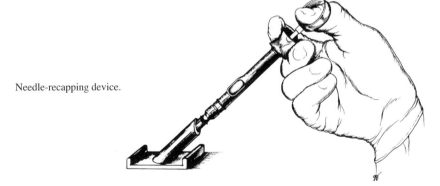

Needle-recapping device.

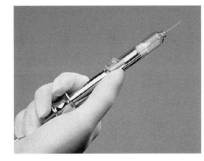

Self-sheathing syringe.

19. What is a work practice control? How does it differ from an engineering control?

Work practice controls are determined by behavior rather than technology. Quite simply, a work practice control is the manner in which a task is performed. Safe work practice controls sometimes require changing the manner in which a task is performed to reduce the likelihood of an exposure incident. For example, in recapping a needle, whether or how you use a device is the work practice. Something as simple as how you wash your hands is a work practice control as well.

20. What is the most appropriate work practice control in cleaning instruments?

Probably the best technique for cleaning instruments is to use an ultrasonic cleaner because of its potential to reduce percutaneous injuries. If an ultrasonic cleaner is not available, the work practice is to select one or two instruments at a time with gloved hands, hold them low in the sink under running water, and scrub them with a long-handled brush. Essentially, the strategy is to clean reusable instruments and items in a manner that minimizes hand contact.

21. What should a proper handwashing agent be expected to accomplish?

At a minimum, it should (1) provide good mechanical cleansing of skin; (2) have the capacity to kill a variety of microorganisms if it is used in a surgical setting; (3) have some residual antimicrobial effect to prevent regrowth of resident bacteria and fungi when used for surgical handwashing; and (4) be dispensed without risk of cross-contamination among workers.

The major concern, exclusive of surgery, is the transient flora on workers' hands. The primary idea is to wash off the flora, not just to kill them in situ with an antimicrobial agent. In surgery, antimicrobial products are the standard of care to address the health care worker's resident flora, which multiply under the glove. Surgical handwashing is used when a direct intent of the medical procedure is to break soft tissue.

22. When should a dental health care worker wash and dry hands before gloving? When should he or she use an antiseptic hand rub agent?

New recommendations from the CDC are outlined in the table on the following page. Hand hygiene recommendations are specific to the type of procedure to be performed, i.e. clean technique or surgical procedure.

23. Can dental charts be contaminated? How can you reduce the risk of cross-contaminating dental charts?

A dental chart may be contaminated if it is in area where it may come in contact with potentially infective fluids. This risk may be minimized if the charts are not taken into a patient or clinical area. If, however, they must be accessible during treatment, they should be appropriately handled with noncontaminated gloves. Overgloves worn atop clinic gloves for handling records is one possibility. Another is to protect the record with a barrier.

PERSONAL PROTECTIVE EQUIPMENT

24. What type of gloves should be worn for different procedures and tasks?

The type of glove must first provide appropriate hand protection for the anticipated exposures such as biological, chemical, and/or physical (sharp). Next, within each procedure/exposure category there are choices of materials based on several factors, including personal health compatibility (allergies and fit). See table on page 258.

25. How do you determine what types of personal protective equipment (PPE) you should use?

The selection of PPE should be based on the type of exposure anticipated and the quantity of blood, blood-derived fluids, or other potentially infective materials that reasonably may be expected in the performance of one's duties. With normal use the material should prevent passage of fluids to skin, undergarments, or mucous membranes of the eyes, nose, or mouth.

26. Do gloves protect me from a sharps exposure?

To a limited degree at best. Some studies indicate that the mechanical action of a sharp passing through the glove may reduce the microbial load. However, even heavy-duty utility gloves do

Hand Hygiene

METHODS	AGENT	PURPOSE	AREA	DURATION (MINIMUM)	INDICATIONS (OSHA 1991, CDC Universal Precautions 1988, CDC HIV 1987, Garner SSI and Hand 1986, Larson 1995, Steere 1995, Larson 2000, Pittet 2000, CDC Hand 2002, Garner 1996, Mangram 1999, Doebbeling 1988)
Routine handwash	Water and non-antimicrobial detergent (e.g., plain soap*)	Remove soil and transient microorganisms	Fingertips to the wrist	15 seconds[†]	• Before and after treating each patient (e.g., before glove placement and after glove removal)
Routine hand antisepsis Antiseptic handwash or	Water and antimicrobial agent/detergent (e.g., chlorhexidine, iodine and iodophors, chloroxylenol [PCMX], triclosan)	Remove or destroy transient microorganisms and reduce resident flora	Fingertips to the wrist at a minimum	15 seconds[†]	• After barehanded touching of inanimate objects likely to be contaminated by blood or saliva • Before leaving the dental operatory[§] • When visibly soiled[§]
Antiseptic hand rub	Alcohol-based hand rub[§]			Rub hands until the agent is dry[§]	• Before regloving after removing gloves that are torn, cut, or punctured
Surgical hand antisepsis	Water and antimicrobial agent/detergent (e.g., chlorhexidine, iodine and iodophors, chloroxylenol [PCMX], triclosan) Water and non-antimicrobial detergent (e.g., plain soap*) followed by an alcohol-based hand rub with persistent activity	Remove or destroy transient microorganisms and reduce resident flora (persistent effect)	Hands and forearms up to the elbows[¶]	2–6 minutes Follow manufacturer instructions for alcohol-based hand rub[§§]	• Before donning sterile, surgical gloves for surgical procedures

*Pathogenic organisms have been found on or around bar soap during and after use (Kabara 1984). Use of liquid soap with hands-free dispensing controls is preferable.
[†]Washing times of 10–15 seconds have been reported as effective in removing most transient flora from the skin. For most procedures, a vigorous, brief (at least 15 seconds) rubbing together of all surfaces of premoistened lathered hands and fingers followed by rinsing under a stream of cool or tepid water is recommended (Steere 1975, Ojajärvi 1981, Garner 1985, Larson 1986, Ayliffe 1992, CDC Hand 2002). Hands should always be dried thoroughly before donning gloves.
[§]60–95% ethanol or isopropanol. Alcohol-based hand rubs should not be used in the presence of visible soil or organic material. If using an alcohol-based hand rub, apply adequate amount to palm of one hand and rub hands together, covering all surfaces of the hands and fingers, until hands are dry. Follow manufacturer's recommendations regarding the volume of product to use. If hands feel dry after rubbing hands together for 10–15 seconds, an insufficient volume of product likely was applied. The drying effect of alcohol can be reduced or eliminated by adding 1–3% glycerol or other skin-conditioning agents (CDC Hand 2002).
[¶]Removal of all jewelry, washing as described in the second footnote, holding the hands above the elbows during final rinsing, and drying the hands with sterile towels (Mangram 1999, Larson 1995, CDC Hand 2002, AORN 2002).
[§§]After application of the alcohol-based product as recommended, allow hands and forearms to dry thoroughly and immediately don sterile gloves (Hobson 1998, Mulberry 2001).
From Centers for Disease Control and Prevention: Draft Recommended Infection Control Practices for Dentistry, 2003. Atlanta, CDC, Feb. 12, 2003.

Types of Gloves

GLOVE TYPE	INDICATIONS	COMMENTS	COMMERCIALLY AVAILABLE GLOVE MATERIALS*	
			MATERIALS	COMMENTS[††]
Patient examination gloves[†]	Patient care, examinations, and other nonsurgical procedures involving contact with mucous membranes	Medical device regulated by the FDA should be labeled as a medical or dental glove Nonsterile and sterile single-use disposable. Use for one patient and discard appropriately	Natural-rubber latex (NRL) Nitrile Nitrile & chloroprene (Neoprene) blends Nitrile & NRL blends Butadiene methyl methacrylate Polyvinyl chloride (PVC, vinyl) Polyurethane Styrene-based copolymer	1,2 2,3 2, 3 1, 2, 3 2, 3 4 4 4, 5
Surgical gloves[†]	Surgical procedures	Medical device regulated by the FDA should be labeled as a medical or dental glove Sterile and single-use disposable. Use for one patient and discard appropriately Orthopedic surgical gloves may be thicker and more resistant to tear than other surgical gloves.	NRL Nitrile Chloroprene (Neoprene) NRL & nitrile or chloroprene blends Synthetic polyisoprene Styrene-based copolymer Polyurethane	1, 2 2, 3 2, 3 2, 3 2 4, 5 4
Non-medical gloves	Housekeeping procedures (e.g., cleaning and disinfection) Handling contaminated sharps or chemicals Do not use during patient care	Not a medical device regulated by the FDA Commonly referred to as utility, industrial, or general purpose gloves and should be puncture- and chemical resistant. Latex gloves do not provide adequate chemical protection Sanitize after use	NRL & nitrile or chloroprene blends Chloroprene (Neoprene) Nitrile Butyl rubber Fluoroelastomer Polyethylene and ethylene vinyl alcohol copolymer	2, 3 2, 3 2, 3 2, 3 3, 4, 6 3, 4, 6

*Physical properties can vary by material, manufacturer, and protein and chemical composition.
[†]Medical or dental patient examination gloves and surgical gloves are medical devices regulated by the FDA. Only FDA-cleared medical or dental patient examination gloves and surgical gloves can be used for patient care.
[††]Material: 1—contains allergenic NRL proteins; 2—vulcanized rubber, contains allergenic rubber processing chemicals; 3—likely to have enhanced chemical and/or puncture resistance; 4—nonvulcanized and does not contain rubber processing chemicals; 5—inappropriate for use with methacrylates; and 6—resistant to most methacrylates.
From Centers for Disease Control and Prevention: Draft Recommended Infection Control Practices for Dentistry, 2003. Atlanta, CDC, February 12, 2003

not block penetration. In addition, blunt instruments pose injury risks for the dental health care worker and patient.

27. Does clinic attire (lab coats) protect me from potentially infective fluid?

The intent of clinic attire is to prevent potentially infective fluids from reaching skin, especially nonintact skin, that can serve as a portal of entry for pathogenic organisms. Putting an effective barrier, such as a lab coat, between your body and these fluids reduces the risk of infection. Such garments are contaminated and should not be worn outside the clinic area.

28. Should clinic attire be long- or short-sleeved?

Because the OSHA standards are performance-based, the dental health care worker must determine whether the procedure is likely to result in contact with patient fluids or materials. If the answer is yes, the potential contact area should be covered.

29. How do you determine whether eyewear is protective?

The best way is to look to the standards of the American National Standards Institute (ANSI). These standards describe protective eyewear as impact-resistant, with coverage from above the eyebrows down to the cheek and solid side-shields to provide peripheral protection. The eyewear should protect not only from fluids but also from flying debris that may be generated during a dental procedure.

30. Is a surgical mask needed under a face shield?

Yes, unless the face shield has full peripheral protection at the sides and under the chin. The mask protects the dental health care worker from splashes and spatters to the nose and mouth.

31. What type of protection do most masks used in dental offices offer?

The masks used in dental offices do not provide definable respiratory protection; their primary design is to protect the patient. However, the physical barrier certainly protects covered areas from droplet scatter generated during treatment. If respiratory protection is indicated, masks must be certified for respiratory protection. Read the product label.

32. How long can a mask be worn?

Basically, you can wear a mask until it becomes wet or torn. You must, however, use a new mask for each patient. Limited research indicates that the duration for use is about 1 hour for a dry field and 20 minutes for a wet field.

33. What is the purpose of heavy-duty utility gloves?

Heavy-duty utility gloves, such as those made of nitrile rubber, should be worn whenever contaminated sharps are handled. They are worn for safe pick-up, transport, cleaning, and packing of contaminated instruments. They also should be used for housekeeping procedures such as surface cleaning and disinfection. Routine cleaning and disinfection are necessary because the gloves also become contaminated. They should not be worn when handing or contacting clean surfaces or items. **Note:** Exam gloves are not appropriate for instrument cleaning or reprocessing or any housekeeping procedure.

How to Select Task-appropriate Gloves

FOR THIS TASK:	USE THIS GLOVE:
Contact with body, as during surgery	Sterile latex gloves
Routine intraoral procedures, routine contact with mucous membranes	Latex exam gloves*
Routine contact with mucous membranes, cases of latex allergy	Vinyl exam or other non-latex gloves
Nonclinical care or treatment procedures, such as processing radiographs and writing in a patient record	Copolymer gloves or over-gloves
Contact with chemical agents, contaminated sharps, and other potential exposure incidents not related to patient treatment	Nitrile rubber gloves

*Latex gloves may be contraindicated in the event of patient or health care worker allergy.

34. What is irritant dermatitis?
It is a nonallergic process that damages superficial layers of skin. It is caused mostly by contact that challenges the skin tissue.

35. What are its symptoms?
In general, the top layer of the skin becomes reddened, dry, irritated, or cracked.

36. What causes of dermatitis are associated with health care workers' hands?
Nonallergic irritant dermatitis is the most common form of adverse reactions. It is often caused by (1) contact with a substance that physically or chemically damages the skin, such as frequent antimicrobial handwash agents on sensitive skin; (2) failure to rinse off chemical antiseptic completely; (3) irritation from corn starch powder in gloves; and (4) failure to dry hands properly and thoroughly.

37. What common types of hypersensitivity symptoms are caused by latex gloves and other latex items?
1. **Cutaneous anaphylactic reaction** (type I hypersensitivity) typically develops within minutes after an allergic person either comes into direct contact with allergens via tissues or mucous membranes (donning latex examination or surgical gloves) or is exposed via aerosolization of allergens. Natural rubber latex proteins adhering to glove powder particles can remain suspended in the air for prolonged periods after gloves are placed on hands and when new boxes of gloves are opened. Wheal and flare reaction (i.e., urticaria, hives) may develop along with itching and localized edema. Coughing, wheezing, shortness of breath, and/or respiratory distress may occur, depending on the person's degree of sensitization. Type I hypersensitivity can be a life-threatening reaction; appropriate medical supplies (e.g., epinephrine) should always be immediately available.

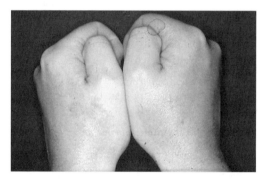

Type I hypersensitivity reaction on the skin of the hands.

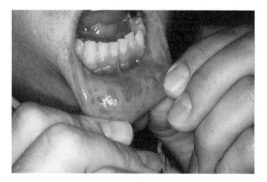

Type IV hypersensitivity reaction in the oral mucosa.

2. **Contact dermatitis** (delayed type IV hypersensitivity) is characterized by a several hour delay in onset of symptoms and reaction that peaks in 24–48 hours. This slow-forming, chronic inflammatory reaction is well demarcated on the skin and is surrounded by localized erythema. Healing may take up to 4 days with scabbing and sloughing of affected epithelial sites.

38. What should be done for health care workers who develop symptoms or reactions that may be due to latex hypersensitivity?

The first step is to determine that you are dealing with a true reaction to latex. The most common type of hand dermatitis is actually nonspecific irritation and not an immunologic response. Nonspecific irritation can have a similar appearance to type I or type IV reactions but often results from improper hand care, such as not drying hands completely before putting on gloves. In addition, allowing dry hands to go untreated, especially during colder seasons, may lead to development of chapped, broken areas in the epithelium.

Definitive diagnosis through clinical and laboratory tests by a qualified health care professional is necessary. Specific treatment and latex avoidance recommendations must be followed by the latex-sensitive/allergic health care worker. Accommodations in products selection and work environment may be required in order for the health care worker to safely return to work. In an alert to health professionals in 1991, the FDA also suggested that persons with severe latex sensitivity should wear a medical identification bracelet in case they require emergency medical care and are unable to alert hospital personnel.

39. What risk factors are associated with latex allergy?
1. Frequent exposure to latex
2. History of surgery
3. Spina bifida
4. Frequent catheterization
5. Allergies to certain food, such as bananas, avocados, kiwi fruit, and chestnuts

40. What are the official recommendations for protection of health care workers with ongoing exposure to latex?

The National Institute for Occupational Safety and Health (NIOSH) recommends the following steps for worker protection:

1. Use non-latex gloves for activities that are not likely to involve contact with infectious materials (e.g., food preparation, routine housekeeping and maintenance).

2. When appropriate barrier protection is necessary, choose powder-free latex gloves with reduced protein content.

3. When wearing latex gloves, do not use oil-based hand creams or lotions unless they have been shown to reduce latex-related problems.

4. Frequently clean work areas contaminated with latex dust.

5. Frequently change the ventilation filters and vacuum bags in latex-contaminated areas.

6. Learn to recognize the symptoms of latex allergy: skin rashes and hives; flushing and itching; nasal, eye, or sinus symptoms; asthma; and shock.

7. If you develop symptoms of latex allergy, avoid direct contact with latex gloves and products until you see a physician experienced in treating latex allergy.

8. Consult your physician about the following precautions:
- Avoid contact with latex gloves and products.
- Avoid areas where you may inhale the powder from latex gloves worn by others.
- Tell your employer(s), physicians, nurses, and dentists that you have latex allergy.
- Wear a medical alert bracelet.

9. Take advantage of all latex allergy education and training provided by your employer.

See NIOSH website (www.NIOSH.gov) for updated information.

41. A patient reports a latex allergy and says that if a glove touches her, she will break out. What type of glove should be used in place of latex?

Newer, better non-latex (synthetic) gloves provide adequate barrier protection and reduce concern for an allergic response. However, depending on the severity of the allergy, more serious responses may occur merely in the presence of latex. You may wish to consult with the patient's allergist for additional recommendations.

42. Why are lanolin hand creams contraindicated with glove use?
   The fatty acids in lanolin break down the latex, causing wicking. This same process can cause a build-up of film on the hands.

BLOODBORNE INFECTIONS AND VACCINATION

43. What are universal precautions?
   Universal precautions, a concept of infection control, assume that any patient is potentially infectious for a number of bloodborne pathogens. Blood, blood-derived products, and certain other fluids that are contaminated with blood are considered infectious for human immuodeficiency virus (HIV), hepatitis B virus (HBV), hepatitis C virus (HCV), and other bloodborne pathogens. Standard precautions are procedure-specific, not patient-specific. In dentistry, saliva is normally considered to be blood-contaminated. The basic principle and implementation of this concept is that gloves (and other PPE as appropriate) should be worn "*universally* with *all* patients, i.e., without regard to whether a particular patient's bloodborne infection state is known."

44. What are standard precautions?
   In 1996 the CDC developed new guidelines that combined the major components of universal precautions and body substance isolation into one set of precautions known as "standard precautions." According to the Oral Health Division of the CDC, they are similar to universal precautions in that they are designed to reduce the risk of transmission of pathogens from both recognized and unrecognized sources of infection to other patients and to health care workers. Standard precautions apply to blood, body fluids, secretions, and excretions (except sweat), regardless of whether they contain blood, to nonintact skin and mucous membranes. Standard precautions should be used in the care of all patients regardless of their infectious status. This expanded set of precautions teaches simply that "if it's a wet body substance and it doesn't belong to you, wear your gloves and other PPE as appropriate to avoid direct contact with it while delivering healthcare to the patient."

45. What is the chain of infection?
   The chain of infection refers to the prerequisites for infection (by either direct or indirect contact):

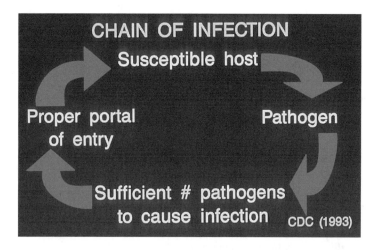

Chain of infection. (From U.S. Department of Health and Human Services, Centers for Disease Control and Prevention: Practical Infection Control in the Dental Office. Washington, DC, DHHS, 1993.)

1. A susceptible host
2. A pathogen with sufficient infectivity and numbers to cause infection
3. An appropriate portal of entry to the host (e.g., a bloodborne agent must gain access to the bloodstream, whereas an enteric agent must enter the mouth [digestive tract])
4. A reasonably efficient physical mode of pathogen transfer from source to host

46. Which factor is easiest to control: agent, host, or transmission?

Agent and host are more difficult to control than transmission. Standard precautions are directed toward interrupting the transfer of microorganisms from patient to health care worker and vice versa.

47. What is one of the single most important measures to reduce the risk of transmission of microorganisms?

Handwashing is one of the most important measures in reducing the risk of transmission of microorganisms. Hands should *always* be thoroughly washed between patients, after contact with blood or other potentially infective fluids, after contact with contaminated instruments or items, and after removal of gloves. Gloves also play an important role as a protective barrier against cross-contamination and reduce the likelihood of transferring microorganisms from health care workers to patients and from environmental surfaces to patients. A cardinal rule for safety is never to touch a surface with contaminated gloves that will subsequently be touched with ungloved hands.

48. Is exposure synonymous with infection?

No. An exposure is a contact that has a reasonable potential to complete the chain of infection and result in disease of the host.

49. What are hepatitis B and delta hepatitis?

Hepatitis B is one of most common reportable diseases in the United States. HBV is transmitted through blood or blood-contaminated body fluids. It is highly transmissible because of the large numbers of virus in the blood of infected persons (about 100 million per ml). Delta hepatitis is caused by a defective virus (hepatitis D virus [HDV]) that relies on HBV for its pathogenicity and can infect only in the presence of HBV. HBV and HDV coinfection, however, results in a fulminant course of liver disease.

50. Why is hepatitis B vaccination so important?

HBV is the major infectious occupational hazard to health care workers. Transmission has been documented from providers to patients and vice versa. In 1982, a vaccine became available to provide protection from HBV infection. The first-generation vaccine was plasma-derived, but the vaccine in current use is genetically engineered. The safety and efficacy of the vaccine are well established, and there is no current recommendation for booster doses. Furthermore, protection from HBV also confers protection from HDV.

51. If you are employed in a dental practice, who pays for the HBV vaccine—you or your employer?

If an employee may be exposed to blood or other potentially infectious fluids during the course of work, it is the obligation of the employer to offer and pay for the series of vaccinations. HBV antibody titer tests are recommended 1–2 months after the completion of the vaccine series to verify that the health care worker is protected. Because this is a USPHS recommendation the employer is expected to pay the cost of the titer test.

52. What if I refuse the vaccination?

In most states, you have a right to refuse the vaccination. You should realize, however, that without the HBV vaccination series or evidence of previous infection you remain at risk for ac-

quiring HBV infection. Because OSHA considers the HBV vaccination one of the most important protections that a health care worker can have, the agency requires the employee to sign a
waiver if the vaccination is refused. Signing the waiver does not mean that, if you change your
mind in the future, the employer does not have to pay.

53. What is the risk of acquiring HBV infection from a percutaneous exposure to blood known to be infected with HBV?

The risk of becoming infected with HBV varies with the presence or absence of HBeAg. If
the sources is e antigen-positive, the risk of 22–30%; if the source is e antigen-negative the risk
is 1–6%. This risk is for an unprotected, nonvaccinated health care worker.

54. What is the risk of HIV transmission associated with percutaneous and/or mucous membrane exposures to blood known to be HIV-positive?

The risk is about 0.3% (1/300) for percutaneous and about 0.09% (1/900) for mucous membrane exposures. Many factors, however, influence the likelihood of transmission (see question
62). Accumulated data from studies involving health care worker exposures suggest a 0.2–0.4%
risk of HIV infection with the worst-case scenario of a severe percutaneous injury involving exposure to blood from a terminal HIV patient.

55. Have injuries to dental health care workers increased or decreased over the past decade?

Injuries have decreased from reports of 12 per year to 3–4 per year by 1991. More recent data
suggest that currently 2–3 injuries are reported per year.

56. Where do most injuries occur?

Most reported injuries occur outside the mouth, mainly on the hands and fingers. Burs have
been cited as the most common source of injury. For oral surgery, wires are frequently cited as
the cause of injury.

57. How do you prevent percutaneous injuries?

1. Use devices with engineered safety features designed to prevent injuries and/or use safer
work practices such as self-sheathing needles, not recapping by hand, not disengaging needles
from a reusable syringe by hand, use of disposable needle systems, and by the use of appropriate
sharps containers.

2. Avoid hand contact with sharps, such as not debriding an instrument by hand with gauze
but rather by using a single hand technique such as cotton rolls taped to a bracket tray or use of a
commercial safe wipe device.

58. What are the elements of a postexposure management program?

1. Wound management
2. Exposure reporting and documentation
3. Medical follow-up

59. How do you assess the risk of infection?

The risk of infection is assessed by type of exposure, body substance involved, and source evaluation. Assessing the type of exposure determines whether it is percutaneous, mucous membrane,
nonintact skin, or bites resulting in blood exposure. Risks also depend on body fluid, with blood or
bloody fluid being a higher risk. Caution is also for potentially infectious fluid or tissue. In terms of
the source evaluation consideration must be given to the presence of HBsAg, presence of HCV antibody, and/or the presence of HIV antibody. If the source status is unknown, a community or practice assessment is indicated.

60. What is the appropriate wound management?

1. Cleaning the wound with soap and water
2. Flushing mucous membranes with water
Note: Bleeding the wound or the use of bleach or caustic agents is not recommended.

61. Are any of these injuries preventable?

Yes. Data indicate that most reported injuries were preventable.

62. What is the major factor in prevention of bloodborne pathogen transmission in health care settings?

Although engineering controls are a major factor in reducing the risk of an exposure, work pracice controls have the greatest impact on preventing bloodborne disease transmission. Over 90% of the injuries leading to disease transmission have been associated with syringes and sharp instruments. Injuries also may be prevented by engineering controls, particularly the use of safer medical devices. A safe device will not prevent an injury unless it is properly used. The overall message is to maintain consistent levels of attention and to take personal care.

Recommendations for Managing Occupational Blood Exposures

Establish written protocols for management of occupational exposures:
- Based on current PHS guidelines
- Review periodically
- Provide training to personnel
  - Prevention and response to occupational exposures
- **Identify a qualified healthcare provider who:**
  - is familiar with current PHS postexposure management recommendations, antiretroviral therapy, bloodborne disease transmission, and the OSHA BBP Standard
  - will ensure prompt evaluation, treatment, management, and follow-up of occupational exposures
  - will provide necessary counseling

Provide immediate care to the exposure site:
- Wash wounds and skin with soap and water
- Flush mucous membranes with water

Immediately report the exposure to the infection control coordinator who should:
- Initiate referral to a qualified healthcare professional
- Complete necessary reports

Include the following information in the postexposure report:
- Date and time of exposure
- Details of the procedure being performed
  - where and how the exposure occurred
  - type of device involved
    - how and when during its handling the exposure occurred
- Details of the exposure
  - type and amount of fluid or material
  - severity of the exposure
- Details about the exposure source (HBV, HCV, HIV)
  - if the source was infected with HIV:
    - note the stage of disease, history of antiretroviral therapy, and viral load, if known
- Details about the exposed person (e.g., hepatitis B vaccination and vaccine-response status)
- Details about counseling, postexposure management, and follow-up

From Centers for Disease Control and Prevention, Division of Oral Health, 2002.

63. If I injure myself while working on a patient or with contaminated instruments from an identifiable patient, can someone call the patient's personal physician for additional medical history information?

In almost all states, a written informed consent is necessary before a physician can release information on a patient. Obtaining information without this consent may be a violation of medical confidentiality. The situation may be discussed with the source patient to ask for consent to obtain additional information about his or her health. Regardless of the answer, an appropriate health care professional should evaluate you as soon as feasible if the injury warrants.

64. What treatment options are available to a health care worker who has been exposed to HBV?

The health care worker may consider having a hepatitis B antibody titer to determine HBV serostatus. However, treatment should be initiated within 24 hours. If the health care worker was not vaccinated against HBV or does not have demonstrable antibody titer against hepatitis B surface antigen (anti-HBsAg), hepatitis B immunoglobulin (HBIG) should be administered as soon as possible. The HBV vaccination series should be initiated at the same time. An exposed health care worker also may need to consider the possibility that HIV and/or HCV exposure may have occurred simultaneously.

The efficacy of HBV PEP is based on perinatal data. These data indicate that if multiple doses of HBIG alone or the vaccine series alone is given within 1 week, the prevention of HBV infection is 70–75%. If a combination of HBIG and the vaccine series is administered, the efficacy increases to 85–95%.

65. How effective is the HBV vaccine?

Anti-HBs titers decline in 30–50% of adults within 8–10 years after vaccination. However, it is believed that the immune memory remains intact for at least 20 years after immunization. Chronic infection has rarely been documented in vaccine responders.

66. Describe postexposure follow-up for HBV.

The major elements are baseline evaluation and testing of the exposed health care worker, consideration of treatment options, and follow-up testing and counseling as indicated. If the exposed person has been vaccinated but the vaccine response is unknown, test for anti-HBs. If, however, the exposed health care worker has not been vaccinated or if the response is known, baseline testing is not necessary.

For health care workers who receive the HBV vaccine, follow-up testing for anti-HBs is indicated at 1–2 months after the last dose. If however, HBIG was also administered, the vaccine response cannot be ascertained until 3–4 months. If the source is not infected, follow-up is not necessary.

67. When must a percutaneous exposure (i.e., needlestick) be reported to OSHA?

Any occupational exposure or injury must be recorded on either OSHA forms or the practice's forms if it is work-related, required medical evaluation and/or follow-up, or resulted in seroconversion. Seroconversion, as the result of occupational exposure, also should be reported to the appropriate state agencies and the Centers for Disease Control and Prevention (CDC).

68. If I am a hepatitis B carrier, can I continue work that involves patient contact?

In many states you may continue clinical care as long as you adhere strictly to standard (universal) precautions. However, you should check with your department of public health, board of registration, or professional association for copies of the guidelines for HBV- or HIV-infected health care workers. Although based on guidelines developed by the CDC, they differ among states.

69. If I am not hepatitis B e antigen (HBeAg)-positive, am I still able to transmit hepatitis B?

Yes. Recently published data about four surgeons who were carriers of HBV and transmitted HBV to their patients indicate that surgeons, even in the absence of detectable levels of HBeAg in the serum, can transmit HBV during surgical procedures involving inapparent exposures of patients to small amounts of infective blood or serum.

70. How is such transmission possible?

In a study of surgeons, a mutation was found that prevented the expression of the e antigen. However, you should not be misled by this study because the e antigen is associated with the highest titers of HBV in the blood, which can range from 100 million to 1 billion/ml as opposed to about 100,000/ml in people who are not e antigen-positive.

71. What is the relationship between hepatitis C and non-A, non-B hepatitis (NANBH)?

The designation NANBH was first used in the 1970s, when sera from certain patients with signs and symptoms of hepatitis were found to be serologically negative for immunologic markers of hepatitis A and hepatitis B virus infection. The occurrence of manifestations typically associated with liver inflammation (i.e., jaundice, dark urine, chalky colored stools) without a defined etiology was exacerbated by the observation that some of the patients showed definite signs of a chronic carrier state. In 1989, investigators isolated the predominant cause of NANBH in the United States, a single-stranded RNA virus designated hepatitis C virus (HCV).

72. How is HCV transmitted? What are the implications for health care workers?

HCV is a blood-borne disease and is spread primarily via a parenteral route; sexual and maternal-fetal (vertical) transmission are minor modes of viral passage. Health care workers should follow standard precautions as indicated. HCV is not efficiently transmitted by occupational exposure. The prevalence among health care workers is about 1–2% (less than in the adult general population) and 10 times lower than for HBV infection. The average risk is 1.8% afer a percutaneous injury from an HCV-positive source.

73. What other information about HCV is important for health care workers?

1. No postexposure prophylaxis is available.
2. No vaccine is available.
3. Health care workers should be educated about risk and prevention.
4. Policies about testing and follow-up should be established.
5. There are no current recommendations for restriction of practice for HCV-infected health care workers.
6. Risk of transmission from health care worker to patient appears low.
7. Appropriate control recommendations for prevention of bloodborne disease transmission should be followed.

74. Does the CDC have specific policy recommendations for follow-up after percutaneous or permucosal exposure to HCV-positive blood?

As of July 4, 1997, the CDC recommends that minimal policies should include the following:
1. For the source, baseline testing for antibody to HCV (anti-HCV)
2. For the person exposed to an anti-HCV-positive source, baseline and follow-up testing (e.g., 6 month) for anti-HCV and alanine aminotransferase activity
3. Confirmation by supplemental anti-HCV testing of all anti-HCV results reported as repeatedly reactive by enzyme immunoassay (EIA)
4. Recommendation against postexposure prophylaxis with immunoglobulin or antiviral agents (e.g., interferon)
5. Education of health care workers about the risk for and prevention of bloodborne infections, with routine updates to ensure accuracy

75. In the absence of postexposure prophylaxis, what other issues should be considered?

The CDC recommends consideration of at least six issues in defining a protocol for the follow-up of health care workers occupationally exposed to HCV:
1. Limited data suggest that the risk of transmission after a needlestick is between that for HBV and HIV. Data for other routes of exposure are limited or nonexistent.
2. Available tests are limited in their ability to detect infection and determine infectivity.
3. The risk of transmission by sexual and other exposures is not well defined; all anti-HCV-positive persons should be considered potentially infectious.
4. Benefit of therapy for chronic disease is limited. Data support use of interferon combination therapy for early infection.
5. Costs associated with follow-up.
6. A postexposure protocol should address medical and legal implications, such as counseling about an infected health care worker's risk of transmitting HCV to others, therapy decisions, and individual worker concerns.

76. What are the elements of postexposure management for HCV?

As with other bloodborne exposures, baseline testing and follow-up testing and counseling are necessary. If the source patient is HCV-positive, the exposed health care worker should be tested for anti-HCV and ALT. If the source is not infected, baseline testing is not necessary. However, if the source is unknown, the risk of infection must be assessed to determine the indicated follow-up.

77. What if the source is HCV-positive?

If the source is HCV-positive, test for anti-HCV and ALT at baseline and 4–6 months after the exposure. For earlier diagnosis of HCV infection, an HCV-RNA test may be done at 4–6 weeks. Positive results should be confirmed with a supplemental

78. What is the relationship between viral load and potential rate of transmission to health care workers for HBV, HIV, and HCV?

Potential Transmission Risks to Health Care Workers

PATHOGEN	CONCENTRATION/ML IN SERUM/PLASMA	TRANSMISSION RATE (%) AFTER NEEDLESTICK INJURY
HBV	1,000,000–100,000,000	6.0–30.0
HCV	10–1,000,000	1.8
HIV	10–1,000	0.3

79. Have there been reports of health care workers-to-patient transmission of HCV?

There have been no reports of transmission in dental facilities. There have been recent reports in the United States of transmission from a cardiac surgeon to at least three patients. According to the CDC, the genetic match was "almost perfect" between the surgeon and the patients. The CDC further indicates that such transmissions are "exceedingly rare."

80. What are the new guidelines for postexposure management for occupational exposure to bloodborne pathogens?

In June 2001 the CDC updated and revised the guidelines for postexposure management to occupational bloodborne exposures to reflect new information and considerations. Since 1998, the FDA has approved new antiretroviral agents and more is known of the safety and efficacy of PEP (postexposure prophylaxis). Concern over resistance has increased as well as concern over when not to use PEP such as for low-risk exposures. This document also consolidates PEP for HBV and HCV to provide a comprehensive guideline.

81. What factors are associated with an increased risk of HIV transmission after a percutaneous injury?

The risk for HIV infection after an exposure to blood known to be infected with HIV is increased if the exposure is to a larger quantity from the source as indicated by either or both of the following:

1. Visible blood on the device
2. A procedure that involved a needle being directly placed into a vein or artery

Risk is also increased if the source has terminal illness, possibly meaning a higher titer of virus in the blood. Studies have demonstrated that more blood is transferred if the injury is deep and if hollow-bore needles are used.

82. What is the rationale for HIV PEP?

The rationale behind the use of PEP is based on the plausibility that infection can be prevented or ameliorated by the use of antiretrovirals. There are indications that if antiretrovirals are given early, the pathogenesis may be affected because systemic infection does not immediately occur. There is a window of opportunity during which antiretrovirals may modify or prevent replication. There is also direct and indirect evidence from human and animal studies that specific agents may work if appropriately used. In addition, retrospective studies of exposed health care workers demonstrated that the use of ZDV after an occupational exposure was associated with a 81% reduction in risk of seroconversion.

83. What does the USPHS recommend for chemoprophylaxis after HIV exposure?

The USPHS recommends that in certain cases health care workers should take ZDV and other antiretroviral drugs* after exposure on the job to reduce the risk of becoming infected. These drugs are recommended for the highest-risk exposures, such as needlesticks contaminated with the blood of a patient in the late stages of AIDS. For lower-risk exposures, such as a blood splash to the eye, drugs should be offered to the worker; however, considerable thought should be given to taking drugs for lower-risk exposures because the possible side effects in healthy (i.e., not HIV-infected) persons are not well known.

84. What antiretrovirals are FDA-approved and appropriate for HIV PEP?

Three classes of drugs are available and approved: nucleoside reverse transcriptase inhibitors, nonnucleoside reverse transcriptase inhibitors, and protease inhibitors. The recommendations are generally to use two- or three-drug combinations, depending on the significance of the exposure. For a more significant exposure a three-drug regimen may be justified. For lower risk exposures, the regimen is uncertain.

85. Have adverse effects been reported in the use of antiretrovirals?

Studies indicate that about half of health care workers report some adverse symptoms, such as nausea, malaise, headache and about 33% discontinue the use because of adverse symptoms. This consideration is important in designing a regimen that can be tolerable. More serious side effects have been reported but are rare.

86. What is the concern over resistance?

Resistance is a concern in the use of antiretrovirals either because of source information about resistance or the potential resistance associated with one of the agents used in PEP. Resistance has been reported with all available drugs as well as cross-resistance within drug classes. Resistance testing of the source is not practical because of the interval until results are available. However, modifications may be made if resistance is known or suspected.

87. What if I am pregnant?

Data are limited about the potential effects on a fetus. Consultation with an expert is advised.

88. When else is expert consultation advised?

Expert consultation is advised if there is a delay in medical follow-up (later than 24–36 hours after the exposure), if the source is unknown and the injury is significant, if resistance is known or suspected to the recommended drug regimen, and if toxicity or adverse symptoms occur.

89. For how long must prophylactic drugs be taken?

The current recommendation is to take the drugs for 4 weeks.

90. Do antiretrovirals prevent occupational infection?

Postexposure prophylaxis does not prevent all occupational infections. There have been at least 21 reports of antiretrovirals failing to prevent infection in health care workers. Factors that may influence failure include antiretroviral resistance, treatment interruption (too short a duration), delayed initiation of treatment, a high titer or inoculum exposure, or host factors. Following current infection control recommendations and using safer needle devices are the primary means of preventing occupationally acquired HIV infection. However, if an exposure occurs, the risk of infection is usually low; when warranted, taking drugs as soon as possible (within 2 hours) after exposure may reduce the risk further.

91. Does the employer have to pay for the antiretroviral drugs?

OSHA has made no official statement. However, because OSHA relies on the most current USPHS recommendations, the agency may well expect the employer to pay for the chemoprophylactic regimen. This rapidly evolving area may change further as the USPHS reviews its recommendations, which are based on surveillance studies demonstrating that antiretroviral therapy is beneficial if taken immediately after a significant exposure incident.

92. What is a prudent course for postexposure chemoprophylaxis?

It is important to discuss the postexposure management options in advance of an exposure incident. The discussion should include the potential risk associated with various injuries, source patient factors, selection of a health care professional, and availability of antiretrovirals, if indicated.

93. Has HIV seroconversion been *documented* among dental health care workers as the result of an occupational exposure?

No, not as of December 2001. There are voluntary reports to CDC of 57 health care workers with documented seroconversion.

94. Have any dental health care workers *possibly* seroconverted as the result of an occupational exposure?

Yes. As of December 2001, about 6 dental health care workers of 138 total health care workers have been reported to the CDC as possible cases of occupational transmission.

95. What is the difference between a documented occupational transmission and a possible occupational transmission of HIV?

The difference is in the testing. A documented occupational transmission requires that the exposed health care worker be tested for HIV at the time of the incident and that the baseline test be negative. If, after a designated time, HIV seroconversion occurs, it is considered to be the result of the exposure incident. In the possible category, health care workers have been found to be without identifiable behavioral or transfusion risk. Each reported percutaneous exposure to blood or body fluids or lab solutions containing HIV, but HIV seroconversion specifically resulting from an occupational exposure was not documented. There was no baseline testing at the time of the incident to prove that the health care worker was HIV-negative before the incident.

96. What is the purpose of baseline testing after an occupational exposure incident?

Baseline HIV antibody and HBV testing allows the health care professional who evaluates the exposed worker to determine whether any subsequently diagnosed disease was acquired as the result of the exposure incident. Blood is tested soon after the injury occurs to determine the health care worker's HBV and/or HIV serologic status.

97. Can an employee refuse baseline testing?

An employee may decline testing or choose to delay testing of collected blood for 90 days. If a delay is chosen, the blood must be drawn but not tested until consent is given.

98. If I consent to baseline blood collection but not testing, then what?

If within 90 days the employee consents to testing of the baseline sample, it should be done as soon as possible. If consent is not given within the 90 days, the sample may be discarded.

99. What is the difference between confidential and anonymous HIV testing?

Confidential testing with consent means that the test results become part of your confidential medical record and cannot be released without your consent and in accordance with state laws. The test results are linked to your name, even if only in your medical record. Anonymous testing refers to a system whereby test results are linked to a number or code and not a name. Therefore, you are the only one who will know the results; they will not be part of your medical record. Whether a coded result will suffice as evidence of baseline testing for the purposes of documenting an exposure incident has not been challenged. If you are reluctant to have any HIV test information in your medical record but are concerned about documenting an incident, you may wish to consider baseline blood collection at both an anonymous and a confidential test site. Have the anonymous sample tested, and store the confidential sample for not more than the 90 days allowed. Thus you have time to consider testing and an opportunity to find out whether you are seronegative.

100. Who pays the cost of HIV testing?

The employer is responsible for the cost of HIV testing under the obligation to provide medical evaluation and follow-up of an exposure incident.

101. Is the employer responsible for costs associated with treatment of disease if transmission occurs?

No. The employer is not expected to pay the costs associated with long-term treatment of disease—only for the immediate evaluation and postexposure prophylaxis as prescribed by OSHA in accordance with USPHS recommendations.

102. What is a sharps injury log?

A sharps injury log is used to record percutaneous injuries from contaminated sharps. The log must be maintained to ensure confidentiality. At a minimum, the log should contain:

1. Type and brand of device involved
2. Work area where the incident occured.
3. Explanation of how the incident occurred

103. How long must an employer maintain employee medical records?

The employer must maintain employee medical records for the duration of employment plus 30 years in accordance with OSHA's Standard on Access to Employee Exposure and Medical Records, 29 CFR 1910.20. An employer may contract with the health care professional to maintain the records as along as they are accessible to OSHA.

104. Who selects the health care professional for postexposure evaluation and follow-up?

The employer has the right to choose the health care professional who will treat exposure incidents.

Postexposure Evaluation and Follow-up Requirements under OSHA's Standard for Occupational Exposure to Bloodborne Pathogens

Exposure incident occurs
↓

Employee	Employer	Health care professional (HCP)
• Reports incident → to employer	• Directs employee to HCP →	• Evaluates exposure incident
	• Sends to HCP:	• Arranges for testing of exposed employee and source patient (if not already known)
	• Copy of standard	• Notifies employee of results of all testing
	• Job description of employee	• Provides counseling
	• Incident report (route, etc.)	• Provides postexposure prophylaxis
	• Source patient's identity and HBV/HIV status (if known) and other relevant medical	• Evaluates reported illnesses (above items are *confidential*)
	• Documents events on OSHA 200 and 101 (if applicable)	
	• Receives HCP's written opinion	← • Sends (only) written opinion to employer: Documentation that employee was
• Receives copy ← of HCP's written opinion	• Provides copy of HCP's written opinion to employee (within 15 days of completed evaluation)	informed of evaluation results and need for any further follow-up and Whether HBV vaccine is indicated and if vaccine was received

Prepared by OSHA (February 1995). This document is not considered a substitute for any provisions of the Occupational Safety and Health Act of 1970 or for any standards issued by OSHA.

105. Does the employer have an obligation to former employees?

OSHA's standard on bloodborne pathogens requires immediate medical evaluation and follow-up of an employee. If an employee leaves the practice, the employer is no longer obligated to meet the obligations in the standard.

106. Does the employer have any obligation to temporary workers under OSHA standards?

The responsibility to protect temporary workers from workplace hazards is shared by the agency that supplies a temporary worker. The agency is required to ensure that all workers have been vaccinated and are provided follow-up evaluations. The contracting employer is not responsible for vaccinations and follow-up unless the contract so specifies. However, the contracting employer is expected to provide gloves, masks, and other personal protective equipment.

107. How accurate is the HIV antibody test?

At 6 months after an exposure incident, the current serum test has the ability to detect the presence of HIV antibody with 99.9% accuracy. After 1 year, it is 99.9999% accurate. In addition to the traditional serum test, a new saliva collection system is available. The accuracy of the saliva test is reported to be comparable to the serum test. The FDA has given preliminary approval to a rapid HIV test that requires "a drop" of blood and can produce results in 20 minutes.

108. What concerns are raised by the rapid test?

First, the test does not detect HIV-2 (a less prevalent strain). Second, there are questions about whether the test can be approved for use in doctor's offices and public health clinics rather than labs.

109. What should you recommend to a health care worker who has been potentially infected with HIV?

The first step is to seek voluntary, anonymous testing and counseling services. Early medical intervention is most important in light of the new multidrug combinations for anti-HIV therapy. In addition, it is important to consult state guidelines for HIV/HBV-infected health care workers, your professional association, or a legal advocate.

110. Have there been any recent reports of HBV transmission from dentists to patients?

Since 1987 there have been no reports of HBV transmission from a dentist to a patient. From 1970–1987, nine clusters were reported in which HBV infection was associated with dental treatment by an infected dental health care worker. Reasons for the current lack of reports of HBV transmission may include the following:

1. Increased adherence to standard (universal) precautions
2. High compliance with HBV vaccination among dental health care workers
3. Reporting bias, incomplete reporting, or failure to correlate HBV transmission with previous dental treatment

Factors that enhanced the transmission of HBV in the past included failure to use gloves routinely during patient care, failure to receive HBV vaccination, noncompliance with universal precautions, and inability to detect disease in dental health care workers.

111. Are the guidelines for preventing transmission of airborne disease different from those for preventing transmission of bloodborne disease?

Yes. In October 1994, the CDC issued their final version of the *Guidelines for Preventing the Transmission of Mycobacterium tuberculosis in Health-Care Facilities*, which emphasize the importance of the following: (1) the hierarchy of control measures, including administrative and engineering controls and personal respiratory protection; (2) the use of risk assessments for developing a written tuberculosis (TB) control plan; (3) early identification and management of persons who have TB; (4) TB screening programs for health care workers; (5) training and education of health care workers; and (6) evaluation of TB infection control programs. No information suggests that bloodborne diseases are transmitted by aerosols.

112. What are specific recommendations for preventing TB transmission in dental settings?

Recommendations for the Prevention of the Transmission of TB in Dental Settings

1. A risk assessment should be done periodically, and TB infection control policies should be based on the risk assessment. The policies should include provisions for detection and referral of patients who may have undiagnosed active TB; management of patients with active TB, relative to provision of urgent dental care; and employer-sponsored health care worker education, counseling, and screening.
2. While taking patients' initial medical histories and at periodic updates, dental health care workers should routinely ask all patients whether they have a history of TB disease and symptoms suggestive of TB.
3. Patients with a medical history or symptoms suggestive of undiagnosed active TB should be referred promptly for medical evaluation of possible infectiousness. Such patients should not remain in the dental care facility any longer than required to arrange a referral. While in the dental care facility, they should wear surgical masks and should be instructed to cover their mouths and noses when coughing or sneezing.
4. Elective dental treatment should be deferred until a physician confirms that the patient does not have infectious TB. If the patient is diagnosed as having active TB, elective treatment should be deferred until the patient is no longer infectious.
5. If urgent care must be provided for a patient who has, or is strongly suspected of having, infectious TB, such care should be provided in facilities that can provide TB isolation. Dental health care workers should use respiratory protection while performing procedures on such patients. (Note: dental facilities may want to research appropriate referral facilities prior to the need for referral).
6. Any dental health care worker who has a persistent cough (i.e., a cough lasting 3 weeks), especially in the presence of other signs or symptoms compatible with active TB (e.g., weight loss, night sweats, bloody sputum, anorexia, and fever), should be evaluated promptly for TB. The health care worker should not return to the workplace until a diagnosis of TB has been excluded or until the health care worker is on therapy and determination has been made that the health care worker is noninfectious.
7. In dental care facilities that provide care to populations at high risk for active TB, it may be appropriate to use engineering controls similar to those used in general use areas (e.g., waiting rooms) of medical facilities that have a similar risk profile.

Centers for Disease Control and Prevention: Recommendations for the prevention of the transmission of TB in dental settings. MMWR 43:(RR-13):52–53, 1994.

113. What is the risk of TB transmission in dental settings?

The risk is probably quite low and is determined by a number of factors, including community profiles and patient population characteristics. TB infection control policies are linked to a facility's level of risk, which is determined by risk assessment.

Elements of a TB Control Program for Dental Facilities

| | RISK CATEGORY* | |
ELEMENT	MINIMAL	VERY LOW
Designate a TB control individual	Recommended	Recommended
Conduct baseline risk assessment	Recommended	Recommended
Review community TB profile	Yearly	Yearly
Written TB control plan	Recommended	Recommended
Reassessment of risk	Yearly	Yearly
Protocol for identifying, managing, and referring patients with active TB (includes providing/referring for urgent dental care but allows delay/referral for elective care)	Recommended	Recommended
Education and training	Recommended	Recommended
Counseling oral health care workers about TB	Recommended	Recommended
Protocol to identify/evaluate oral health care workers with signs/symptoms of active TB	Recommended	Recommended
Baseline purified protein derivative (PPD) testing of oral health care workers	Optional	Recommended

(continued)

Elements of a TB Control Program for Dental Facilities (Continued)

	RISK CATEGORY*	
ELEMENT	MINIMAL	VERY LOW
Periodic PPD screening of oral health care workers	Not applicable	Yearly
Protocol for evaluating and managing oral health care workers with positive PPD tests	Recommended	Recommended
Protocol for managing oral health care workers with active TB	Recommended	Recommended
Protocol for investigating PPD conversions and active TB in oral health care workers	Recommended	Recommended
Protocol for investigating possible patient-patient transmission of TB	Recommended	Recommended

Note: In addition, for dental facilities in a low-risk category, all of the above apply, but there are stronger recommendations for engineering controls and respiratory protection programs.

*Risk categories are determined by a number of factors, including community profile and patient population. If, after a review of the community profile and the patient profile, it is determined that there are no TB patients in a facility or community, then a "minimal" risk classification is indicated. However, if a review indicates the presence of TB patients, then further analysis is necessary to complete the risk assessment including evaluation of health care worker screening. If screening is negative, no TB patients were identified in the previous year, and a plan is in place to refer patients with suspected or confirmed TB to a collaborating facility, the classification is "very low" risk.

Adapted from the Centers for Disease Control and Prevention: Guidelines for Preventing the Transmission of *Mycobacterium tuberculosis* in Health-Care Facilities. Atlanta, Centers for Disease Control and Prevention, 1994, pp 12–15.

INSTRUMENT REPROCESSING AND STERILIZATION

114. What is the difference between sterilization and disinfection?

Sterilization is a process capable of killing all forms of microorganisms on an instrument or surface, including high numbers of highly resistant bacterial spores if they are present. **Disinfection** is the process of destroying pathogenic organisms, but not necessarily all organisms.

115. List some methods of sterilization common for dentistry.

Saturated steam, saturated chemical vapor, dry heat—rapid transfer, dry heat—convection, ethylene oxide gas, and chemical immersion.

116. Describe the types of heat sterilization procedures.

1. Steam under pressure, or autoclaving, is the most widely used method.

2. Dry-heat sterilization involves placing instruments in a dry heat sterilizer cleared for marketing as a medical device by the FDA. Instruments must remain in the unit for a specified period of heating at a required temperature.

3. Unsaturated chemical vapor sterilization uses a specific chemical solution, which, when heated under pressure, forms a sterilized vapor phase with a low concentration of water.

Note: Manufacturer's directions for each sterilizer must be followed closely.

117. How do you select the appropriate sterilizer?

Consider your facility and the types of instruments and devices that you use. You may need more than one type of sterilizer to accommodate your needs. The size of the practice, instrument inventory, and space considerations may influence your choice.

118. What is an elementary doctrine in choosing a method of sterilization?

Do not disinfect or "cold-sterilize" what you can sterilize with a heat-based process: "Don't dunk it, cook it." If an item or instrument is heat-stable, it should be heat-sterilized. No other methods (e.g., gases or liquids) have equivalent economy, potency, and safety assurance.

119. According to the Spaulding classification, what are critical, semicritical, and noncritical items?

CDC/Spaulding Classification of Surfaces

	DESCRIPTION	EXAMPLES	DISEASE TRANSMISSION RISK	REPROCESSING TECHNIQUE
Critical instruments	Pointed/sharp Penetrates tissue Blood present	Needles Cutting instruments Implants	High	Sterile, disposable Heat sterilization
Semicritical instruments	Mucous membrane or broken skin contact No tissue penetration	Medical "scopes" Nonsurgical dental instruments Specula Catheters	Moderate	Heat sterilization High-level disinfection
Noncritical instruments	Unbroken skin contact	Face masks Clothing Blood pressure cuffs Diag electrodes	Low	Sanitize (no blood) Intermediate-level disinfection (blood present)
Environmental surfaces	Indirect to no direct patient contact during treatment			Sanitize (no blood) Intermediate-level disinfection
Medical equipment	Indirect contact	Knobs, handles x-ray machine Dental units	Moderate to low	
Housekeeping	No contact	Floors, walls Countertops	Least	

Table incorporates the expansion of Spaulding's classic "critical, semicritical, noncritical" surface classification, as described by Favarro and Bond, 2001.

Because the vast majority, if not all, of dental instruments are heat-stable, they should be sterilized using a heat-based method (e.g., autoclaving). High-level disinfection using liquid chemical/sterilant germicides is *not* the current standard of practice in dentistry.

120. How are critical and semicritical items treated after use?

If reusable, all heat-stable critical and semicritical instruments should be sterilized with a heat process. Semicritical items require either heat or chemical-vapor sterilization.

121. To what does the term "cold sterilization" refer in dentistry?

In dentistry, cold sterilization refers to the past practice of immersion (liquid chemical) disinfection used to reprocess reusable semicritical instruments or items for patient care. The practice was not sterilization per se and is no longer considered appropriate for reprocessing heat-stable medical instruments. Virtually every reusable dental instrument in current use is heat-stable and should be appropriately cleaned, wrapped, and sterilized between uses with a heat-based, biologically monitored process such as a steam autoclave. Accordingly, the near universal heat stability of dental instruments creates little justification or economic utility for use of other "low-temperature" sterilization procedures (e.g., with gasses such as ethylene oxide or vapor-phase hydrogen peroxide).

122. What is the appropriate use of a glutaraldehyde solution in a dental operatory or laboratory?

There is little appropriate use in dentistry for this or any other sterilant/disinfectant liquid chemical product. Some workers feel the need and prefer the use of $2^+\%$ glutaraldehyde solutions to disinfect dental impression material. Others may have a few select reusable heat-sensitive critical or semicritical instruments or devices that require sterilization or high-level disinfection, respectively, between uses. To "sterilize" using such a product requires procedures such as meticulous precleaning of the item, total immersion (no bubbles anywhere) for up to 10 or more hours in (preferably) fresh solution at the indicated temperature, aseptic retrieval of the item with *sterile* forceps (preferably in a laminar flow safety cabinet to minimize extraneous contamination), thorough rinsing with *sterile* water, drying with *sterile* towels (workers wearing *sterile* gloves), and packaging in a *sterile* container unless the item is used immediately. The practical probability of delivering a *truly sterile* item (probability of contamination of one in one million—a probability impossible to validate or confirm by post-process sampling and culturing) to the patient under such circumstances is virtually nil. For high-level disinfection of a heat-sensitive item using a similar procedure (the chemical agent is the same as for "sterilization"), the only change in the process is significantly less time of exposure to the liquid chemical agent (minutes instead of hours).

Whatever the target case (sterilization or high-level disinfection), before purchasing and using any chemical agent for these purposes, the workers should perform a carefully considered inventory of instruments or devices appropriate for being reprocessed using a "cold" or "low-temperature" procedure. Further, recognizing the toxic nature and use patterns of these agents (especially the liquid chemicals that require the use of trays or other open containers of the product) workers should closely consider the label-directed procedures for agent containment, worker protection, and agent disposal. Under no circumstance should this class of chemical be used for any purpose other than what is listed on the product label. For example, a glutaraldehyde-based sterilant/disinfectant (or any other immersion-type liquid chemical agent in that class) is *never* appropriate for wipe downs of environmental surfaces, no matter the perceived level or type of contamination. These chemicals have little utility in dentistry.

123. What is the best way to reprocess a handpiece?

The best way is to follow the manufacturer's instructions, which should indicate that a handpiece must be heat-treated between patients. The manufacturer's instructions also should outline clearly the steps for cleaning and lubrication and the most appropriate heat-treatment method. All handpieces manufactured since the late 1980s are heat-stable; older units, if still in working condition, may be modified to withstand heat sterilization. If not so modified, their uses should be discontinued.

124. What is the only function of a so-called glass bead sterilizer?

The glass bead sterilizer is used during endodontic procedures to decontaminate endodontic files while they are used on the same patient. It is not a sterilizer, and this designation is a long-standing misnomer in FDA classification. Recently, these devices have been recalled by the FDA for submission of supplemental data to substantiate or refute classification as sterilizers. These data have not been forthcoming.

125. Can a disposable saliva ejector be reprocessed and reused?

No. It is a single-use item impossible to adequately reprocess and should be disposed of accordingly after a single use.

126. How must a reusable air-water syringe tip be reprocessed?

The only acceptable methods of reprocessing are first, thorough cleaning followed by wrapping and then sterilizing with either steam under pressure, dry-heat, or unsaturated chemical vapor.

127. What is the minimal temperature required for sterilization by an autoclave?

121° Celsius. Manufacturer's instructions should be followed closely.

128. Discuss the advantages and disadvantages of an autoclave.
   Advantage
   • It is the gold standard for sterilization—nothing better is available to the dental setting.

Disadvantages
- Instrument cutting surfaces and burs may become dulled.
- Carbide-steel items may corrode.
- Time is spent precleaning and wrapping instruments.

129. What is the method of choice for sterilizing burs and diamonds?

If burs are not discarded after use, dry heat is the least expensive sterilization method and does not corrode or dull cutting edges. If you must use an autoclave for burs, they should be dipped into a 1% sodium nitrite emulsion preparation to prevent corrosion.

130. In a forced-air dry heat oven preheated to 160–170° C, how long does it take to sterilize instruments?

Sterilization is achieved in 2 hours in a properly working unit. However, additional time may be necessary for cool down before metal items can be used.

131. What are the advantages and disadvantages of dry-heat sterilizers?
Advantages
- They do not dull or otherwise corrode instruments.
- They are equivalent to a steam autoclave in germicidal potency in a completed cycle.

Disadvantages
- Cycle time is long
- Most plastics, paper, and fabrics char, melt, or burn and cannot be sterilized in this manner.

132. Can a dental handpiece withstand dry-heat sterilization?

Currently, it cannot, and manufacturers do not recommend dry-heat sterilization. Handpieces, however, may be appropriately sterilized by saturated steam under pressure or unsaturated chemical-vapor sterilization.

133. Which federal agency is responsible for regulating handpieces?

The FDA, Center for Devices and Radiological Health, Office of Device Evaluation, Dental and Medical Services Branch, in accordance with the Safe Medical Devices Act, clears medical devices, including sterilizers, for marketing. The user, however, must be aware that clearance to market proves neither efficacy nor manufacturer's claims.

134. What packaging material is compatible with autoclaves?

The most suitable material for use in an autoclave is one that the steam can penetrate; for example, paper or certain plastics. It is best to read the manufacturer's instructions and follow them precisely.

135. What packaging material cannot be used in dry-heat sterilizers?

The manufacturer's instructions specify that you cannot use most of the plastics (pouch or wrap) and paper wrap commonly used for steam autoclaves. They melt or burn at high temperatures.

136. What packaging material is compatible with unsaturated chemical-vapor sterilizers?

The manufacturer's instructions make clear that perforated metal trays and paper are suitable for use in chemical-vapor sterilizers. The vapor must be able to penetrate the material. Chemical-vapor sterilizers also rely on high levels of heat and pressure for efficacy.

137. What is an easy method to demonstrate that sterilization conditions have been reached in a cycle?

Process indicators and other chemical integrators demonstrate that some conditions to achieve sterilization were reached.

138. What is the definition of sterile?

The state of sterility is an absolute term: an item is either sterile, or it is not sterile. Sterility is the absence of all viable life forms, and the term reflects a carefully designed and monitored process used to ensure that an item has a very low probability of being contaminated with anything at time of use. For surgical instruments, this probability is one in one million—i.e., a sterility assurance level (SAL) of 10 to the minus 6th.

139. What are the most common reasons for sterilization failure in an autoclave?

1. Inadequate precleaning of instruments
2. Improper maintenance of equipment
3. Cycle time too short and/or temperature too low
4. Improper loading or overloading
5. Incompatible packaging material
6. Interruption of a cycle to add or remove items

Multiple investigations have found that the most frequent cause of sterilizer failure is human error.

140. What types of sterilization monitoring are available?

1. Mechanical/electronic
2. Chemical indicators (color change integrators)
3. Biologic indicators (spore tests)

141. What is a mechanical or electronic control?

These devices consist of observation of gauges and indicators on the sterilization equipment (cycle monitors). They measure time, temperature, and pressure, for example.

142. What is the difference between chemical indicators and biologic (spore) monitors?

Biologic spore monitors more precisely reflect the potency of the sterilization process by directly measuring death of high numbers of highly resistant bacterial endospores, whereas simple chemical indicators merely reflect that the temperature of sterilization has been reached. Other chemical indicators (i.e., integrators) are becoming more sophisticated and reflect both time and temperature during the process. There are insufficient data to indicate whether the two processes are equivalent. Current recommendations suggest that simple chemical indicators be placed in the center of every individual instrument pack to show the user that the package went through a heating process. In using any process monitor, the instructions provided by the monitor manufacturer or the monitor testing service should be followed precisely. Process monitors perform exactly as their name indicates. They monitor specific parameters of the sterilization process. Neither of the two "proves" that the end product of a sterilization process is, in fact, sterile. That proof was included in the laboratory design and validation of the particular sterilizer and its sterilization process.

143. What should be done if the spore test is positive?

A positive spore test indicates a failure. Recall implantable devices, but not necessarily all instruments. Reprocess any instrument that you can recall from the suspect load if a second spore test remains positive.

144. In biologic monitoring of sterilization equipment, which nonpathogenic organisms are used for each type of unit?

For autoclaves and chemical-vapor sterilizers, *Geobacillus stearothermophilus,* formerly *Bacillus stearothemophilus,* spores are used. For dry-heat and ethylene oxide units, *Bacillus atrophaeus,* formerly *Bacillus subtilis,* is used. Placement of the monitor in a load is critical; manufacturer's instructions should be followed closely.

145. How often should biologic monitoring of sterilization units be performed?

At a minimum, on a weekly basis.

Indications for More Frequent Biologic Monitoring of Sterilization Units

1. If the equipment is new and being used for the first time
2. During the first operating cycle after a repair
3. If there is a change in packaging material
4. If new employees are using the unit or being trained in use of equipment or procedure for monitoring
5. After an electrical or power source failure
6. If door seals or gaskets are changed
7. If cycle time and/or temperature is changed
8. Waste shall not be processed in an instrument sterilizer.
9. For all cycles to render infectious waste as noninfectious, as mandated by state law*
10. If the method of biologic monitoring is changed

*This may not apply in all states; contact the appropriate state agency.

146. What is the rationale for use of a holding solution?

A holding solution is a good idea if the circumstance warrants; for example, when it is not possible to clean instruments or items immediately after patient use. It is easier to clean the instruments safely and efficiently if the material is not dried. The intent of a holding solution is only to keep debris moist; if it dries, cleaning becomes more difficult. Holding solutions are not intended for disinfection, and chemical disinfectants should not be used as holding solutions. Chemical disinfectants, in particular, sterilant/disinfectant agents such as glutaraldehyde, should not be used as holding solutions. Even beyond the fact that such use is off label, glutaraldehyde, for example, is a protein fixative agent, and immersion of soiled instruments in it will only "fry" (fix) the protein to the items, making them difficult to clean.

147. Do instruments need to be cleaned before sterilization?

Instruments must be cleaned thoroughly before sterilization. Two methods of instrument cleaning are ultrasonic cleaning and handscrubbing. Ultrasonic cleaning is the method of choice, because it minimizes hand contact with contaminated sharps and may clean more thoroughly than handscrubbing. If an ultrasonic unit is not available, handscrubbing must be done in a safe manner to avoid injury. The preferred method is to clean one or two items at a time, holding them low in the sink under running water and scrubbing them with a long-handled brush. Regardless of cleaning method, contaminated instruments should be handled only while wearing reusable, heavy-gauge, industrial, or housekeeping gloves. Vinyl or Latex gloves are not appropriate.

148. What are the methods for cleaning contaminated instruments?

Ultrasonic cleaning, washer/disinfector, or manual handscrubbing.

149. How do you ensure that an ultrasonic cleaning unit is in proper working order?

A function test may be performed on a routine basis, according to the manufacturers' instructions. In general, a function test requires that fresh solution be activated in the unit, that a piece of aluminum foil of specified size be cut and placed vertically into the activated solution for exactly 20 seconds, and that the foil be removed and examined under a light source. A functional unit causes holes and/or pitting in the foil; if no holes are present or a uniform pitting pattern is not evident, the unit is not working properly and should be repaired.

USE AND MISUSE OF LIQUID CHEMICAL GERMICIDES

150. Which federal agencies are involved in the regulation of liquid chemical germicides?

The FDA regulates chemical germicides if they are used for terminal reprocessing of reusable medical devices. The Environmental Protection Agency (EPA) regulates and registers chemical germicides used to disinfect environmental surfaces. The FDA also regulates the instruments themselves, including autoclaves, dry-heat, and other sterilizers.

151. Upon what does the efficiency of a disinfectant depend?

1. The amount of organic material (bioburden) left on surfaces and the proportionately higher numbers and types of microorganisms contained in and being protected by the organic material. Organic material can also rapidly inactivate certain germicides before they have opportunity to work against microorganisms. Soiled instruments are the absolute bane of liquid chemical disinfectant efficacy.

2. Proper concentration of the disinfectant

3. Length and temperature of exposure

4. Accuracy with which the operator follows specific instructions on the product label or inserted in the product package

152. Why is the destruction of *Mycobacterium tuberculosis* required by the EPA as a benchmark for testing chemical disinfectants on environmental surfaces?

The question is typically asked in the context of the additional statement, "We are not really as concerned about tuberculosis being spread from the countertops as we are about hepatitis B and C viruses and HIV." That line of thinking is correct because *M. tuberculosis* is not transmitted via inanimate surfaces such as countertops. It is transmitted through the inhalation of infectious microdroplet nuclei created from infectious aerosols. This vegetative, acid-fast bacillus serves as the resistance standard for disinfectants solely because of its resistance to germicidal chemicals. According to the EPA classification, an approved label claim of "hospital disinfectant" assures the purchaser that the product has a demonstrated ability to kill *Staphylococcus aureus, Pseudomas aeruginosa,* and *Salmonella choleraesuis.* An additional claim for "tuberculocidal" activity provides the level of microbial inactivation appropriate for contaminated surfaces in health care facilities—intermediate-level disinfection. The ability to destroy the more resistant tubercle bacilli leads to the consistent inactivation of less resistant vegetative bacteria, fungi, and viruses. Chemicals such as phenols, chlorine compounds, iodophors, and alcohol-containing products are tuberculocidal and are suitable for disinfecting environmental surfaces.

153. Give practical guidelines for performing the tasks required for surface disinfection.

The same fundamental principle that applies to asepsis and aseptic technique also applies to environmental surface disinfection: clean it first. As straightforward and logical as this statement appears, exaggerated product claims, time constraints between patient appointments, and the need to accomplish multiple tasks rapidly have created confusion about the potential for environmental surface-mediated disease transmission and disinfection.

154. Have problems of chemical efficacy and potential toxicity challenges developed only since the introduction of newer classes of disinfectants in the 1970s?

No. Many of the same issues concerning the use of chemical disinfectants and antiseptics have confronted health care professionals since they were introduced in the 19th century. Early on people began to notice irritation and toxicity problems. Unfortunately, when health care workers are exposed to high concentrations of aerosolized disinfectants over time, as a result of overspraying germicides, multiple health hazards develop—from mucous membrane irritation to dermatitis and severe respiratory allergic reactions. These reactions are observed even with quartenary ammonium compounds. "Spray zealots" can do harm to themselves, to others in the practice, and to equipment repeatedly exposed to harsh chemicals.

155. What are Spaulding's classifications of biocidal activity?

1. **Sterilization** is a process that kills all microorganisms, including high numbers of highly resistant bacterial spores.

2. **High-level disinfection** is a process in which chemical sterilants are used in a manner that kills vegetative bacteria, tubercle bacillus (mycobacteria), lipid and nonlipid viruses, and fungi, but not all bacterial spores, if they are present in high numbers. Hot water pasteurization is also high-level disinfection. The application of high-level disinfection in dentistry is limited because virtually all dental instruments are heat-stable and can be sterilized in an autoclave.

3. **Intermediate-level disinfection** kills vegetative bacteria and fungi, tubercle bacillus, and lipid and nonlipid viruses. These agents (phenols, chlorine compounds, iodophors, and alcohol-containing products) are designed for disinfecting environmental surfaces, or medical equipment, but *not* for critical or semicritical medical instruments.

4. **Low–level disinfection** kills only vegetative bacteria, some fungi, and lipid viruses, but not tubercle bacillus. These products (mostly quaternary ammonium compounds) are designed for use on housekeeping surfaces.

156. What special considerations apply to handling contaminated instruments?

First is to use the appropriate PPE such as puncture-resistant gloves. The next concern is the safe transport of the instruments in an appropriate container. Another is not to handle contaminated instruments unnecessarily in the operatory; instruments should be transported to the reprocessing area of the facility.

157. Is household bleach acceptable for surface decontamination?

OSHA's Instruction CPL 2-2.44C, "Enforcement Procedures for The Occupational Exposure to Bloodborne Pathogens Standard," states that disinfectant products registered by the EPA as tuberculocidal are appropriate for the clean-up of blood-contaminated surfaces. Although generic sodium hypochlorite solutions are not registered as such, they are generally recommended by the CDC as an alternative to other proprietary germicides for disinfection of environmental surfaces. A dilution of 1:100 with water (approximately 500 ppm chloride) is acceptable after proper precleaning of visible material from surfaces. A usable approximation of this dilution can be achieved by mixing 1/4 cup of household sodium hypochlorite bleach in a gallon of water. It is best to renew the dilution at least weekly and to dispense from a clearly labeled spray bottle. Use bleach dilutions with caution, because they are corrosive to metals, especially aluminum.

158. When and how should laboratory items and materials be cleaned and disinfected?

Items should be cleaned, disinfected, and thoroughly rinsed with fresh, potable tap water after handling and certainly before placement in a patient's mouth. Before disinfecting, read the manufacturer's directions for specific material compatibility or contraindications for use. In general, an intermediate-level tuberculocidal hospital disinfectant with an EPA registration number on the label is a suitable choice.

159. Do I have to keep an environmental surface wet for 10 minutes for a disinfectant to be effective?

The user should follow the label instructions as closely as possible. The label of an environmental germicide requires testing that reflects the worst-case situation of an uncleaned surface. In a practical sense, if a surface has been thoroughly precleaned of organic material and moistened with fresh, uncontaminated germicide, whenever it dries, it is "safe"—provided all other appropriate hygienic and aseptic procedures are firmly in place. Precleaning is of utmost importance.

160. What type of microorganisms do EPA-registered, tuberculocidal hospital disinfectants generally claim to kill?

Under EPA registration, the kill claim is for *Mycobacterium tuberculosis, Salmonella* spp., staphylococci, and *Pseudomonas* spp. Obviously, a wide variety of other types of less resistant microorganisms, including many pathogenic varieties, also are killed. A specific microorganism kill claim (e.g., HIV, HBV, or antibiotic-resistant strains) should not be a primary criterion for purchase or use. Such claims are printed on labels primarily for marketing purposes; most pathogens of contemporary concern have no unusual resistance levels and are susceptible to a wide range of germicidal chemicals.

161. What are the categories under which a manufacturer may apply for registration of a hospital disinfectant?

Under the disinfectant heading, a manufacturer can apply for four separate categories for registration: bactericidal, virucidal, pseudomicidal, and tuberculocidal activity. Other specific genera and species also may be listed in the label claim; however, the first four categories are the most important to determine the general potency spectrum of a product.

162. In choosing a chemical disinfectant, which would be the more potent or broad-spectrum claim—tuberculocidal or HIV-specific?

The more important claim is *M. tuberculosis,* which is one of the more resistant microbial forms. If mycobacteria are killed, all microorganisms of lesser resistance are assumed to be killed also. HIV is a highly sensitive microorganism and is easily killed by many, if not all, proprietary germicides. Neither of these potency indicator organisms is transmitted by surfaces.

163. Do EPA tests of germicidal chemicals indicate efficacy?

No. The EPA tests reflect a spectrum of potency, not efficacy. The EPA tests are standardized lab tests for comparing the potency of one germicide with another and are based on descending order of general microbial resistance to germicides. Efficacy is established by inference according to the potency of the germicide and the manner in which the product is used by the worker.

164. How do you determine use and reuse life of a surface disinfectant?

The EPA requires that use and reuse life information be obvious on a label. As a general rule, it is important to follow the manufacturer's instructions for use.

165. What are the minimal label requirements for a disinfectant product to be appropriate for use in a dental setting?

For surfaces frequently contaminated by patient material (e.g., light handles, prophy trays, and other environmental surfaces that come in contact with contaminated instruments), registration as an EPA hospital disinfectant with additional label claim for tuberculocidal activity (under the Spaulding classification scheme, an intermediate-level disinfectant). For general housekeeping, such as floors or countertops in nonclinical areas, the label claim for hospital disinfectant alone is adequate.

166. What is an antiseptic?

An antiseptic is a chemical agent that can be applied to living tissue and can destroy or inhibit microorganisms. Examples are antimicrobial handwash agents and antimicrobial mouth rinses.

167. How does an antiseptic differ from chemical sterilants and disinfectants?

Chemical sterilants and disinfectants cannot be applied to living tissue, whereas antiseptics are designed for use on tissue rather than on environmental surfaces or medical instruments.

168. Should a disinfectant be used as a holding solution?

No. It is not necessary. The purpose of a holding solution is merely to keep debris moist on hand instruments until they can be cleaned and sterilized. Holding solutions cannot disinfect or sterilize. Presoaking in a disinfectant does not disinfect; it only adds unnecessary time and expense because the items still need to be cleaned, wrapped, and heat-sterilized before use.

169. What is the preferred holding solution?

Soapy water, using a detergent that is noncorrosive or low in corrosives, is effective. Clinicians also may choose the ultrasonic solution used in their practice as an instrument holding solution. These solutions should be changed at least daily or as directed by the manufacturer.

170. What is the best source for safety information about a hazardous product?

The Material Safety Data Sheet (MSDS) provides the most comprehensive product information and is the best source for safety information as well as precautions, emergency procedures, and personal protective equipment requirements. The MSDS must be provided by the manufacturer or distributor of the product if it is covered under the Hazard Communication Standard (HazCom). The product label is also a good source of information, but it is not as complete as an MSDS.

171. If I transfer a chemical agent from its primary container to a secondary container, must I label the secondary container?

No—not if it is for your immediate use during the same work day. If, however, it is intended for use by other employees, it must be appropriately labeled.

172. What ventilation requirements are indicated during use of liquid chemical germicides?

All chemical agents are toxic to varying degrees and should be used in well-ventilated areas. Additional ventilation is not necessary (if the product is used according to instructions provided by the manufacturer) unless indicated by the manufacturer.

173. What are the special ventilation requirements for surface disinfectants?

Again, all chemical agents should be used in well-ventilated areas. The manufacturer's instructions, label, or MSDS may indicate special requirements or personal protective equipment.

174. Is a chemical exposure incident a reportable injury?

Yes. If it results in the need for medical follow-up, chemical exposure should be reported in accordance with OSHA standards.

175. What personal protective equipment is indicated during use of chemical agents?

At a minimum, protective eyewear, a mask, and task-appropriate gloves, such as heavy-duty utility or nitrile gloves, should be worn for handling of chemical agents. The key point is barrier protection of skin and mucous membranes from potential contact with hazardous or caustic chemical agents.

HANDLING AND DISPOSAL OF DENTAL WASTE

176. Who regulates dental waste?

OSHA regulates how the waste is handled in a dental facility. Federal, state, and local laws govern the disposal itself.

177. What is the intent of the Resource Conservation and Recovery Act (RCRA) of EPA?

The intent of the RCRA is to hold the generator of a hazardous waste responsible for its ultimate disposal or treatment and for any clean-up costs associated with improper disposal. Each dentist, therefore, is responsible for ensuring proper disposal of waste, and improper disposal by an unscrupulous company is ultimately the responsibility of the dentist.

178. What is potentially infective waste?

It is waste contaminated by patient material and should be handled and disposed of accordingly.

179. Does the term "contaminated" refer to wet or dry materials or both?

Contaminated refers to both wet and dry materials. For example, HBV can remain viable in dried materials for at least 7 days and perhaps longer. However, HBV is easily killed by moderate levels of heat or by a wide variety of chemical germicides, including low-level germicides.

180. Is all contaminated waste potentially infective waste?

No—but all infective waste is contaminated by definition. Some contaminated waste, although it contains potential pathogens, may not have sufficient quantity or type to pose a reasonable threat of infection transmission.

181. What is toxic waste?

Toxic waste is capable of causing a poisonous effect.

182. What is hazardous waste?

Hazardous waste poses peril to the environment.

183. Is all hazardous waste toxic?

No. It may not have a poisonous effect.

184. If potentially infective waste is autoclaved, must you biologically monitor the cycle?

If you use heat-sterilization equipment to treat potentially infective waste, most state regulations mandate that you must biologically monitor each waste load to ensure that the cycle was successfully completed. Each load must be labeled with a date and batch number so that if a sterilization failure occurs, the load can be retreated. Although required by many states, the merits or necessity for this degree of monitoring is highly controversial among experts.

185. What method should be used to dispose of potentially infective items such as gauze, extracted teeth, masks, and gloves?

Blood-soaked gauze, extracted teeth, and any other material that is contaminated by patient fluids, saliva, or blood should be considered potentially infective waste and disposed of according to federal, state, or local law. Masks, provided they are not blood-soaked, can be disposed of as ordinary trash. Contaminated gloves should be disposed of as potentially infective waste.

186. What is the most appropriate method for disposal of used needles and sharps?

Although needles may be recapped by a one-hand technique or mechanical device, they should not be bent or broken or otherwise manipulated by hand. An appropriate sharps container should be used for disposal of all spent sharps and needles.

DENTAL WATER QUALITY

187. Is there concern about the microbial biofilm known to populate dental unit water lines?

Biofilm contamination of dental unit water lines (DUWLs), although not a new phenomenon, has received widespread attention from the media and scientific community. There are few current data on which to formulate recommendations to control biofilm accumulation or to establish safe levels of microorganisms in dental unit water used for nonsurgical (restorative) procedures. The American Dental Association released a statement recognizing the microbial levels in DUWLs and urging improvement of the amplified microbiologic quality of water through research, product development, and training. Other organizations, such as the CDC and the Organization for Safety and Asepsis Procedures (OSAP), have issued guidelines for DUWLS.

188. Have there been any documented cases of infection or disease in dental health care workers from microorganisms in DUWLs?

Some published reports suggest increased exposure of dental health care workers to legionellae from aerosolized dental unit water. DUWL water from an unmaintained dental unit may contain literally millions of bacteria and fungi per ml (many of them potential clinical pathogens); the lack of specific epidemiologic studies has prevented accurate assessment of the potential effect on public health. To date, however, a major public health problem has not been identified.

189. What is biofilm?

Microbial biofilms are found virtually anywhere that moisture and a suitable solid surface for bacterial attachment exist. Biofilms consist primarily of naturally occurring slime-producing bacteria and fungi that form microbial communities in the DUWL along the walls of small-bore plastic tubing in dental units that deliver coolant water from high-speed dental handpieces and air-water syringes. As water flows through the microbial matrix, some microorganisms may be released. Dental plaque is the best-known example of a biofilm.

190. Where do the microorganisms come from?

The vast majority are indigenous to house water mains. Patient microorganisms may be transient "tourists" in the biofilm.

191. What conditions facilitate biofilm formation?

Low numbers of microbes continually enter the dental unit water lines. They can be affected by nutrients in the incoming water, stagnation in the tubing, and the low flow rate near tubing walls. In addition, the small inside diameter of the dental unit waterlines results in a large surface-to-volume ratio, which presents optimal conditions for the growth of biofilm microorganisms, especially in times when the water sits stagnant.

192. What are some suggested control measures?

You can use independent reservoirs, chemical treatment, filtration, sterile water delivery systems, or combinations of these. The first and perhaps most effective measure is routine monitoring (culturing) coupled with a regimen of chemical disinfection of the lines. Other augmentative strategies include improvement of the incoming water quality (e.g., sterile water in independent water reservoirs, heating, ultraviolet irradiation, filtering, constant low-level chemical treatment of incoming tap water) or only by controlling the microbial levels in the output water (e.g., filters).

193. What is the purpose of flushing water lines?

Current recommendations are to flush water lines for at least 3 minutes at the beginning of the clinic day and for at least 15–20 seconds between patients. This process does not remove biofilm, but it may transiently lower the levels of free-floating microorganisms in the water. Control of water line contamination requires a number of steps, such as chemical disinfection of the lines, a sterile water source, a specific filtration system in the water line, or a combination of these treatments. Only a chemical disinfection regimen done on a routine basis will remove/control biofilm formation. Filters, for instance, remove only the free-floating microorganisms that originate from the biofilm.

194. What is the purpose of an antiretraction valve?

To prevent aspiration of patient material into water lines and thereby reduce the risk of transmission of potentially infective fluids or patient material from one patient to another.

195. What should be done with the water supply on a dental unit when local health authorities issue a "boil water notice" after the quality of the public water supply is compromised?

Use of the dental unit should be stopped if it is attached to the public water supply or if tap water is used to fill the bottle of an isolated water supply to the unit. Immediately contact the unit manufacturer for instructions on flushing and disinfecting the water lines. Use of house water should not resume until the boil water notice is lifted by the local authorities.

RESOURCES

Centers for Disease Control and Prevention (CDC) World Wide Web/Internet Resources
www.cdc.gov
For hepatitis information, www.cdc.gov/ncidod/diseases/hepatitis/index.htm
For hospital infections, www.cdc.gov/ncidod/hip/default.htm
For HIV information, www.cdc.gov/nchstp/hiv_aids/dhap.htm
CDC Health Care Quality with guidelines, www.cdc.gov/ncidod/hcq
CDC Oral Health with templates on evaluated needle safety devices, <http://www.cdc.gov/
OralHealth/infection_control/forms.htm

Samples Resources for Infection Control Guidelines and Documents

Advisory Committee on Immunization Practices: http://www.cdc.gov/nip/ACIP/default.htm
American Dental Association: http://www.ada.org/
Association for Professional in Infection Control and Epidemiology, Inc.:
http://www.apic.org/resc/guidlist.cfm
CDC Division of Healthcare Quality Promotion: http://www.cdc.gov/ncidod/hip/
CDC Division of Oral Health, Infection Control:
   http://www.cdc.gov/OralHealth/infection_control/index.htm
CDC Morbidity and Mortality Weekly Report: http://www.cdc.gov/mmwr/
CDC Recommends . . . Prevention Guidelines System:
   http://www.phppo.cdc.gove/cdcRecommends/AdvSearchV.asp
Food and Drug Administration: http://www.fda.gov
Immunization Action Coalition: http://www.immunize.org/acip/
Infectious Diseases Society of America: http://www.idsociety.org/PG/toc.htm
National Institute for Occupational Safety and Health: http://cdc.gov/niosh/homepage.html
National Library of Medicine: http://hazmap.nim.nih.gov/
Occupational Safety and Health Administration, Dentistry:
   http://www.osha.gov/SLTC/dentistry/index.html
Organization for Safety and Asepsis Procedures: http://www.osap.org/
Society for Healthcare Epidemiology of America, Inc.: http://www.shea-online.org/PositionPapers.html

Referenced Guidelines for Infection Control for Health-Care Settings

DOCUMENT TITLE	YEAR	ADVISORY AUTHOR	COMMITTEE
Guidelines for Handwashing and Hospital Environmental Control	1985	Garner	None
Recommendations for Preventing Transmission of Human Immunodeficiency Virus and Hepatitis B Virus to Patients During Exposure-Prone Invasive Procedures	1991	CDC	None
Guidelines for Preventing the Transmission of *Mycobacterium tuberculosis* in Health-care Facilities	1994	CDC	None
Guideline for Hand Washing and Hand Antisepsis in Health-Care Settings	1995	Larson	APIC*
Guideline for Isolation Precautions in Hospitals	1996	Garner	HICPAC[†]
Guideline for Selection and Use of Disinfectants	1996	Rutala	APIC*
Immunization of Health-Care Workers	1997	CDC	ACIP[§]/HICPAC[†]
Guideline for Infection Control in Health-Care Personnel	1998	Bolyard	HICPAC[†]
Guideline for Prevention of Surgical Site Infection	1999	Mangram	HICPAC[†]
Recommendations for Infection Control for the Practice of Anesthesiology	1999	ASA[#]	None
Updated US Public Health Service Guidelines for the Management of Occupational Exposures to HBV, HCV, and HIV and Recommendations for Postexposure Prophylaxis	2001	CDC	HICPAC[†]

(continued)

Referenced Guidelines for Infection Control for Health-Care Settings (Continued)

DOCUMENT TITLE	YEAR	AUTHOR	ADVISORY COMMITTEE
Draft Guideline for Environmental Infection Control in Health-Care Facilities	2003	Chinn, Sehulstor	HICPAC[†]
Draft Guideline for Cleaning, Disinfection, and Sterilization in Health-Care	2003	Rutala	HICPAC[†]
Guideline for Hand Hygiene in Health-Care Settings	2002	CDC	HICPAC[†]
Guidelines for the Prevention of Intravascular Catheter-Related Infections	2002	CDC	HICPAC[†]

*Association for Professionals in Infection Control and Epidemiology, Inc.
[†]Healthcare Infection Control Practices Advisory Committee, formerly the Hospital Infection Control Practices Advisory Committee (national advisory committee to CDC).
[§]Advisory Committee on Immunization Practices (national advisory committee to CDC).
[#]American Society of Anesthesiologists.

REFERENCES

1. American Association of Infection Control Practitioners (APIC): www.APIC.org.
2. Block SS (ed): Disinfection, Sterilization and Preservation, 5th ed. Philadelphia, Lea & Febiger, 2001.
3. Bolyard EA, the Hospital Infection Control Practices Advisory Committee: Guidelines for infection control in health care personnel, 1998. Am J Infect Control 26:289–354, 1998.
4. CDC: Guideline for hand hygiene in health-care settings: Recommendations of the Healthcare Infection Control Practices Advisory Committee and the HICPAAC/SHEA/APIC/IDSA 2868 Hand Hygiene Task Force. MMWR 51(No. RR-16):1–46. 2869, 2002.
5. CDC: Hepatitis B virus: A comprehensive strategy for eliminating transmission in the United States through universal childhood vaccination. MMWR 40(No. RR-13), 1991.
6. CDC: Recommendations for preventing transmission of human immunodeficiency virus and hepatitis B virus to patients during exposure-prone invasive procedures. MMWR 40(RR-8):1–9, 1991.
7. CDC: Recommended infection-control practices for dentistry, 2003. Atlanta, CDC, Feb. 12, 2003.
8. CDC: Guidelines for preventing the transmission of *Mycobacterium tuberculosis* in health-care facilities, 1994. MMWR 43(RR-13):1–132, 1994.
9. CDC: Public Health Service guidelines for the management of health-care worker exposure to HIV and recommendations for post exposure prophylaxis. MMWR 47(No. RR-7):1–33, 1998.
10. CDC: Recommendations for prevention and control of hepatitis C (HCV) infection and HCV-related chronic disease. MMWR 47(RR-19):1–38, 1998.
11. CDC: Immunization of health-care workers—recommendations of the Advisory Committee on Immunization Practices (ACIP) and the Hospital Infection Control Advisory Committee (HICPAC). MMWR 46(RR-18):1–42, 1997.
12. CDC: Updated U.S. Public Health Service guidelines for the management of occupational exposures to HBV, HCV, and HIV and recommendations for postexposure prophylaxis. MMWR 50(No. RR-11), 2001.
13. Farero MS, Bond WW: Chemical disinfection of medical and surgical instruments. In Block SS (ed): Disinfection, Sterilization, and Presentation, 5th ed. Philadelphia, Lippincott Williams & Wilkins, 2001, pp 881–917.
14. Fisher J: Training for development of innovative control technology project. San Francisco, San Francisco General Hospital, 1999.
15. FDA medical device safety alerts. www.fda.gov/cdrh/safety.html www.fda.gov/medwatch.
16. FDA Safety Alert: Needlestick and Other Risks from Hypodermic Needles on Secondary I.V. Administration Sets Piggyback and Intermittent I.V. Rockville, MD, FDA, 1992.
17. FDA Supplementary Guidance on the Content of Premarket Notification [510(K)] Submissions for Medical Devices with Sharps Injury Prevention Features. Rockville, MD, FDA, 1995.
18. Garner JS, Favero MS: Guidelines for Handwashing and Hospital Environmental Control, 1985. Atlanta, U.S. Department of Health and Human Services, Public Health Service, Centers for Disease Control, 1985.
19. FDA, NIOSH, OSHA: Glass Capillary Tubes: Joint Safety Advisory About Potential Risks. Rockville, MD, Food and Drug Administration: <www.cdc.gov/niosh/capssa9.html>. Date accessed: May 28, 1999.
20. Garner JS, Hospital Infection Control Practices Advisory Committee: Guideline for isolation precautions in hospitals. Infect Control Hosp Epidemiol 17:53–80, 1996.

21. Larson EL, Association for Professionals in Infection Control and Epidemiology Guidelines Committee: APIC guideline for hand washing and hand antisepsis in health care settings. Am J Infect Control 23:251–269, 1995.
22. Mangram A, Horan T, Pearson M, et al: The Hospital Infection Control Practices Advisory Committee: Guideline for prevention of surgical site infection, 1999. Infect Control Hosp Epidemiol 20:247–278, 1999.
23. Miller CH, Palenik CJ: Infection Control and Management of Hazardous Materials for the Dental Team, 2nd ed. St. Louis, Mosby, 1998.
24. National Institute of Occupational Safety and Health (NIOSH) www.cdc.gov/niosh. For needlestick injuries, call 1-800-35-NIOSH (1-800-356-4674).
25. NIOSH. Selecting, evaluating, and using sharps disposal containers. Cincinnati, OH, U.S. Department of Health and Human Services, Public Health Service, Centers for Disease Control and Prevention, National Institute for Occupational Safety and Health, DHHS (NIOSH) Publication No. 97-111, 1998.
26. National Institute for Occupational Safety and Health. Alert: Prevention of Needlestick Injuries in Health Care Settings. Department of Health and Human Services (NIOSH) publication number 2000–108, 1999.
27. Occupational Safety and Health Administration (OSHA) www.osha.gov. For needlestick information, www.osha-slc.gov/SLTC/needlestick/index.html (or call the OSHA Publications Office at 202-593-1888).
28. OSHA Exposure to Bloodborne Pathogens Final Rule, December 6, 1991 (29 CFR 1910.1030) Booklet. Controlling Occupational Exposure to Bloodborne Pathogens in Dentistry, OSHA Publication No. 3129, 1992.
29. Post-Exposure Evaluation and Follow-up Requirements under OSHA's Standard for Occupational Exposure to Bloodborne Pathogens. A Guide to Dental Employer Obligations, 1997.
30. OSHA Compliance Directive CPL 2-2.44D: Enforcement Procedures for the Occupational Exposure to Bloodborne Pathogens, Nov. 5, 1999.
31. OSHA: How to Prevent Needlestick Injuries: Answers to Some Important Questions. Washington, DC, U.S. Safety and Health Administration, OSHA, #3217 [revised], 1999.
32. OSHA Exposure to Bloodborne Pathogens Final Rule, December 6, 1991 (29 CFR 1910.1030). Revised January 18, 2001 as published in the Federal Register. The updated rules became effective April 18, 2001.
33. Rutala WA, Weber DJ, HICPAC: Draft Guideline for Cleaning, Disinfection, and Sterilization in Healthcare. HICPAC, 2002.)
34. Sehulster L, Chinn R: Guideline for environmental infection control in healthcare settings. MMWR 52, 2003 [in press].
35. Strausbaugh L, Jackson M, Rhinehart E, Siegel J, HICPAC: Guideline to Prevent Transmission of Infectious Agents in Healthcare Settings, 2002 [in development].
36. Training for Development of Innovative Control Technology Project (TDICT): www.tdict.org.

BIBLIOGRAPHY

Preprocedural Mouth Rinse
Reduction of Patient Bacteremia
1. Brown AR, Papasian CJ, Shultz P, et al: Bacteremia and intraoral suture removal: Can an antimicrobial rinse help? J Am Dent Assoc 129:1455–1461, 1998.
2. Fine DH, et al: Assessing pre-procedural subgingival irrigation and rinsing with an antiseptic mouthrinse to reduce bacteremia. J Am Dent Assoc 127:641–646, 1996.
3. Larsen PE: The effect of chlorhexidine rinse on the incidence of alveolar osteitis following the surgical removal of impacted mandibular third molars. J Oral Maxillofac Surg 49:932–937, 1991.
4. Lockhart PB: An analysis of bacteremias during dental extractions: A double-blind, placebo-controlled study of chlorhexidine. Arch Intern Med 156:513–520, 1995.
5. Tzukert AA, Leviner E, Sela M: Prevention of infective endocarditis: Not by antibiotics alone. Oral Surg Oral Med Oral Pathol Oral Radiol Endod 62:385–388, 1986.
Microbial Contamination of Aerosols
6. Fine DS, Yip J, Furgang D, et al: Reducing bacteria in dental aerosols: pre-procedural use of an antiseptic mouthrinse. J Am Dent Assoc 124(5):56–58, 1993.
7. Litsky BY, Mascis JD, Litsky W: Use of an antimicrobial mouthwash to minimize the bacterial aerosol contamination generated by the high-speed drill. Oral Surg Oral Med Oral Pathol 29:25–30, 1970.
8. Logothetis DD, Martinez-Welles JM: Reducing bacterial aerosol contamination with a chlorohexidine gluconate pre-rinse. J Am Dent Assoc 126:1634–1639, 1995.
Saliva Ejectors
9. Barbeau J, Bokum L, Gauthier C, Prevost AP: Cross-contamination potential of saliva ejectors used in dentistry. J Hosp Infect 40:303–311, 1998.

10. Mann GLB, Campbell TL, Crawford JJ: Backflow in low-volume suction lines: the impact of pressure changes. J Am Dent Assoc 127:611–615, 1996.
11. Watson CM, Whitehouse RLS: Possibility of cross-contamination between dental patients by means of the saliva ejector. J Am Dent Assoc 124:77–80, 1993.

Handwashing
12. Conly J, et al: Handwashing practices in an intensive care unit: The effects of an educational program and its relationship to infection rates. Am J Infect Control 17(6):330–339, 1989.
13. Zaragoza M, Salles M, Gomez J, et al: Handwashing with soap or alcoholic solutions? A randomized clinical trial of its effectiveness. Am J Infect Control 27:258–261, 1999.

Jewelry/Artificial Nails
14. Salisbury DM, et al: The effect of rings on microbial load of health care workers' hands. Am J Infect Control 25:24–27, 1997.
15. Hedderwick SA, McNeil SA, Lyons MJ, Kauffman CA: Pathogenic organisms associated with artificial fingernails worn by healthcare workers. Infect Control Hosp Epidemiol 21:505–509, 2000.

Gloves: General Recommendations
16. Adams D, Bagg J, Limaye M, et al: A clinical evaluation of glove washing and re-use in dental practice. J Hosp Infect 20:153–162, 1992.
17. Allen AL, Organ RJ: Occult blood accumulation under the fingernails: A mechanism for the spread of blood-born infection. J Am Dent Assoc 1982;105:455–459, 1982.
18. Gonzalez E, Naleway C: Assessment of the effectiveness of glove use as a barrier technique in the dental operatory. J Am Dent Assoc 117:467–469, 1988.
19. Martin MV, Dunn HM, Field EA, et al: A physical and microbiological evaluation of the re-use of non-sterile gloves. Br Dent J 165:321–324, 1988.
20. Olsen RJ, Lynch P, Coyle MB, et al: Examination gloves as barriers to hand contamination in clinical practice. JAMA 270:350–353, 1993.

Glove Perforation Studies
21. Avery CME, Hjort A, Walsh S, Johnson PA: Glove perforation during surgical extraction of wisdom teeth. Oral Surg Oral Med Oral Pathol Oral Radiol Endod 86:23–25, 1998.
22. Burke F JT, Baggett FJ, Lomax AM: Assessment of the risk of glove puncture during oral surgery procedures. Oral Surg Oral Med Oral Pathol Oral Radiol Endod 82:18–21, 1996.
23. Burke FJT, Wilson NHF: The incidence of undiagnosed punctures in non-sterile gloves. Br Dent J 168: 67, 1990.
24. Patton L, Campbell TL, Evers SP: Prevalence of glove perforations during double-gloving for dental procedures. Gen Dent 43:22–26, 1995.
25. Schwimmer A, Massoumi M, Barr C: Efficacy of double gloving to prevent inner glove perforation during outpatient oral surgical procedures. J Am Dent Assoc 125:196–198, 1994.
26. Upton LG, Barber HD: Double-gloving and the incidence of perforations during specific oral and maxillofacial surgical procedures. J Oral Maxillofac Surg 51:261–263, 1993.

Sterile Surgical Gloves vs. Nonsterile Exam Gloves
27. Giglio JA, Roland RW, Laskin DM, Grenevicki L: The use of sterile versus nonsterile gloves during outpatient exodontia. Quint Int 24:543–545, 1993.

Types/Materials of Gloves
28. Checchi L, Montebugnoli L, Boschi S, Achille CD: Influence of dental glove type on the penetration of liquid through experimental perforations: A spectrophotometric analysis. Quintessnce International 25:647–649, 1994.
29. Chua KL, Taylor GS, Bagg J: A clinical and laboratory evaluation of three types of operating gloves for use in orthodontic practice. Br J Orthod 23:115–220, 1996.
30. Jordan SLP, Stowers MF, Trawick EG, Theis AB: Glutaraldehyde permeation: choosing the proper glove. Am J Infect Control 24:67–69, 1996.
31. Monticello MV, Gaber DJ: Glove resistance to permeation by a 7.5% hydrogen peroxide sterilizing and disinfecting solution. Am J Infect Control 27:364–366, 1999.
32. Rego A, Roley L: In-use barrier integrity of gloves: Latex and nitrile superior to vinyl. Am J Infect Control 27:405–410, 1999.

Dental Material Compatibility
33. Richards JM, Sydiskis RJ, Davidson WM, et al: Permeability of latex gloves after contact with dental materials. Am J Orthod Dentofac Orthop 103:224–229, 1993.

Surgical Masks (Not to Prevent Inhalation of Aerosols)
34. Pippin DJ, Verderame RA, Weber KK. Efficacy of face masks in preventing inhalation of airborne contaminants. J Oral Maxillofac Surg 45:319–323, 1987.

Personal Barrier Protection - Gowns
35. Huntley DE, Campbell J: Bacterial contamination of scrub jackets during dental hygiene procedures. J Dent Hyg 72(3):19–23, 1998.

Instrument Cleaning
36. Bettner MD, Beiswanger MA, Miller CH, Palenki CJ: Effect of ultrasonic cleaning on microorganisms. Am J Dent 11:185–189, 1998.
37. Macdonald G: Can the thermal disinfector outperform the ultrasonic cleaner. J Am Dent Assoc 127: 1787–1788, 1996.

Sterilization/High-level Disinfection of Instruments
38. Farero MS, Bond WW: Chemical disinfection of medical and surgical instruments. In Block SS (ed): Disinfection, Sterilization, and Preservation, 5th ed. Philadelphia, Lippincott Williams & Wilkins, 2001, pp 881–917.

Environmental Disinfection (Intermediate/Low-level)
39. Agolini G, Russo A, Clementi M: Effect of phenolic and chlorine disinfectants on hepatitis C virus binding and infectivity. Am J Infect Control 27:236–239, 1999.
40. Griffiths PA, Babb JR, Fraise AP. Mycobactericidal activity of selected disinfectants using a quantitative suspension test. J Hosp Infect 41:111–121, 1999.
41. Sagripanti JL, Eklund CA, Trost PA, et al: Comparative sensitivity of 13 species of pathogenic bacteria to seven chemical germicides. Am J Infect Control 25:335–339, 1997.
42. Weber DJ, Barbee SL, Sobsey MD, Rutala WA: The effect of blood on the antiviral activity of sodium hypochlorite, a phenolic, and a quaternary ammonium compound. Infect Control Hosp Epidemiol 20:821–827, 1999.

Dental Handpieces: Precleaning and Sterilization
43. Anderson HK, Fiehn NE, Larsen T: Effect of steam sterilization inside the turbine chambers of dental turbines. Oral Surg Oral Med Oral Pathol Oral Radiol Endod 87:184–188, 1999.

Evidence of Internal Contamination (Need to Sterilize)
44. Checchi L, Montebugnoli L, Samaritani S: Contamination of the turbine air chamber: a risk of cross infection. J Clin Periodontal 25:607–611, 1998.
45. Epstein JB, Rea G, Sibau L, et al: Assessing viral retention and elimination in rotary dental instruments. J Am Dent Assoc 126:87–92, 1995.
46. CDC: Recommended infection control practices for dentistry, 2003. Atlanta, CDC, Feb. 12, 2003.
47. Lewis DL, Boe RK: Cross-infection risks associated with current procedures for using high-speed dental handpieces. J Clin Microbiol 30:401–406, 1992.

Sterilization Methods
48. American Dental Association: Infection control recommendations for the dental office and dental laboratory. J Am Dent Assoc 116:241–248, 1988.
49. Leonard DL, Charlton DG: Performance of high-speed dental handpieces subjected to simulated clinical use and sterilization. J Am Dent Assoc 130:1301–1311, 1999.
50. Kolstad RA. How well does the Chemiclave sterilize handpieces? J Am Dent Assoc 129:985–991, 1998.
51. Silverstone SE, Hill DE: Evaluation of sterilization of dental handpieces by heating in synthetic compressor lubricant. Gen Dent 47:158–160, 1999.

Ethylene Oxide
52. Parker HH 4th, Johnson RB. Effectiveness of ethylene oxide for sterilization of dental handpieces. J Dent 23:113–115, 1995.
53. Pratt LH, Smith DG, Thornton RH, Simmons JB, Depta BB, Johnson RB. The effectiveness of two sterilization methods when different precleaning techniques are employed. J Dent 27:247–248, 1999.

Low-speed handpiece
54. Miller CH, Waskow JR, Rigen SD, Gaines DJ: Justification for heat-sterilizing air-driven slow-speed handpiece motors between patients. J Dent Res 75 (IADR abstract #3181):415, 1996.

Radiographs
55. Hokett SD: Assessing the effectiveness of direct digital radiography barrier sheaths and finger cots. J Am Dent Assoc 2000.
56. Hubar JS, Oeschger MP: Optimizing efficiency of radiograph disinfection. Gen Dent Jul 43:360–362, 1995.

13. COMPUTERS AND DENTISTRY

Elliot Feldbau, D.M.D., and Harvey Waxman, D. M.D.

Since the last edition of this text, the use of computers in the dental office and in dental education has become the standard of practice. Mobile and miniature devices have replaced standard textbooks, paper databases, even live lectures, and redefined the learning process itself. The question is no longer whether to use computers in dental practice, but how to best implement and facilitate these rapidly evolving technologies into the office environment. This chapter focuses on the highlights of integrating computerized technology into dental practice, and the information needed to make them useful.

DENTAL MANAGEMENT APPLICATION SOFTWARE

1. What constitutes the digital dental office?

The concept of high-tech electronic and fully digitized systems to manage a dental office and integrated clinical tasks is becoming the standard model of current practice. The near future will see systems that genuinely integrate with one another. To this end the Dental Informatics Committee of the ADA (www.ada.org/prof/prac/stands/) is developing uniform standards to ensure that systems from different manufacturers are interoperable. This has been a major limitation of many newer technologies. Currently, some vendors' digital devices and software may not link with an office's network to allow full usability across all workstations. With the acceptance of these uniform standards seamless integration should be the norm.

2. What skills are becoming prerequisite for establishing a high-tech dental office?

1. First and foremost is an adequate level of computer literacy regarding the basic skills of the computer operating system and computer networks.
2. A knowledge of how to use the internet for research and communication.
3. Familiarity with basic word-processing, database applications, and spreadsheets.
4. How to use and manage images and graphic presentation software.
5. How to edit and publish web pages.

3. What is the first step to develop the digital dental practice?

The installation of a computer-based practice management software system is the initial step in establishing the so-called technology infrastructure. These turnkey systems integrate all aspects of dental office and clinical management into one seamless program application. Companies provide hardware, software, full data input, training, and support.

4. List basic requirements of the dental management software application.

1. The company should be well known with a track record of longevity and, most importantly, should have satisfied customers for reference.
2. Training, local support, and periodic updates should be available.
3. The application should conform to current computer operating systems (Win2000, NT, XP or MAC OS X).
4. The program should include charting, treatment planning, and progress and treatment notes and integrate with voice activation for probing and charting
5. The program should integrate well with intraoral cameras, digital radiography, and image management.
6. The application should have multifeatured scheduling, referral, and recall tracking
7. The program should feature full office accounting, electronic insurance claims, and billing submission and tracking.

8. The program should integrate with word processing, mail merge, e-mailing, and database management.

9. The program should have personal digital assistant (PDA) integration and graphic case presentation (i.e., PowerPoint) capability.

10. The program should allow for tracking of laboratory cases and coordination with scheduling.

5. What is internet-based practice management software?

A rapidly developing management product is the internet-based software provided by an application service provider (ASP). This product exists in two different platforms: web-hosting and web-enabled. Neither form requires software or data storage to be installed on the dental office computer. Rather, the software vendor essentially sets up the supercomputer to run the office management software applications and store all data. A dental office then contracts to use this software service. Access to this service requires only a secure internet connection.

6. What is the difference between web-hosted and web-enabled?

Both forms of application have data and programs residing on a computer system outside the dental office.

Web-enabled programs are JAVA- and HTML-based. Java is a general purpose programming language with a number of features that make the language well suited for use on the World Wide Web. Small Java applications are called Java *applets* and can be downloaded from a web server and run on your computer by a Java-compatible Web Browser, such as Netscape Navigator or Microsoft Internet Explorer. Web-enabled programs require that a small program be downloaded for each screen that is displayed on the office computer. For this reason, a high-speed internet connection (DSL/cable) is necessary.

A **web-hosted application** does not download any applets but runs the entire program on the host computer. Because only the computer screen information is sent, this application is usually much faster in operation. Furthermore, much less computing power is required with the web-hosted application, and even a 56k modem internet connection can be fast enough for most operations.

7. What are the advantages of internet-based management software?

1. There are no substantial start-up costs to purchase software. Because the management application resides on a vender's supercomputer outside the office, there are only monthly fees for usage (usually per terminal), support, and electronic claims submission. This model often is more compatible with the cash-flow needs of a small business.

2. The data can be accessed from anywhere with an internet connection—home, satellite office, or even on vacation.

3. The practice data are very secure, with guaranteed back-ups maintained in power-safe and secured physical structures. Indeed, data are far more secure than in any dental office environment.

4. There is no software installation locally, and hardware requirements are less demanding. Any internet-capable computer can access the software. This minimizes the need to upgrade hardware as often, and any operating system will perform (Windows, Mac, Linux).

5. Software updates are automatic, provided by the vendor, without interruption, and usually without additional cost.

6. Programs are usually Windows-based and therefore familiar to use.

8. What are the disadvantages of internet-based management software?

1. There is less flexibility in everyday usage of internet-based systems.
2. Total control of data is given to a third party.
3. The office is completely dependent on another party and an internet connection.
4. Less likely to be able to customize applications.

9. What precautions should one consider before adopting a web-based management system?

Generally references from satisfied clients and the support and reliability of the vendor govern the decision. The contract should be open-ended, allowing cancellation without penalty. Most importantly, there should be the ability to export the dentist's data files in a format that is usable by other software programs. This ensures against loss of data if a company discontinues service or support.

10. Give a short list of current computer management software.

- Ciraden (www.ciraden.com), a web-based application management product; 100 installations.
- Dentrix (www.dentrix.com), comprehensive dental office management software; 17,500 installations.
- EagleSoft (www.eaglesoft.net), office management software by Patterson Dental Supply; 10,000 installations.
- Easy Dental (www.easydental), small office-oriented; 22,000 installations.
- MOGO (www.mogo.com); 1600 installations.
- PracticeWorks (www.practiceworks.com; 19,000 installations.
- Softdent (www.softdent.com); 13,000 installations.

See also the ADA Guide to selecting software. Available at www.ada.org/prof/prac/manage/software/selectguide/general.html and in the Buyer's Guide to Dental Software in *Dentistry Today,* Sept 2002, p 124.

11. What is the next step in developing the high-tech dental office infrastructure?

After the basic front office and business office network is in place, the extension of the network to treatment room-based computers creates the ability to have full electronic transfer and storage of clinical data and information. Such information includes progress and treatment notes, digital x-rays, intraoral images, treatment charts, and pre- and posttreatment imaging. Once entered into the computer this "paperless" format allows transfer to administrative areas and third parties, such as patients, insurance carriers, and referral sources.

12. What adjunct dental applications are currently available?

1. Automated appointment confirmation systems read the management software confirmation lists and place phone calls within designated parameters. These packages, offered by Tel-A-Patient (www.telapatient.com) and others, use a USB telephone-dialing module and proprietary software to make confirmation calls effortlessly. The software allows reading of patient names, the date, time, and location of the appointment, and custom messages. It also allows patients to leave voice messages. The report logs completely track all messages and list any failures to connect, allowing manual follow-up.

2. Patient education applications use DVD or CD-ROM multimedia presentations to offer information about all aspects of dental treatment. Typical before-and-after treatments and even postoperative instructions can be presented in the operatory or waiting room. Excellent sources are Casey Education Systems (www.casey.com) and the Smile Story (www.smart-technology.net).

3. Case presentation software allows professional multimedia presentations of specific treatment plans. PowerCase, a SoftDent program from PracticeWorks (www.softdent.com), takes treatment plan information from its charting module and creates MS PowerPoint slide shows for display and presentation.

4. Dental stone model scanning and analysis software allows web-based, computerized laser scanning of traditional plaster models. These three-dimensional models may then be viewed, manipulated, and analyzed from an internet-based application. This allows safe, efficient storage and accessibility of models and highly accurate space analysis operations. Excellent sources are e-Models from Geodigm Corp (www.dental models.com) and OrthoCAD (orthocad.com).

5. Dental supply and inventory management software is available from most dental supply companies. Ordering, price comparisons, and product information is available 24 hours per day,

7 days per week, via web or direct dial-up connections. Detailed records of past orders, setting up frequently ordered lists, and even MSDS (Material Safety Data Sheets) information are available. One program, Aruba (www.henryschein.com), allows dedicated dial-up via modem for ordering and maintains full inventory analysis from past orders.

13. What diagnostic applications are available?

1. Digital shade-taking systems such as ShadeVision by X-Rite (http://207.242.38.14/), ShadeScan by Cynovad (http://www.dentalmatic.com/shadescan_p.htm), ShadeEye NCC by Shofu (www.shofu.com), and SpectroShade by MHT International (www.mhtint.com/spectro. htm) allow dentists to digitally map teeth with all variations of hue, value, and chroma and send this information to the lab via e-mail, CD, or Flashcard. The software then calculates the shades of porcelain to be layered to achieve the proper match.

2. Caries detection by Digital Imaging Fiber-Optic Transillumination is now approved by the FDA. DIFOTI (www.Difoti.com) uses safe white light for the detection of incipient, frank and recurrent caries. It instantly creates high-resolution digital images of occlusal, interproximal, and smooth surfaces without radiation. It enables dentists to discover or confirm the presence of decay that cannot be seen radiographically, visually, or through use of an explorer.

3. Periodontal probing instrumentation, such as the Florida Probe (www.floridaprobe.com), automates clinical data collection. The system can record the main parameters of a periodontal exam, including recession, pocket depth, bleeding, suppuration, furcation involvement, mobility, and plaque assessment. The pocket depth and bleeding sites are called out automatically by the user's choice of either a female voice or sound effects from the computer. The patient thereby hears the results from the computer and can watch the exam on a color monitor with color-coded digital readouts—green, black, and red—to identify the risk stages of disease.

14. What nondental software applications are valuable in the office environment?

1. An office suite, such as Microsoft's Office application, includes word processing (Word), spreadsheets (Excel), e-mail and newsgroup client (Outlook and Outlook Express), database management (Access), graphics presentation (PowerPoint), and a web browser and editor (Internet Explorer).

2. General bookkeeping software for payroll and banking such as QuickBooks by Intuit (www. quicken.com).

3. An image management application (see imaging section).

4. A multimedia presentation application such as Windows Media Player or QuickTime.

5. An unzipping application to expand compressed downloads from file transfer applications. (www.winzip.com).

6. A general modem/internet communications application such as Symantec's PCAnywhere. (www.symantec.com/pcanywhere/). This application allows remote access to the office computer with total security.

7. An Antivirus application such as those from McAfee or Symantec.

8. CD-burning software allows creating CDs for archiving and transfer. Products such as Easy CD Creator (www.roxio.com) and Nero (www.nero.com) allow all format recording.

9. Scanning/document management software allows orderly storage and management of documents, minimizing paper transfers. An excellent application is PaperPort (www.scansoft. com).

15. How can a computer function as an analytical tool for practice analysis and business planning?

The computer is unsurpassed as an analytical tool. Management software builds databases in a variety of categories:

- Registration data: name, addresses, phone numbers, date of birth, insurance.
- Patient medical history data: all significant positive elements, medications.
- Production data by category: provider, ADA code, insurance plan.

- Laboratory fee data: by laboratory, patient, provider.
- Treatments by material type, product, technique
- Inventory usage data
- Equipment maintenance logs

By allowing rapid retrieval of data in a meaningful way, the computer can help in making management decisions, in business planning, aid in quality assurance assessments, and analyze treatment outcomes and morbidity. Often a report can be generated by category or key word searching to allow solving a variety of interesting problems. Consider answering the following questions:

- How should a fee schedule be adjusted to account for a 5% increase in laboratory costs and a 7.5% increase in consumables? How will this adjustment affect net production? How many patients have insurance plan B ? What is the income from this group? What would be the impact on production figures if they left the practice?
- How does the productivity of each hygienist compare? How should fees be adjusted to allow a 7.5% salary increase?
- What is the cancellation (broken appointment) rate for each of the operators? What time of day has the highest rates?

Such data are difficult and time-consuming to retrieve and calculate manually. With most report generators in current management applications, they are retrievable at will, with no extra effort since the relevant data are entered routinely for every patient and continually updated. Projections can be easily made by applying the data to a spreadsheet analysis.

16. How can a computer help in clinical consulting?

This relatively new application for dentistry has been used in medicine for several years. By having an internet connection to another clinical facility, one can transmit data and images that can be seen by a consultant. If a video camera is connected to the computers as well, true real-time video conferencing can be accomplished. The benefits for the patient and doctor are obvious.

17. How can a computer be helpful in clinical diagnosis?

Expert systems are software applications that provide a logical process for establishment of a differential and clinical diagnosis. Using data supplied by a clinician in a carefully ordered sequence, the system analyzes the data, branching to the appropriate next series of questions until a differential diagnosis can be established and eventually, a most likely diagnosis with an estimated percentage of reliability. One such internet-based system is ORAD II (www.orad.org), an oral radiographic differential diagnosis application that assists in generating a differential diagnosis from data input from the clinician. It compares data from over 130 of the most common lesions on the maxilla and mandible.

18. How can a management application improve quality assurance?

An analysis of key subject themes can be addressed by organized database reports. Using category and key word searching, patients can be selected by topics of interest. For example, in a review of the compliance with the office protocol for patients with a medical history of a heart murmur, one may find all patients in this group, determine the percent that received follow-up letters to their physicians about the need for prophylactic coverage, and evaluate the percent that received premedication. Such timely evaluations can greatly enhance quality assurance studies. Another example is the frequency of full-mouth and bitewing x-ray exams based on clinical diagnosis, age group, or other clinical variables.

19. How can risk management analysis improve with an office database?

A computer database can provide for easy adverse event reporting. This database can be used in the collation of types of events, methods of resolution, and analysis outcomes. Such reports may help identify opportunities to prevent future untoward events and thus improve the quality of care

20. How can the office database be of benefit in clinical research studies?

As years of clinical procedures accumulate in a practice database, interesting analysis can begin to be performed to shed some light on the treatment outcomes and product performance, incidence of disease, and other clinical inquiries. Consider answering some of the following questions:

- What is the length of service in this practice of full-coverage crowns, indirect porcelain onlays, posterior composite restorations, and amalgams?
- How does postoperative sensitivity compare using various luting cements?
- What types of complications arise after implant placement? How do different fixture designs compare relative to these types?

COMPUTER HARDWARE

21. What governs the choice of hardware?

After choosing the management software application, one usually follows the advice of the vendor to meet specific requirements. However, also important is the office physical space, which determines the optimal number and location of workstations, printers, and communication port distribution (wall outlets). The location, number, and type of monitors in office areas and treatment rooms as well as cabinetry design and operatory equipment come into play for the final decision.

22. Compare Mac vs. Windows

Nearly all dental programs are based on Windows 95/98, 2000/NT, but several Mac programs are available. Remember that most manufacturers of dental hardware and applications do not develop updated drivers (auxiliary software that allows interaction of the application with various peripherals, especially printers) for their products as quickly as the operating systems evolve. There may be a lag time of 2 or more years. Therefore, when upgrading an operating system (i.e., Windows XP or Mac OS X), be careful to check with all of your vendors to ensure that the appropriate drivers are available.

23. Give a short list of hardware components.
Main CPU
- Intel Pentium or AMD at the highest speed you can afford (minimal: 1.8GHz); L2 cache (onboard chip memory bank) should be maximized (512KB).
- RAM (random access memory) SDRAM, min 512MB.
- Hard Drives: 60–100 GB; adding two will serve for backups.
- Video graphics: AGP with 64-MB video RAM and multiple input/output: S-video; composite video; VGA output or digital (DVI) for digital LCDs.
- CD-ROM, DVD writers or burners.
- Zip drive: 250 USB.
- Sound card with multiple input/output; speakers 10/100 NIC card; 56-K modem.

Networking devices
- Server: dual CPU; redundant power supplies; multiple hard disk. disk drives; tape back-up; network adapters.
- Switching device; hubs; routers; category 5 wiring.
- UPS back-up power supply.
- Wireless devices: access point; wireless adapters.

Data entry devices
- Keyboards, touchpad, mice (wired or wireless).
- Scanners for graphics or optical character recognition.
- Bar code readers.
- Light pens or touch screen.
- Headsets for voice activation.
- Intraoral video and imaging devices.

Data back-up and Storage
- Tape drive (20–40GB).
- Removable cartridge: Zip (100–250MB); Jazz 1–2 GB.
- Compact Flash/Smart Media Reader (up to 1 GB).
- CD-R, CD-RW (650–700MB), DVD-R (4–16 GB).
- USB/Firewire removable hard disk drives (up to 120 GB).

Communications resources
- Modems 56 K.
- Cable/DSL modems; routers to share internet connections.
- T1 lines for large installations.
- Cameras for video conferencing.

Ports
- Parallel, serial for legacy devices.
- Multiple USB with additional hubs to connect up to 256 devices.
- SCSI for high speed scanners.
- Firewire, I-link, or IEEE 1394 (fast 400 MB/s) for newer cameras, scanners,
- External hard drives

Monitors
- 15–21 inch CRT (flat screen) usually has best image quality and color matching for digital photo applications at resolutions of up to 1600 × 1200 with 0.25 dot pitch or less. A standard 17 inch is a good general purpose monitor.
- For space savings 15–18 inch TFT LCD (analog and digital) flat panels have bright, sharp images at 1024 × 768 resolutions. For critical viewing of x-rays, medical grade LCD screens are available. LCDs with touch screen and sealed front panels are very desirable for the operatory because they can be disinfected.

Printers
- Inkjet. High-output and photo quality units are excellent for graphic and printing x-rays and photo and routine documentation. Printer cost is low, but paper and inks are costly.
- Laser printers are definitely faster for the office output and have a lower cost over time. Printer cost is higher than inkjet. Both can be networked so that multiple workstations can be directed to any printer.
- Dye Sublimation: very high-quality archival prints.

NETWORKS

24. What is a computer network?

Two or more computers connected together running software that allows them to communicate with one another are called a network. They may form a LAN (local area network) when connected via wireless devices or directly with cables. When several distant sites are linked in this way, such as dormitories in a university, the network is termed WAN (wide area network). The computers may share files, applications, internet access, and a host of peripheral devices such as printers, scanners, and digital cameras. Each device connected in this network is called a node, and there may be unlimited numbers of nodes in a network.

The most common LAN architecture is termed Ethernet and is usually categorized by how fast it can move data; 10 Mbps (megabits per second) and 100 MBps are Standard and Fast Ethernet, respectively. Soon 1 GB (gigabit, 10 × 100 Mbps) will be common. Most connection devices, such as hubs, switches, and network adapters, are autosensing in that they adjust to the transmission speed automatically.

25. Define server and client.

A **server** is a computer that runs software (Windows 2000 Server, Windows NT, Novell Netware, Unix) that controls access to a network and its resources. The server acts as a centralized source for storing and sending data and files to other computers on the network. It is the infor-

mation provider. Usually it is a robust computer with fast hard disks. Built for reliability and durability, servers usually possess dual processors, dual hot swappable power supplies, and multiple
high-speed (15,000 rpm) redundant disk drives to ensure protection of valuable data.

A **client** (or workstation) is an information requestor. It is connected to the server and receives data and files via its network connection from the server. The clients are usually located in
the principal areas of service, reception area, business offices, and operatories.

26. How are computers wired together in a network?

The most reliable and direct method is with category 5 wire cables. They consist of four
twisted pairs of wire (total of eight wires) and terminate in an RJ 45 connector, which is a larger
version of RJ11 (the standard telephone plug). Sometime called 10/100baseT, these are the back
bone of a reliable network. Each computer on the network needs a network adaptor (NIC) that receives the RJ45 connector. From there, cables go to connectors called hubs, switches, and routers.
These are the central points in the network and help transfer data across the network.

Generally **hubs** are slower devices that share their bandwidth. If a 100 Mbps hub has 10 ports
that connect 10 computers, each port can only transfer 10 Mbps. Hubs are also half-duplex, meaning that they can only alternate sending and receiving data.

Switches are much more capable of handling larger numbers of ports or connections at higher
data transfer rates. A 100 Mbps switch with 24 ports can connect 24 devices and transfer data at
a full 100 Mbps at each port. Furthermore switches are full-duplex, sending and receiving data simultaneously at a full 100 Mbps, making the full speed 200 Mbps. Although more costly, switches
are a better investment when growth in network traffic is anticipated.

A **router** works much like a switch in terms of file sharing and general networking but is
more like a bridge that allows the exchange and sharing of different protocols. This is why routers
are able to share an internet connection (with an ISP) between multiple computers. A router also
allows an increased level of internet security by selectively blocking unwanted intrusions with its
intrinsic firewall protection capability (see internet security).

27. Describe an office client/server with internet access.

A DSL or cable router feeds internet access to a dedicated server. PCs have local devices, and
a laser printer and wireless access point are available on the network. All connections to PCs are category 5 cable. Peripheral devices may be USB, Firewire, parallel or serial port, or by SCSI cable.

28. What types of cables do you need to connect computers and peripherals on a network?

Category 5 cables terminated in RJ45 connectors are the common cable connectors for all
Ethernet devices. These cables come in a variety of lengths or in bulk rolls for custom wiring applications.

USB cables have dedicated A and B ends and are used for connecting external devices such
as printers, modems, Ethernet NIC cards, digital cameras and camcorders. They are usually limited in length to 10 feet and can support up to 12-Mbps transfer rates.

Serial cables are shielded cable that connect devices to a computer's serial port. They usually have a plug at one end, the other being directly attached to the device.

SCSI cables commonly have A and B ends for parallel connections of peripherals to a dedicated terminal on an added computer card (i.e., an Adaptec SCSI PCI card). They provide fast
(up to 80 Mbs in the Wide Ultra 2 version) connections that can daisy-chain several devices off
a single port. Scanners, external hard drives, and the Gendex digital x-ray scanner use SCSI cable attachments. Important to note is that SCSI devices may employ different types of connectors; it is imperative to know the type of cable that a particular device requires.

Firewire cables have dedicated A and B ends and are used to attach external peripherals such
as scanners and video camcorders to a computer with fast data transfer rates of up to 400 Mbps.
Depending on the manufacturer, these cables are known as the generic IEEE 1394 cable, iLink,
Lynx, or Firewire.

Parallel cables are commonly used for printers and are terminated in a 25-pin connector called type DB-25 (formerly Centronics). Newer parallel cables are called extended capabilities port (ECP), a parallel-port standard for PCs that supports bidirectional communication between the PC and attached devices (such as a printer). ECP is about 10 times faster than the older Centronics standard.

Other coaxial cables commonly used for video hookups are shielded S-video and RCA cables. These connect to video capture cards such as those from ATI, NVIDIA, and Matrox.

29. What are alternatives to hard wire cabling?

Wireless connections are the fastest growing type of networking (termed 802.11 standards or Wi-Fi). They lack the restrictions and difficulty of installing cables. Depending on whether the wireless network has to share data or peripherals with a wired network, two different modes may be set up: **infrastructure** and **ad-hoc.** If the computers need to share data with a wired network, the mode is set up as an Infrastructure around a central transmitter called the access point. Access point transmits data to PCs with wireless network adapters. There is a limit to the range, but this system allows laptops to move freely while maintaining a network or internet connection. If the wireless network needs to share only with other computers on the wireless network, the Ad-hoc mode is used. Each laptop needs only a wireless adapter; no access point is needed. Many access point devices and wireless adapters use the 2.4-GHz bandwidth. This is the same frequency used by wireless home digital phones and wireless video transmitters (Sony's Digital Doc intraoral camera). Interference is not uncommon. A phone call can shut down a wireless internet connection.

Two additional connection modes use **existing building wiring:** PhoneLine Networking and PowerLine Networking (www.linksys.com). Although having the advantage of using existing cables within a structure rather than running new cables throughout, both methods may be better suited to home and small network applications because of their limited bandwidth (14 Mbps) and their lower reliability with DSL or cable internet access.

Finally, devices with a well-standardized form of local wireless communication capability will be forthcoming using the **Bluetooth** technology (www.bluetooth.com). This system represents a set of specifications for short-range radio links that can be incorporated into all sorts of devices, such as electronic perio probes, intraoral cameras, or basically any device that may transfer data without cables or wires. With an appropriate Bluetooth receiver, a Bluetooth-enabled device may make effortless transfers of data and information.

30. Compare the two major Ethernet configurations used in dental offices.

For small offices with fewer than 10 computers, the **peer-to-peer network** is usually the least expensive, easiest to maintain, and most efficient. All of the computers are connected to send and receive data and thus are used as client/servers. Typically data are stored on a single computer, and the other computers in the network can communicate with it to retrieve data and share peripherals. All Microsoft operating systems from Windows 98 and up have peer-to-peer network software applications as part of the operating system. This system allows any computer on the network to share the disk drives, peripherals, printers, and files of any computer on the network. For example, if terminal 1 has a hard disk C drive, and terminal 2 is configured to have its entire C drive and local printer as shareable, the user of terminal 1 will have a C and D drive (user 1's D drive is actually terminal 2's C drive), and the printer is available to either. Folders in a directory structure may be similarly shared. Because drives are easily shared, applications may be installed on only one computer and used by the others. Back-up copies of one computer's data may be saved to another computer for security. This route is by far the easiest and least expensive for the small network.

In the **dedicated server network,** one PC is designated as the server and handles all network tasks. All files are stored on this centralized, high-speed computer, and the other PCs (clients) depend on the server for network connections. The advantages of this configuration are that larger arrays of computers (10 or more) can access and transfer data at much higher rates, growth of the practice computing needs is not limited, and, unlike a peer-to-peer array, more than one computer can access a particular database or application at a time. This system comes at a cost. Client-server networks are more expensive, require more technical support to maintain, and occupy more space.

31. How is a printer shared in a client/server network?

Printing from one or more PCs to a single laser printer, for example, is handled by a print server. It may be an actual computer with the printer physically attached to it or a small box attached directly to a printer and the network cabling. When a user sends a print job, it travels over the network cabling to the file server, which then transfers the file to its attached printer. This system allows several front office computers to use one high-speed laser printer or a dedicated label printer. Similarly, operatory computers may send image data to a single high-resolution photo quality printer stocked with glossy paper, whereas routine color dental charting may go to a general-purpose color inkjet printer.

32. How is security achieved on a network?

When computers have access to the internet, there is a danger of intrusion by hackers or viruses attached to e-mail or web pages. Antivirus software installed on each computer effectively protects all local applications and any incoming mail from unwanted viruses (www.norton.com; www.mcafee.com). But the simplest and probably most effective way to block intrusion is to install an Internet firewall (a network shield against intrusions), which is included in most hardware routers. The router is installed between the internet connection (either a DSL or cable modem) and the rest of the network. The router becomes the only visible device to the outside world, making individual computers on the network virtually invisible. Some routers even have firewall software built into their internal chipsets to make it even more difficult to decode the routers data (www.linksys.com; www.belkin.com).

33. What is an uplink port?

An uplink port is usually an RJ45 port used to connect hubs, switches, and routers and is located on the back of any of the units. The uplink port can help increase the number of ports available to your network. Options can include sharing wireless capabilities, Internet access, print servers, and numerous other devices.

34. What is a MAC address?

The Media Access Controller (MAC) is associated with MAC addresses. All networking devices, such as network adapters (NICs), hub, switches, and routers, have a unique identification number assigned by their manufacturer and registered by the FCC for licensure. Since these numbers do not change and are permanently attached to the device that they describe, they become useful for managing which devices are allowed access to a network, thus increasing network security. Many routers allow selective filtering of MAC addresses.

35. What is SSID?

On a wireless network, the **service set identifier** (SSID) is an identification name that wireless devices use to make connections. For devices to communicate, they must all be set to the same channel and have the same SSID. If one uses an access point (a wireless transmitter adapter) to connect two computers, both must be on the same channel and have a common SSID.

36. What is WEP?

Wired equivalent privacy (WEP) is a process of data encryption to provide security in wireless communication. When two wireless devices communicate, they first establish a code through exchanging a shared key, then an encryption process begins either at 64- or 128-bit levels. This gives a high level of security but also consumes added bandwidth and may affect performance.

37. Describe devices that protect against power fluctuations.

Slight voltage fluctuations occur frequently and may have a harmful effect on data files. **Surge protectors** are inexpensive devices that filter small- to medium-voltage surges; however, they do not protect against voltage drops.

Uninterruptible power supplies (UPS) will protect against both major voltage surges and voltage drops and are an excellent investment, at least for the main server. These devices instantly switch to battery power in the event of an electrical drop or complete failure, allowing several minutes of back-up power to safely turn off the computer. Higher-capacity systems have enough reserve power to allow backing up the files before automated shutdown. Software for UPS systems automatically saves data and powers down the computer when a preset threshold of battery reserve power has been reached (www.apc.com).

HANDHELD COMPUTERS IN DENTISTRY

38. What are PDAs?

The acronym PDA refers to personal digital assistants. PDAs are small, multifeatured minicomputers in two general body styles: handheld-sized and palm-sized. The former are larger (4 $\times$ 7 inches) units with small keyboards, generally color TFT screens, and expansion card slots. The latter are smaller (3 $\times$ 5 inches), fitting into the hand, and use a stylus and touch screen for data entry.

39. What are the choices in operating systems (OS) for PDAs?

There are two market leaders: the Palm OS developed for Palm computers and the Microsoft Pocket PC (formerly Windows CE). Which system to choose is likely to be based on the system used by your office management software. For example, SoftDent has a full-featured palm organizer application, called Practigo, that synchronizes with the Palm OS; Dentrix uses DX Mobile for the Palm OS, and Dental.com's OffSite is designed for the MS Pocket PC.

40. Describe the features of the palm and handheld PDA.

Because they are larger, the handheld devices from HP, NEC, Casio, and others often feature the MS Pocket PC OS with scaled-down features of the Windows OS and MS Office. They come with wireless modems, multiple ports, and expansion card options and generally are a substitute for a full-fledged laptop computer. But the market leader in this group is the palm-sized PDAs. Brands from Casio, HP, Palm, Visor, Compaq, NEC, Sony, and Blackberry give a vast array of choices and features at many price levels. They also have wireless features, expansion card options, and office suite applications as well as and mobile phone, internet connection, and e-mail ability.

All PDAs feature calendar/appointment/address books, note taking, to-do listing, clocks and calculator functions. The full-featured devices add word processing, database management, spreadsheets, web browsers, e-mail applications, image display, and audio and even video display. In addition, e-book readers allow whole texts and books to be downloaded and read off the PDA.

The versatility of PDAs is their feature of synchronizing to the PC (HotSync), usually via a USB cradle. This allows bidirectional transfer of files from the PC databases (i.e., Outlook) to the handheld database and visa versa. It also allows the installation of software application and web content to the PDA.

41. What functions specific to dentistry do PDAs perform?

Dental management software applications feature HotSync function to a variety of file databases:

- Appointment schedules
- Patient lists and phone numbers
- Financial data
- Pharmacy lists
- Notes, messages, and call-back requests
- Referring doctor lists

All of these features are bidirectional, allowing information to go from the mobile device to the management software and back. The transfers may even be made via wireless or infrared portals. A dentist may receive a phone call message, phone in a prescription for a patient, reappoint the patient, schedule treatment remotely, and then transfer this information into the office PC the next day.

42. What web databases are available for the PDA devices?

One of the most useful databases is the equivalent of the drug index for the *Physicians' Desk Reference* and the *Merck Manual*. Websites such as www.epocrates.com (free) and www.lexi. com have vast clinical databases for drug and formularies, diagnostic aids, and informational content that updates automatically with each hot sync operation. Another site (www.palmdmd.com) is a useful resource for all PDA information and applications in clinical dentistry. There is even an excellent PDA version of an oral pathology text at www.dentalmedsoft.com. The site www. avantgo.com allows custom selection of web content that updates each time that you cradle your PDA to sync. Useful pages include ADA codes, fluoride concentration calculations, and regional fee schedules.

43. What is a Smart Display?

A Smart Display is a wirelessly connected, instant-on, touch-screen monitor that allows access and use of a work station computer and most of its applications. Its light weight, superior portability, and long battery life may allow some fascinating dental applications. Examples include viewing of digital images (both x-ray and photo) as one walks from room to room as well as direct data entry into the primary patient database. No longer would one have to have full workstations in each operatory. Currently these products employ an 802.11 wireless connection and require the Windows XP Professional OS.

44. What is a Tablet PC?

Tablet PC are super-sized PDAs with more functionality through the Windows XP Tablet PC OS. With no disk drives and touch screens, they are highly portable and light-weight and have long battery life. They are more closely related to the notebook computer but feature handwriting and speech recognition and may be docked to other peripherals

DENTISTRY AND THE INTERNET

45. How can one connect to the internet?

One can connect to the internet via a broadband modem (Cable, DSL, satellite) and Ethernet cable (RJ45 connector) or via a conventional dial-up modem and a standard telephone line (RJ11 connector). These connections may be hard-wired or wireless. An internet service provider (ISP) provides subscription-based service, usually for a monthly fee based on speed and type of connection.

Some ISPs are free but offer limited services. The best known, Net Zero and Juno, are for Windows only. These services provide e-mail only and include some commercial material with each e-mail received and sent.

A comprehensive listing of free or low cost ISP's can be found at the following sites: <http://www.all-free-isp.com/> and <http://cheapandfreeisp.com/>.

Computers on the internet communicate using transmission control protocol/internet protocol (TCP/IP) on client/server architecture. Thus the remote server computer sends files and information to local client machines. Your browser allows you to view these displays.

ACCESS LOCATION	TYPE OF CONNECTION	HARDWARE	SPEED (BPS)	RELATIVE COST
Home/office	56 K modem	Phone line jack	56 K	+
	ISDN modem	Phone line jack	128 K	+++
	DSL modem	Ethernet RJ 45/USB	2–8 M	++
	Cable modem	Ethernet RJ 45/USB	2–10 M	++
	Satellite dish	Phone + custom	400 K	++
Institution	T1	Ethernet RJ 45	1.5 M	++++
	T3	Ethernet RJ45	45 M	+++++++
Remote access	56 K Modem	Phone line jack	56 K	
	Wireless	Cell phone	19.2 K	
	Wireless LAN	8012.11a/b/g adaptor	11 M–54 M	

For a complete list of ISPs, consult: <http://thelist.internet.com>.

46. What questions should you ask in choosing an ISP?
- What modem types/speeds do you support?
- Do you support router or switch applications for multiple workstations?
- What is the monthly charge? Is there a choice of monthly charges depending on amount of use or number of workstations?
- Do you offer any proprietary services such as chat lines or informational databases?
- How many mailboxes can I have with my account?
- What e-mail utility do you offer? Can I send files through my e-mail account? Is there a limit to the file size?
- If I can set up a web page, how much space is provided?
- Do you offer spam filters to help cut down on junk mail?
- What is the charge to set up a web page?
- What kind of set-up help do you offer?
- Is there an 800 number I can call from out of town?

47. What is broadband?
Broadband refers to transfer rates that are faster than conventional dial-up speeds. Modems that use normal telephone lines are the slowest methods of transmission, ranging from 300 bps (bits per second) to 57.6 Kbps (thousand bps). Transmission rates greater than these are considered broadband:
- Cable modems are available that offer 2 Mbs rates. Data are delivered over existing cable lines with an appropriate splitter to separate the internet signal from the television signal.
- T1 is dedicated phone connection supporting data rates of 1.544 Mbits per second.
- ISDN is an international communications standard for sending voice, video, and data over digital telephone lines or normal telephone wires. ISDN supports data transfer rates of 64 Kbps. ISDN lines offered by telephone companies provide two lines at once, one line for voice and the other for data, or you can use both lines for data to give you data rates of 128 Kbps, three times the data rate provided by the fastest modems.
- Digital subscriber lines (DSL). DSL technologies use sophisticated modulation schemes to pack digital data onto copper wires at frequencies where voice signals are not used. Both data and voice can travel over the same wires. They are sometimes called last-mile technologies because they are used only for connections from a telephone switching station to a home or office, not between switching stations.

DSL TYPE	DESCRIPTION	DATA RATE DOWNSTREAM; UPSTREAM	APPLICATION
SDSL	Symmetric DSL	1.544 Mbps duplex (U.S. and Canada); 2.048 Mbps (Europe) Same upstream and downstream	Used for internet and web access, motion video, video on demand, remote LAN access
ADSL	Asymmetric digital subscriber line	1.544–6.1 Mbps downstream; 16–640 Kbps upstream	Used for Internet and web access, motion video, video on demand, remote LAN access
HDSL	High bit-rate digital subscriber line	1.544-Mbps duplex on two twisted-pair lines; 2.048-Mbps duplex on three twisted-pair lines	T1/E1 service between server and phone company or within a company; WAN, LAN, server access

48. How are individual servers and locations found?
Two kinds of addresses locate all computers on the Internet, IP addresses and domain names. Each computer on a network has a unique internet protocol (IP) address, which has the form of numbers separated by dots (e.g., 140.147.2.12, the IP address for the Library of Congress). This number is primarily read by computers and is composed of 4 octets totaling 32 bits. It functions just like a telephone number to identify a region, network, and server computer, but is not very user-friendly. A more easily remembered address scheme is the domain name system (DNS).

49. How does the DNS work?

A domain name is a unique address that represents an IP address. Computers called "name-servers" match or translate domain names into their IP addresses so that connections can be established. Domain names are organized into hierarchies describing the country of the network (with the exception of the U.S.), what kind of organization owns it, and other information. A domain name has a number of categories and is usually read from right to left and separated by dots. Thus, <rubens.anu.edu.au> is the name of a computer in Australia (the geographically based domain is .au) in the educational category (.edu) at the Australian National University (anu) and on the computer named "rubens". The domain name <bics.bwh.harvard.edu> is the server at Harvard University (harvard.edu) for Brigham and Women's Hospital (bwh) and the computer named "bics."

There are presently six top-level domain categories:

    com (commercial internet user)
    org (organization, often nonprofit)
    edu (university or other educational institution)
    gov (government user)
    net (network)
    mil (military user)

There are also two-letter geographical domain designations that append to the name. Because the system began in the United States, no U.S. country designation is allowed. Common country designations include:

.uk (United Kingdom)	.de (Germany)
.ca (Canada)	.it (Italy)
.il (Israel)	.su (Sweden)
.fr (France)	.ar (Argentina)
.jp (Japan)	

50. What is a URL?

Each server or computer document has a unique address called a uniform resource locator (URL). Thus, to go to a specific document on a server, one simply enters a URL into the software program (browser) to initiate the connection.

51. Define the elements in the following URL: *http://www.ada.org/prof/govt/dentistryworks/ fluoride.html.*

The first part of a URL defines the internet protocol or tool used to read the document (*http://www*), signifying that it is hypertext transfer protocol for the world wide web. Next comes the domain name and category, which identify the computer—in this example, *ada.org* for the American Dental Association server.

Finally, the name of the document itself. In the example, the actual filename is *fluoride.html* located in the directory *dentistryworks,* which is in the directory *govt* in the directory *prof.* If the path to the document is unspecified, a default or index document will open.

Using a URL greatly simplifies locating documents via the internet, because a long series of numbers is replaced with a logical path name.

52. What are the basic components of the internet?

- E-Mail. Using an e-mail application such as Microsoft Outlook Express, AOL mail, Eudora, or Netscape Messenger, text and graphics may be sent using SMTP (simple mail transport protocol) and received using POP (post office protocol) worldwide.

Helpful adjunct utilities that compress large files so that they transmit faster include Adobe Acrobat (PDF file), WinZip (Windows), and Stuffit (Mac and PC) . The recipient then can view these upon receipt usually with automatic decompression. Wireless handheld (Blackberry.com) devices expand e-mail access to near universal availability as effortlessly as a cell phone call. A comprehensive e-mail explanation and tutorial can be found at <http://www.acsa.edu.au/internet/ email_home.htm>.

- world wide web (WWW). These servers support the use of hypertext transfer protocol

(HTTP) and also support all other protocols in a user-friendly environment. To read such information one needs only a browser such as Internet Explorer, Netscape, or Opera. The received information may be text, graphics, or multimedia radio and television; by using automatic "push" technology, such as Java and Visual Basic, dynamic content is relayed.

- Telnet (Telnet protocol) allows remote logon to a computer host such as a library catalog or an on-line database. Your remote computer then issues commands that allow searches on the host computer. Access usually requires a username and password.
- FTP (file transfer protocol) is a program and protocol to transfer text or binary files between an FTP server and client. These remote sites contain every imaginable form of information (e.g., books, software, games, multimedia).
- Usenet (Network News Transfer Protocol or NNTP) distributes Usenet news articles derived from topical discussions on newsgroups that are stored on central computers. Rather than receiving messages by e-mail, as with Listserv, one must connect to a Usenet group to read or download messages and use a newsreader (Outlook Express or Netscape Messenger) to view these messages.

Most ISPs have a list of newsgroups on their servers, or you may go to a newsgroup search engine such as <http://www.google.com/grphp> to find topics and subscribe. Dental newsgroups include the following:

- IDF (Internet Dental Forum) at http://www.internetdentalforum.org/
- Student Doctor at http://www.medstudents.net/links/newsgroups.html
- Newsgroup about dental issues at <news:sci.med.dentistry>. Support group for TMJ/TMD sufferers at <news:alt.support.jaw-disorders>. For more information, see <http://www.faqs.org/faqs/usenet/what-is/part1/>.

53. What software applications are used in each component?

- E-mail: software that can transmit and receive text and images using an internet connection. Eudora <http://www.eudora.com/> offers free and paid versions for Mac and Windows. Outlook Express <http://www.microsoft.com/windows/oe/> offers versions for Mac and Windows.
- Browser: an application that can decode and display pages found on the world wide web. When connected to the internet, a browser has the tools necessary to move from one web page to another with a simple click of a mouse. Examples include Internet Explorer (free) at <http://www.microsoft.com> for Mac and Windows; Netscape (free) at <http://www.netscape.com/> for Mac and Windows; Opera (demo available) at <http://www.opera.com/> for all OSs; and iCab (MAC only, demo available) at <http://www.icab.de/index.html>.
- Newsreaders: applications that allow connection to newsgroups to send and receive messages from newsgroups. Netscape has newsreader capabilities built in to the application and Internet Explorer uses linked software to connect to newsgroups. A comprehensive listing of available software for all platforms can be found at <http://www.newsreaders.com/>.
- FTP software stands for file transfer protocol and is the software used to transfer files from a computer to the server (uploading) that hosts a website. Several packages are available for low or no cost.

Some of the editing software as well as some browsers have FTP functionality built in. Titles include:

1. Internet Neighborhood (Windows) at <http://www.deerfield.com/products/internet_neighborhood/>
2. Fetch (Windows, MAC) at <http://www.fetchsoftworks.com/>.
3. Transmit (MAC) at <http://www.panic.com/transmit/>
4. Robo-FTP (Windows) at <http://www.robo-ftp.com/>
5. CoffeeCup direct FTP (Windows) at <http://www.coffeecup.com/software/>

    6. AbsoluteFTP (Windows) at <http://www.vandyke.com/products/absoluteftp/>
    7. QueueFTP (Windows) at <http://www.eesoft.com/qftp/>

54. Discuss practical applications of the basic internet systems.

- E-mail discussion groups or mailing list (Listserv) are topical discussion forums distributed by e-mail. When one subscribes by sending a message to a listserv computer, messages from all other subscribers are sent to your electronic e-mailbox. Many active discussions of academic interest are exchanged in this manner. Majordomo and Listproc are software that handle e-mail discussion groups.
- Chat refers to a type of instant bulletin board. Using chat software, groups of people can send messages to the entire group immediately. A message appears on all users' screens the moment the sender sends it. Chat rooms are usually organized by subject of interest and are frequently part of a website service.
- Instant messaging is more like immediate e-mail. Similar to chat, it is between individuals rather than groups. The participants need to have compatible messaging software on both computers. The best-known example is AOL's Instant Messenger. ICQ (http://web.icq.com/) is another similar program available for both MAC and Windows platforms. See Yahoo at <http://chat.yahoo.com/> or AOL at <http://groups.aol.com/>.
- FAQ (frequently asked questions) are postings to Usenet groups that contain specific information related to a topic of the newsgroup. See <http://www.faqs.org> for a collection of web-based resources.
- The web conference is a discussion between a group of people that takes place on the web. This form of e-groups is becoming quite popular because there is no need to use extra software, such as a newsreader, and it does not clog up the e-mail in-box, as an active mailing list can do. Web conferences can do everything that a mailing list and newsgroup can do and more. Services such as Yahoo! Groups have made it easy for people to set up their own conferences and are gaining in popularity.

Comparison of Internet Discussion Groups

	MAILING LIST	NEWSGROUP	WEB CONFERENCE
Software needed to access	E-mail program: Netscape, Eudora, Outlook Express.	Newsreader program: Netscape, IE, Free Agent, or other. Also possible to access newsgroups over the web through service such as the Google Groups service.	A Web Browser— Netscape, IE, Opera or other
Subscription	Required in order to read and post.	Depends. If you are accessing the newsgroups with a newsreader it is free to read and post messages. Some web-based services are subscription based, others are not.	Most web conferences can be read in guest mode. Subscription is required to post comments.
Reputation	Tend to be more scholarly and professional in content.	There are some excellent newsgroups, but also many that are unmitigated trash.	Most often associated with a website that is for a specific community such as teachers, readers, investors, web searchers.
Involvement	Fairly private.	Quite public.	Can be private

Source: <http://www.websearchguide.ca/discuss/egrodiff.htm>.

55. How do I subscribe to a mailing list?

To subscribe to a mailing list, send an e-mail to the listserv address. Leave the subject area blank, and in the body of the text type the following: subscribe {listname}{your first name}{your last name} without the brackets. E-mail software automatically includes your return address. For example, to subscribe to the Buffalo Board of Oral Pathology send an e-mail to <Listserv@ubvm.cc.buffalo.edu>. In the body of the message type: subscribe bboplist elliot feldbau. This begins e-mails on topics of oral pathology. To terminate your subscription, type the word *unsubscribe* in place of subscribe. Other mailing lists may be addresses as LISTPROC or MAJORDOMO. A summary of common LISTSERV commands follows:

- Subscribe <listname> <your first name> <your last name>
- Subscribe digest <listname> causes the program to send all of the day's messages in one mailing per day rather than individual messages as they are written throughout the day.
- Unsubscribe <listname>
- Set nomail <listname>. When this is received, the listserver will not send you mail.
- Set mail <listname> resumes mail delivery
- Set conceal <listname> hides your name on the subscription list
- Info Refcard <listname> causes the listserv program to send a list of commands.

A sample of interesting dental listservs:

- AMALGAM: information about mercury poisoning at <listserv@vm.gmd.de>.
- BROPLIST: oral pathology, discussion groups at <listserv@ubvm.cc.buffalo.edu>.
- CALCIF-L: biomineralization in calcified tissues at <listproc@usc.edu>.
- CBR-L: craniofacial biology reasearch at <majordomo@po.cwru.edu>.
- CCIS_SE: dental software at <listproc@bite.db.uth.tmc.edu>.
- D-ORAL-L: oral microbiology/immunology at <listserv@nihlist.bitnet>.
- D-PERIO: periodontal disease program discussion at <listserv@nihlist.bitnet>.
- DENTALART at <listserv@dental.stat.com>.
- DENTALIB at <for dental librarians, oral health issues listproc@usc.edu>
- DENALIC: infection control in dentistry at <listproc@sparky.uthscsa.edu>.
- DENTALMA: dentistry-related articles, reports, and techniques at <listproc@list.cren.net>.
- DENTAL_CE: continuing education, seminars at <listproc@bite.db.uth.tmc.edu>.
- DENTAL-DRUGS: drug therapeutics in dentistry at <listserv@dental.stat.com>.
- DENTAL-LAB: dental lab discussion group at <listserv@dental.stat.com>.
- DENTAL-MARKETING: at <listserv@dental.stat.com>.
- DENTAL-PUBLIC-HEALTH at <majordomo@list.pitt.edu>.
- DENTAL-SLEEP: sleep breathing disorders at <listserv@dental.stat.com>.
- DENTAL-WEB: dental-related world wide web and dental-related infosystems in at general at <listproc@bite.db.uth.tmc.edu>.
- DENTIST-L: discussion of internet uses for dental information at <listserv@vm.temple.edu>.
- DENTISTRY: dental professionals discussion group at <david@stat.com>.
- DBLIST: databases for dentistry at <listproc@list.ab.umd.edu>.
- EXPATH-L: oral pathology at <listproc@usc.edu>.
- IMPLANTOLOGY: at <listserv@home.ease.1soft.com>.
- MANAGED-CARE: at <listserv@dental.stat.com>.
- ORADLIST: oral radiology discussion group at <listserv@grizzly.ucla.edu>.
- ORTHOD-L: orthodontics discussion group at <listproc@usc.edu>.
- PERIODONT: moderated periodontal discussion groups at <periodont@krypta.snafu.de>.
- PGD: at <listserv@lists.acs.ohio-state.edu>.

For a comprehensive list of dental related Listserv's see <http://www.lib.umich.edu/hw/dent/communication.htm>.

E-MAIL IN THE DENTAL OFFICE AND SECURITY

56. What are some essential uses of e-mail for dental practice?

With over 150 million people using e-mail in the U.S., it is becoming the communication medium of choice. Benefits include the ability to send out recall notices, billing statements, e-mail newsletters, and promotional and marketing materials and to receive communications from patients without tying up valuable phone-line resources.

57. How is e-mail supported?

Most Windows-based systems have integrated e-mail through Outlook or Outlook Express as long as there is an internet connection, either dial-up or broadband. These are MAPI-compliant. The Mac OSX has integrated mail capabilities as well, and other applications are available, including Eudora, for both platforms in a free and paid version.

58. What is MAPI?

MAPI is an acronym for messaging application programming interface (Windows). It is a standardized set of functions placed into a code library known as a dynamic link library (DLL). Having a standard library of messaging functions allows Windows application developers to take advantage of the Windows messaging subsystem, supported by default with Microsoft Mail. By writing to the generic MAPI interface, any Windows application can become mail-enabled. Since MAPI standardizes the way messages are handled by mail-enabled applications, each such application does not have to include a vendor-specific code for each target messaging system.

Some very popular e-mail services, such a AOL and Hot Mail, are not MAPI-compliant, and your computer application cannot send e-mail directly to these services. Cutting and pasting into these e-mail services is necessary.

59. How may images be shared with colleagues?

Once an image is transferred from camera or scanner to a hard drive it can be sent with e-mail, either as part of the e-mail itself or as an attachment. In the latter case, the recipient receives two files, the e-mail message and the image. The advantage of the attachment method is that the image can be more easily opened and manipulated by the recipient with appropriate software.

60. Discuss the differences among image formats.

- TIFF (tagged image file format) provides a high level of detail (up to 600 dpi or 4,800 × 6,600 pixels for a letter-sized page). TIFF format should be used for archival files because there is no compression and the file sizes can be very large.
- JPEG (joint photographic experts group) is a lossy (some information lost) compression format well-suited for screen and print presentation. It is supported by all major computer platforms and by internet web browsers. The advantage is that file sizes are much smaller, and image quality is very good in most cases.
- GIF (graphics interchange format) is a lossless compression format well-suited for low-resolution (only 256 colors supported) screen display of images. GIF is often used for image thumbnails and screen versions of text documents and is supported by all major computer platforms and internet web browsers.
- PNG (portable network graphic format) is expected to provide a higher-quality replacement for the GIF, particularly for images delivered to world wide web browsers.
- PDF (Adobe Acrobat portable document format) provides a convenient way to view and print images at high resolution and may also be used to group several files into chapters and books. Both file specifications and viewer software are freely distributed and recognized by all operating systems.

61. How is patient privacy protected when sending images over the Internet?
Patient privacy must be preserved. It is important to realize that identifiable images can be embarrassing and may violate patient confidentiality laws.
- Use patient initials or ID number in place of names
- Mask portions of the image to conceal identity
- Close-ups excluding all but the immediate area.
- Get patient permission in writing before transmission.

62. List benefits of sending images to the dental laboratory.
Shading. It is often helpful to include a photo along with a prescription for prosthetic cases. An image with a shade tab next to a tooth can provide the laboratory technician with an excellent frame of reference to compare value, hue, and saturation. "A little darker than B-2" takes on new meaning when a B-2 tab is held next to the tooth to be matched.
Surface: With good technique one can demonstrate subtle characteristics in a photo far better than by narrative alone. Close collaboration with the laboratory is essential to take full advantage of this technique.
Design. Frameworks for removable bridges drawn directly on photographs of a patient's mouth can reduce ambiguity.

63. Are data at risk when connected to the internet?
The answer is maybe. Several issues effect vulnerability on the internet. While a determined and skilled hacker can certainly do mischief, many things can be done to protect data from attack.

64. What are viruses and worms?
A virus is a program or piece of code that is loaded onto a computer without one's knowledge and that runs against one's wishes. Viruses that replicate themselves are known as worms. All computer viruses are manmade, and a simple virus that can make a copy of itself over and over again is relatively easy to produce. Even such a simple virus is dangerous because it can quickly use all available memory and bring the system to a halt.
An even more dangerous type of virus is one capable of transmitting itself across networks and bypassing security systems. It is highly advisable to install and run security software and update it frequently to be sure that the latest virus protection is always available.

65. How are data protected?
1. Never open a file that is sent with an e-mail (an attachment) from an unknown source. Damaging data (viruses, worms) are most often sent to remote computers as small programs or macros attached to innocent e-mail. Unopened mail is essentially harmless.
2. Antivirus software can detect and remove infected files before they can do damage, but it must be kept up to date to be most effective. Most companies provide automatic update features to ensure that the latest protection against the most current viruses is always available. VirusScan by McAfee (http://www.mcafee.com/) and Norton Antivirus by Symantec (http://www.symantec.com) are just two of several such products.
3. Firewall protection. A firewall is software (or hardware) that filters information before it gets to the computer.
4. Destroy unsolicited mail before opening it. Spam, the internet equivalent of junk mail, is becoming a major problem and can be a source of virus contamination. It is a good policy to filter mail that is not specifically addressed to the intended recipient from a known source and inspect it with virus software before opening it.

66. What security issues are related to a cable (Ethernet) connection?
This a serious consideration when setting up networks, either local (LAN), such as within and office, or wide area (WAN), such as an internet connection. With a dial-up account a computer is essentially connected to the internet as an individual connection, similar to any telephone

call between parties. An Ethernet connection is more like a party line, with many computers sharing a connection to the internet and using the same "node." Thus, it is much easier for security to be breached, and it is prudent to take common sense precautions. The following suggestions are not meant to be a primer on security but should serve to make one aware of the issue and to seek detailed help if necessary.

- Password protection to prevent unauthorized intrusion
- Firewalls and other isolation methods using hardware (routers) or software
- Establishing a network policy that clearly defines levels of access and privileges
- Encrypting data and communications with access via secure certificate or key

Most people agree that the much greater communication speed of Ethernet is well worth the extra effort.

USING THE INTERNET FOR RESEARCH IN DENTISTRY

67. Discuss differences between searching for information on the internet and at a library.

Because of the immense size and rapid growth of offerings on the internet, there is no single complete guide to the material. Furthermore, because there is no central control or standard of organization, it is hard to know if any search is complete or even if material will be available in a particular field. A library, on the other hand, is a statement of organization, collecting, and planning. National standards exist for cataloging the contents of every library (e.g., Library of Congress, the Dewey system), and each university library usually has complete collections for the specialty schools that comprise its academic fields. The library also supports reference professionals to guide you in a literature search.

However, as unorganized as the collections of information may be on the www, there are some important areas in which internet research may provide an advantage. The internet represents both a storage resource and a communication tool. Subscribing to discussion groups on topics of interest provides a wealth of opinions, comments, and suggestions for finding answers to clinical and professional problems. Both Listserv and Usenet newsgroups fulfill these inquiries.

Many libraries, museums, government agencies, and commercial entities have digitized their archives and collections, and the volume and quality of offerings continue to grow. The result is incredible accessibility. Health resource data from the NIDR, the World Health Organization, and the NIH are readily available online. Access to medical journal databases, such as Medline, Paperchase, and OVID, allow the convenience of searching from one's office, and graphical collections are readily downloadable. There are also electronic journals and library catalogues available online, so that locating specific reference works is convenient. To use the internet for searching the www, a working knowledge of searching tools is invaluable.

68. What makes a productive web search?

With billions of documents available and no standard of organization, finding web documents of specific interest requires knowing how to use what are commonly termed *searchable directories and indexes*. These tools use some standard but slightly different criteria to search for information on the internet. The ability to create close matches between terms of interest and words or phrases used in web pages determines how closely you get to your chosen subject.

69. How do search tools work?

Web search services find documents matching the user criteria by searching their database of URLs, texts, and descriptions selected from the whole www. Their "robot" computers, called spiders, scan the web 24 hours per day, updating their databases or indexes where the resource information is stored. Thus, each search tool may be different, depending on the organization of its database. Some search services' yields are first edited or reviewed, whereas others are a mere gathering of the robotlike computers, transferring data directly into the database. The final component is the search engine software, which allows the user to submit requests to the database for sites of interest.

A search generates a list of hypertext links from the engine's database to documents that fulfill the user's search criteria. Clicking on a link sends one to that document on the web. Every search tool's list will vary, based on the features of its search mode, the size of the database, and the selectivity of the organization of the database.

70. How do search engines return results?

Generally some schematic order is applied to the inquiry. It may be a relevancy rating determined by the unique search engine and may include search terms in the title, URL, first heading, or even the number of times that the search term appears in the document. This is called "on the page" ranking and has been used on most first-generation search services.

Newer search engine technologies, termed second generation, organize results by peer ranking, concept, site, or domain rather than by relevancy. This type of search looks at "of the page" information to order the results. (Examples include <www.DirectHit.com>, <www.Guidebeam.com> and <www.surfwax.com>.

71. Describe horizontal presentation search tool.

Although most search tools present long lists of results, some use concept processing to return results in a horizontal organizational format rather than a long list. By viewing the first listing you can review categories before retrieving results within a particular category. Examples of this concept-clustering search tool include <www.Guidebeam.com>, <www.queryserver.com>, and <www.vivisimo.com>.

72. What is "results grouping" in search engine logic?

When multiple results are returned from a single search, because they contain the same search terms, the list can be overwhelming. Some search engines group all of the results from one site into a single cluster to make fewer returned results, but ensuring that they are unique sites. (Examples include <AltaVista.com>, <Excite.com>, and <HotBot.com>.

73. Discuss the major categories of resources for locating material on the internet.

1. **Subject directory:** a service that offers collections of links on the internet submitted by site creators or evaluators and organized into subject categories. The selectivity varies according to service. Bear in mind that there are both academic or professional directories such as Infomine (http://infomine.ucr.edu/), the Internet Public Library (www.ipl.org), or Subject Guides A to Z (http://www2.lib.udel.edu/subj/), and commercial directories, such as Yahoo (www.Yahoo.com) and the Open Directory Project (http://dmoz.org). These are useful when you have a general topic and wish a collection of sites recommended by experts. Thus, if you are looking for the general concept of "evidenced-based treatment," a subject directory is a good place to start.

2. **Search engine:** a searchable database collected by a computer program that enables users to query the index and usually ranks the collection by relevancy. These services consist of three parts, the program or spider, which that traverses the web 24 hours/7 days/week link to link and reads pages; the index, which is the database containing a copy of each page found; and the software search agent, which enables the user enquiry. These are most useful when you have a specific topic, site, or type of information that is well defined. An example is the search for "evidence-based treatment in dentistry" or the site of the American Academy of Cosmetic Dentistry. Examples include: <Google.com>, <HotBot.com>. <AltaVista.com>, <AllTheWeb.com>, <Ask Jeeves.com>, and <Lycos.com>. Medical/dental search engines include:

- Medline at <http://www.healthgate.com/default.asp?page=search&section=13> at <http://www.medscape.com/index.html?>
- Merck Manual at <http://www.merck.com/!!tBTIx1ZmxtBTIx1Zmx/pubs/mmanual/html/sectoc.htm>
- University of Michigan School of Dentistry at <http://informatics.dent.umich.edu/>
- U.S. National Library of Medicine (NLM) at <http://www.nlm.nih.gov/>
- New England Journal of Medicine at <http://www.nejm.org/content/index.asp>

3. **"Deep Web"** refers to information stored on searchable databases and accessible by user enquiry. These are generally not indexed by spiders, but many search services offer separate search options to locate these files. The file types may be varied, multimedia, images, and portable document format (PDF). The information in these databases may be rapidly changing and highly current. Examples of these databases include CompletePlanet (www.completeplanet.com), Invisible Web (www.invisibleweb.com), Invisible-web.net (www.invisible-web.net), and ProFusion (www.profusion.com). Dental-specific databases include oral pathology image database (www.uiowa.edu/~7Eoprm/AtlasHome.html) and Der Web image library (www.derweb.ac.uk).

4. **FTP search tools:** engines that search sites that store computer files and programs. They may use keywords, file names, or theme types such as Windows, Linux, or sound files. Examples are FtpFind (www.ftpfind.com), Ftpsearchengines (www.ftpsearchengines.com), and Oth Net (www.oth.net).

5. **Multimedia and images search tools** locate specific files of sound, video, or still photography. Examples are AltaVista Photo Finder (www.altavista.com/sites/search/simage), FindSounds.com (www.findsounds.com), and TimePix (www.thepicturecollection.com).

6. **Search engine collections:** group hundreds of engines in categories for easy and fast access. An example is Search Engine Colossus (www.searchenginecolossus.com).

7. **Domain name search tools:** specifically search for the availability of a domain name. This tool is useful for creating a new dental office website. Examples are <checkdomain.com> and <namedroppers.com>.

74. What is a meta search engine?

Meta search engines simultaneously search multiple search engine sites (redundant). They are useful when you have obscure topics or simple searches or expect a small number of relevant results. There are two types: those with no collation of results so that you get a large number of separate lists from each engine, such as Dogpile (www.dogpile.com) or Webtaxi (www.webtaxi.com), and those that generate a single list with duplicates removed for viewing from its own website. Examples of the latter with collated results are Iquick(www.ixquick.com), Copernic (www.copernic.com), and MetaCrawler (www.metacrawler.com).

75. How does one use a search engine for dental research?

Dental search engines provide a text box into which the term or terms of interest are entered. Results can be restricted by date, whether abstracts are available, or by language (e.g., English only). Searches can be based on keywords such as general topics, specific subjects, or proper names. The most efficient way to search by subject is to enter relevant terms and, at the same time, exclude terms that may produce irrelevant results. Terms that are too specific may miss important material, whereas terms that are too general can return far too many results to be useful.

For example, one may want the latest information about the use of prophylactic antibiotics for dental patients with knee replacements. Entering "knee replacement" in the Google (google.com) search engine text box returns the following results: *Display the first ten matches of about 202,000. Search took 0.06 seconds.* The search term is too general, and too many articles are listed to be useful. Refining the terms, such as "knee replacement dental prophylaxis," produces the following results: *Display the first ten matches of about 748. Search took 0.23 seconds.*

Most of the first ten links in this actual search yielded precise dosages and indications, whereas other links provided references to more comprehensive articles. Often the abstract alone is sufficient to answer the question that prompted the search. Hard copies, downloads, or online access to the full text are available usually only to subscribers who pay a fee.

76. What is boolean searching?

Boolean searching is an advanced search technique and refers to the use of operators or conjunctions, such as AND, OR, NOT, that instruct the search engine how to use the terms in doing a search. For example, one may be interested in finding the best method of sealing an access cavity in a porcelain crown after endodontic treatment has been completed. Typing *dental adhesion* in a search engine such as Google yielded 15,000 items in 0.05 sec.—from a CE web cast on adhesion to a report on "Evaluation of Dental Adhesion and Durability by Means of the Microbond Test" on the National Institute of Standards and Technology web page. Entering *dental adhesion porcelain* produced 1,060 in 0.1 seconds. Several links also dealt with enamel, however. To further limit this result, one may enter the following using the advanced search capability: *dental adhesion porcelain* exclude *enamel*. Google then returned 560 results in 0.19 seconds with no reference to enamel.

The use of quotation marks is also a useful technique to keep in mind. Entering *dental secrets* into Google produced 71,700 references, the majority having nothing to do with the book *Dental Secrets*. Entering *Dental Secrets* however, yielded 170 listings, each relevant only to this book title.

77. What are advanced search options?

Search engines frequently offer instructions about the way boolean searching should be conducted. Google, for example, ignores NOT and requires the use of its input template under advanced options. The advanced option also allows one to select the age of references to exclude references that were older than a year, for example. This increases the likelihood that only the latest material appears in the results list. For a complete tutorial on boolean searching see: <http://library.albany.edu/internet/boolean.html>.

78. How can newsgroups be helpful in research?

The importance of evidence-based treatment has been revived in recent months. It is important that treatment be based on sound science, part of which is to assimilate clinical evidence. There is simply no other way to be able to discuss clinical experience to the extent available through newsgroups, forums and e-mail lists.

In addition, professionals who participate in these groups share their experiences, positive and negative, with materials, techniques, services (such as insurance companies), website designers, management consultants, and office designers. Information of this type is simply not available from any other source.

DENTAL OFFICE WEBSITES

79. What are the benefits of an office web page?

Marketing. Web advertising is becoming more and more common. Although relatively few dentists have their own websites, the number is growing and those who have them are enthusiastic.

Information. Websites can provide prospective patients with a sense of your dental practice philosophy and values. Office hours, insurance policies, financial policies, directions and maps to the office, personnel bios, and photos are but some of the information that can be made available.

Education. Long-time patients can benefit from informative articles on new technologies, new materials, and general educational materials. It is an opportunity to make patients aware of continuing education courses taken and areas of special interest or expertise.

Motivation. One also has the opportunity to motivate and inform with before-and-after pictures from one's own practice. These can be effective marketing tools if used with skill and good taste.

Examples of professionally created pages can be found at <http://www.dallasartists.com/new_pages/web_portfolio.htm>.

80. What is web hosting?

The most practical way to ensure that a website is available at all times is to use a commercial server that provides a directory on its hard drive to store the website's files. Most ISPs provide free space for each customer for personal use. Although these personal directories can be used for a web page, they can be accessed only by typing in the complete path name to the directory, such as <http://members.yourisp.com/yourdirectoryname/>. It is much more professional for a dental office to have a distinct and easy to remember URL or domain name. When a unique domain name resides on an ISP's server, the ISP is said to be "hosting" the website.

81. What is a domain name? (See question 46.)

A domain name is a unique address that refers to a specific IP address, the numerical identifier of one particular computer (server). When a URL is entered into the address space of a browser, the information is sent first to a computer called a "nameserver." It will match or translate the domain name into the IP address of the hosting computer so that a connection can be established.

82. How can I get my own domain name?

Companies, called domain name registries, determine the availability of a name and register it for an annual fee (typically $12-$35 per year).
- Checkdomain.com searches for name availability
- Network Solutions—http://www.netsol.com/en_US/
- Register.com - http://www..com/
- US domain registry—http://www.nic.us/

If Dr. Jones registers a name—"BestDentist.com," for example—as part of the registration process, it can be linked to the IP address of an existing server. Thus, in the above example, when the URL "BestDentist.com" is typed into a browser, the nameserver will match the domain name to the appropriate IP address and the ISP's server's software will direct all queries for "Best Dentist.com" to the appropriate directory on it's hard drive: <http://members.yourisp.com/yourdirectoryname/>.

If Dr. Jones changes ISPs, the registry must be notified, and the address is relinked to the new host server's IP address. When a patient enters "BestDentist.com" as the URL, the nameserver will match the URL to the new IP address; the user will be sent to an entirely different location but never notice a difference. The address remains the easy-to-remember "BestDentist. com".

83. What are the costs of having a web page?

The website needs to be made available at all times. For that reason it is best to have the site hosted on a commercial server. Cost for this service currently varies from free to as much as $100 per month. A deluxe site offers services such as e-mail forwarding, forms processing, technical support, and hosting your own domain name. Free services provide limited disk space on the server and little else; typically they do not host a personal domain name.

84. Do I have to create my own website?

Absolutely not. Design firms specialize in dental office web design. Costs vary significantly and depend on the services supplied, such as website hosting, e-mail forwarding, pager functions, number of web pages needed, special effects (e.g., multimedia), support, and maintenance. Examples include:
- Elance: at <http://www.elance.com>
- Dental*Website* at <http://www.dentalwebsearch.com/getwebsite.html>.
- TNT Dental Solutions at <http://www.tntdental.com/>; many samples are available.
- WebSite Design at <http://www.websightdesign.com/index.cfm>.
- Udent at <http://www.udent.com/proservices.asp>.

85. What software is needed to create a web page?

1. **Editing software.** Although one can use any word processor to produce a web page, most people do not want to learn html, the mark-up language used by browsers to view pages on the www. Excellent applications make creation of sophisticated websites well within the abilities of anyone interested to devote some learning time:
- Adobe PageMill, Adobe GoLive (http://www.adobe.com/)
- FrontPage, Microsoft (http://www.microsoft.com),
- Fusion, NetObjects (http://www.netobjects.com/)
- SoftQuad (http://www.softquad.com/top_frame.sq),
- HotMetal Pro (http://www.hotmetalpro.com),

- CyberStudio (http://www.cyberstudio.com.au/)
- Dreamweaver, (http://www.macromedia.com/software/dreamweaver/),
- Netscape Communicator, a popular browser (http://www.netscape.com), has a basic editor (Composer) built in.

These titles were available at print time for both Mac and Windows platforms. Many vendors have free demos for download and prices range from $100 to $700.

2. **FTP software** stands for file transfer protocol and is the software used to transfer files (uploading) from a computer to the server that hosts a website. Several packages are available for low or no cost. Some of the editing software as well as some browsers have FTP functionality built in. Titles include,

- Internet Neighborhood (Win) at <http://www.deerfield.com/products/internet_neighborhood/>
- Fetch (Windows, Mac)at <http://www.fetchsoftworks.com/>
- Transmit (Mac) at <http://www.panic.com/transmit/>
- Robo-FTP (Windows) at <http://www.robo-ftp.com/>
- CoffeeCup direct FTP (Windows) at <http://www.coffeecup.com/software/>
- AbsoluteFTP (Windows) at <http://www.vandyke.com/products/absoluteftp/>
- QueueFTP (Windows) at <http://www.eesoft.com/qftp/>

86. What steps are taken to create a web page?

1. Create a design for the opening page after viewing several existing websites.

2. Create a navigation scheme for each page; this scheme directs the user from page to page within the site.

3. Create one master folder or directory for the entire website.

4. Create one folder for images and one for text, and place both in master folder.

5. Create text pages to be used for each page in the website and store in text folder.

6. Gather all images and design elements that will be used and store them in the image folder(s).

7. Place images or other design elements on the pages created in step 5.

8. Create links to images and other site pages as dictated by navigation scheme in step 2

9. Create hyperlinks to other websites as needed.

10. Test the website in as many browsers as possible in both Mac and Windows systems, if possible.

11. Upload the master folder containing all files to the correct directory on the server when satisfied that the pages work as expected.

12. Retest the site over an internet connection.

13. Publicize the site. Type "publicize your web site" into any search engine and get thousands of links to help.

87. What additional considerations should be kept in mind for office websites?

1. Number of visitors or "hits." This useful information can help when making strategic decisions about the efficacy of different features and the value of the website as a whole to the practice. Free "counters" are available to add this function to any web page (www.digits.com, www.prtracker.com/FreeCounter3.html, www.escati.com www.jellycounter.com www.thecounter.com).

2. Security. If a website offers sensitive information or on-line patient scheduling features, it is important to provide effective security. Personal information must always be given the highest priority.

3. Timeliness. Information must be updated frequently to provide patients and prospective patients with the most up-to-date information. This responsibility must be given to one person to be certain that the website reflects precisely what is intended and expected.

4. Children's pages. Pages of games and puzzles are an excellent way to entertain young people while teaching them (and their parents) the important points of dental health. It may also prove to be an excellent marketing tool.

88. Discuss common uses of dental imaging.

Captured images of patients by traditional film, digital camera, or streaming intraoral video allow increased documentation of preexisting conditions. By using imaging applications, it is possible to archive, insert images into patient charts, and communicate with dental labs and other dental specialists. But probably the most exciting use is the cosmetic smile make-over. Closing spaces and changing the length, shape, form, and color of smiles digitally allows the dentist and patient to see before-and-after diagnostic possibilities. One would expect an increased level of case acceptance with this improved mode of patient communication. Major developers of dental-specific cosmetic imaging software applications include Scican's Image FX (www.scican. com), Integra Medical's Vipersoft (www.vipersoft.com), and Practice Works' DICOM Imaging (www.practiceworks.com).

89. Discuss specifications and advantages of the intraoral camera.

The intraoral camera, often similar in size to a dental handpiece, is a live videocam. It generates a live analog, full-motion (30 frames/second) color video stream. The images are shown on a TV monitor and may be captured as still images using a printer. Allowing patients to see pictures of their own mouths is a great tool in educating patients and demonstrating treatment needs. Whether in the hygiene room to illustrate plaque accumulations and periodontal pocket defects or in the treatment operatory to reveal defective and cracked restorations, patients can see their problems in a very dramatic and convincing way. Further, communication with insurance companies on the need for onlays or full coverage is often more convincing than traditional radiographs alone. Finally, intraoral cameras are much easier to use than dental imaging systems in that the equipment is often a self contained camera, light source, and simple USB or S-video connection to a computer and/or TV monitor. However being an analogue signal, managing the images for archiving or manipulation requires input to a computer. Some manufacturers in this area are: Integra Medical's Vipercam (www.vipersoft.com), Dentsply/Gendex's AcuCam (www. gendexxray.com), and Cygnus Technologies' CygnaScope (www.cygnus-technologies.com).

90. How is a digital image created?

Digital picture making can be thought of as a 3-step process:

Image Capture involves using a digital camera, or scanner to capture light information, convert it into digitized data, and then storing the data as a picture file.

Image Processing involves using computer software to alter the stored images, controlling such things as brightness, contrast, color, sharpness, and cropping.

Image Output involves displaying the images on a monitor, creating color prints with any number of color printer options or transmitting the image to another location via email.

91. How can live streaming videos be captured?

Live analogue images may be captured by a video camera and transmitted to a computer with the aid of a video capture card. These common cards (ATI, Winnov, Hauppage, Integral) are either added to a PC or may be part of a video-ready machine. Using RCA or S-video inputs allows the analogue signal to be converted to a digital file that a computer may read, allowing storage on a disk, archiving and manipulation just like any digital image.

Current consumer digital video cams (mini DVD) use faster FireWire (i-Link, IEE 1394) input to directly enter a digital signals, but only one dental cam (Cygnus) is currently FireWire enabled. A capture card will generally display 14–30 frames per second, 24fps being the limit for the human eye for live video. And since the cards display video directly to the screen, bypassing the CPU, the display is fast. The out put from cards may be directly sent to a TV monitor in addition to a computer monitor, allowing over head viewing by the patient. The Integral Flashpoint 3D card even allows external triggers such as foot switches to start, stop, and grab single frames (/www.integraltech.com) For any transfer of video or audio files, the fastest speed is best.

BUS INTERPHASE	TRANSFER SPEED
USB	12 MBps
FireWire IE 1394	1.2 GBps
USB 2	480 MBps
1994b	3.2 GBps

Any video signal passing through current generation cards has a resolution of VGA (640 × 480 pixels) at a 24 bit color depth. Even with a digital video stream with FireWire IE 1394 input, current dental software systems capable of video capture still use 640 × 480 resolution; thus, it may be best to get a camera based on the best-quality image using s-video until more products are developed in the dental field.

92. What are the resolution depths of current capture cards and dental software?

MPEG is a standard for compressing sound and movie files into an attractive format for downloading—or even streaming—across the Internet. The MPEG-1 standard streams video and sound data at 150 kilobytes per second—the same rate as a single-speed CD-ROM drive. It manages the data by taking key frames of video and filling only the areas that change between the frames. Unfortunately, MPEG-1 produces only adequate quality video, far below that of standard TV. MPEG-2 compression improves quality dramatically. With MPEG-2, a properly compressed video can be shown at near-laserdisc clarity with a CD-quality stereo soundtrack. For that reason, modern video delivery mediums, such as digital satellite services and DVD, use MPEG-2. MPEG-4 files, based on MPEG-1 and MPEG-2 and Apple QuickTime technology, are smaller than JPEG or QuickTime files, are designed to transmit video and images over a narrower bandwidth and can mix video with text, graphics and 2-D and 3-D animation layers. MPEG-4 was standardized in October 1998

AVI is the file format used by Video for Windows, one of three video technologies used on personal computers. (The others are MPEG and QuickTime.) In AVI, picture and sound elements are stored in alternate interleaved chunks in the file.

MOV is a file for QuickTime, a method of storing sound, graphics, and movie files. Although QuickTime was originally developed for the Macintosh, player software is now available for Windows and other platforms. If you do not have a QuickTime player, you can always download versions for either Mac or PC from Apple's website.

93. List popular storage media for digital images.
- Compact Flash Card (up to 1 GB)
- Smart Media Card (up to 128MB)
- Memory Stick (Sony)
- Secure Digital (SD up to 128MB)

These devices are termed nonvolatile because they do not require power to retain recorded data. Generally they are removed from a camera and placed in card readers (USB, PCMCIA) to store onto a computer or to print directly to a compatible printer.

94. Define digital image, pixel, and image file.

When a **digital image** is formed, the digitization process divides an image into a horizontal grid of very small regions called "picture elements," or pixels. In the computer this digital grid or "bitmap" represents the image. Each pixel is identified by its position in the grid, as referenced by its row (x) and column (y) number. In most systems, pixels are referenced from the upper-left position of the bitmap, which is considered position 0,0 (row 0, column 0). Each pixel has a different color or grayscale value and together they form a representation of the image. As the single point in a graphic image or bit map, the pixel represents an RGB (red, green, blue) data value. An 8-bit byte contains one of 256 numeric values (2 to the 8 power), 0–255; 0 is the least and 255 is the brightest, In a 24-bit color image 255 is the maximum value for R, G, or B (256 × 256 × 256 = 16.7 million combinations of colors). Three 8-bit numbers are used to create 24-bit true color so that (255,255,0) equals yellow; (0,255,0) equals green; (0,0,0) equals black; and (255,255,255) equals white. In grayscale images, only one 8-bit data value is associated with each pixel (0,255), equaling 256 shades of gray.

An **image file** becomes simply an organized array of data in rows (width) and columns (height) for every RGB pixel. Expressed in each location in the grid, three values of RGB are stored. The viewing software arranges these data to form an image.

95. Define pixel intensity, hue, saturation, brightness, and contrast.

Intensity refers to the amount of light reflected or transmitted from a scene. In a grayscale image, intensity represents the shades of gray, from zero brightness (black) to full brightness (white).

Hue controls the color spectrum from red to yellows, greens, blues, and violets.

Saturation controls the purity of the color, or how washed out the color is with white light. For example, a hue of red can have numerous saturation levels from deep red to pink and finally white.

Brightness controls how bright the color appears. It is similar to intensity, but whereas intensity refers to the amount of reflected color of the original (physical) scene, brightness refers to the intensity value after the image has been acquired. Sometimes brightness is called lightness, in which case the HSB scale (hue, saturation, brightness) becomes the HSL scale (hue, saturation, lightness).

Contrast refers to the degree of difference in frequency values of pixels in the image. An image with low contrast appears as a tightly grouped mound of pixels occupying a small dynamic range of the grayscale spectrum. An image with high contrast occupies a large spectrum of the grayscale. In particular, pixels that are close together should have significant differences in frequency values.

96. Discuss major characteristics of video displays.

Video monitors are generally of two types: cathodray (CRT) tubes that display RGB signals and flat-panel liquid crystal (LCD) displays made of back-lit, active, matrix-thin film transistors (TFT). A new generation of flat panels includes the organic light emitting diode (OLED) displays that promise large screens at much less cost than current TFT LCDs. Screens are rated by their contrast ratio or dynamic range, which is the ability to display dark enough blacks without a loss of detail in dark image areas. The second feature is the screen's resolution, or the ability to display fine detail as specified by the number of horizontal and vertical (columns and rows) pixels across the entire screen area. The highest numbers give the most detail. Monitors are designated by their display resolution.

VGA 640 × 480	=	0.30 million pixels (on a 15 inch monitor, 43dpi)
SVGA 800 × 600	=	0.48 million pixels
XGA 1156 × 864	=	1 million pixels
SXVGA 1280 × 1024	=	1.3 million pixels (on a 20 inch monitor, 64 dpi)

For viewing full-size images on a monitor screen, the captured image size should approximate the display monitor resolution in total pixels. An image of 500 pixels remains only 500 pixels, regardless of the screen resolution, but the size of the image depends on the screen size. A video monitor does not see "inches"—only pixels. If it is larger, parts of the image will not be visible; if it is smaller, it will not fill the screen. For example, MS PowerPoint presentation images need be only large enough to fill the desired size of the display screen. Larger files simply waste space rather than improve quality. Software applications generally resample files to make them full-screen compatible.

97. List the digital sensors used for digital images capture.

Capture devices typically use one of three direct digital receptors, whether they be flat-bed scanners, cameras, or digital x-rays. The CCD (charged-coupled device) is common for wired x-ray sensors and flat-bed scanners; the CMOS (complementary metal oxide semiconductor) is commonly used in cameras because of its lower power consumption; and the PSP (photostimu-lable phosphor plate) is used in the wireless Gendex DenOptex x-ray system. A good review on the technical issues in digital dental imaging can be found at <www.learndigital.net>.

98. Define dpi and ppi.

Dpi and ppi are standard ways of measuring how the data in an image file are organized. They tell you the resolution of scanners, printers, and photo files (which is entirely different from the optical resolution of a photo based on the film and lens). Dpi means dots per inch and refers to the number of dots (or pixels) of a photo image that fit into an inch. Strictly speaking, it is a printer rating. Ppi refers to the number of pixels per inch and is a measure of image resolution. The two terms are often used interchangeably but are context-particular. If the context pertains to images or printing pixels, dpi means pixels per inch. If it pertains to printer ratings, dpi means ink dots per inch on paper. Both dpi and ppi can change to fit different needs (different printing de-vices need different dpi's)—scanners can be set to different resolutions, and photo files can be changed for different purposes. If you compare two photos of equal size but at different dpi, the one with more dots in an inch allows more detail to be displayed (it has a higher resolution). Dpi affects the way a photo is captured by a scanner and how it looks when printed.

99. What is the general rule for how much resolution to set for scanning?

Scan resolution in dpi or ppi is chosen strictly for the needs of the output device, normally a printer or monitor. When scanning for output on a printer, the scan resolution should match the intended output as closely as possible, taking into account the size of the original and the printed reproduction. If the original and print are to be the same size, simply scan at the printers average output (generally 300 dpi inkjet or 600 dpi laser). But if they are different, adjustments are nec-essary. For example, you may want to insert a 1.5×1-in. periapical x-ray film image into a let-ter at the increased size of 3×2. Your printer has a resolution of 300 dpi. If the film were scanned at 300 dpi, the image would have 450 pixels horizontally (1.5×300 dpi) and 300 pixels verti-cally (1×300 dpi). Enlarging the printed image to the intended 3×2 inches would reduce the effective resolution to 150 dpi because the 450 pixels would be spread over 3 inches on paper ($450/3 = 150$), and the same is true for the vertical dimension. This is only one half of the printer's output quality of 300 dpi. To maximize the picture quality on your inkjet printer, scan at 600 dpi.

Similarly, if the intent is to decrease the image size of the original, you must decrease the scan resolution. For instance, you may wish to view a scanned image of a Panorex for e-mail only on a monitor. The original is 10×5in., and the web browser should display it at full size. Com-puter monitors generally have a resolution of 72–90 dpi. Scanning at 72 dpi gives 720×360 pix-els, which is larger than a 640×480 VGA monitor and nearly full screen for a 800×600 SVGA monitor. One can easily scan at 36 dpi with no any loss in quality.

The following formula can be used to calculate the relationship of scan resolution to desired image size:

$$SR = (DR \times DW) / OW$$

where SR = ideal scanning resolution, DR = resolution of final display device, DW = width at which image will be printed or displayed in inches, and OW = width of original being scanned.

Fortunately, photo-editing software makes this process as easy as picking the destination goal. The application then adjusts many of these values automatically.

100. How do photo editors and publishing application display picture files?

A photo editor program *resamples* images that are too large so that they fit a program's win-dow size (as in dental imaging software). We see a smaller copy on the monitor, not the original pixels, and can zoom in or out to change the image size. The original data are unaffected unless the image is saved with the same name, thus overwriting the original.

A page layout program (MS Word, Publisher) designs and prints paper documents and shows image replicas on the screen. These applications *scale* the pixels on paper to print the desired sizes.

101. Discuss the meaning of resolution in images.

When scanning an image, resolution determines the spacing of pixel samples taken from the original object. If we have a 6 × 11 inch Panorex and scan at 100 dpi, the object will be 600 × 1100 pixels on the output. On the video screen, the scanned resolution has meaning only for size. The image of 600 pixels will be 600 pixels wide and 1100 pixels long. If the screen resolution is 800 × 600 pixels, the image is too large for the screen, and one must scroll to see it all. For printing, the scanning resolution is a number that a printer driver will use to determine the spacing of pixels on paper; 600 pixels at 100 dpi will print 6 inches at the same size as the original Panorex film. If we scale the image to 200 dpi on paper, the new size will be 3 inch × 5.5 inch or if 300 dpi, 2 inch × 3.75 inch. Printers have a preference for a particular resolution to print at the maximum quality. Too few pixels result in a low-quality image, whereas too many are discarded. Printing then generally acts the opposite of video display.

The printer drivers and software function to fill a page or scale down an image to size. When photo programs import scans, the scans are printed in real size from a File/Print command. Resolution does not determine image size on a printer as it does for a video display. The size of the original scan area determines printer size on paper. Higher resolutions look better than lower, but the size will be the same at any scan resolution. The scanner's TWAIN driver (the de facto interface for all scanners) scales 100% to make the same dpi for printing and scanning.

Comparison of Properties of Video Screen Images and Printed Images

PRINTED IMAGES	VIDEO SCREEN IMAGES
Image size measured in inches/mm	Image size measure in pixels
Image size does *not* vary with scanned resolution	Image size *does* vary with scanned resolution
Image size modified on paper by *scaling*	Image size modified on screen by *resampling*
Image pixels are spaced on paper using specified scan resolution	Image pixels are located at each screen pixel location one for one
Several printer ink dots are used to represent one image pixel	One screen pixel location contains one image pixel of any RGB value.

102. List common printer types and discuss their uses.

Inkjet printer: A nonimpact printer. Liquid ink is heated or vibrated into a gaseous state and then sprayed through holes in a print head. The quality of inkjet technology is now excellent, but printers can still be relatively slow in high-quality modes. Results vary dramatically with different paper types. For photo quality, glossy film paper can produce near darkroom-like results. For general duty color printing, inkjet and bubblejets are the most cost-beneficial. Some models have compact flash and/or smart media readers that allow direct printing of stored digital images without the use of a computer.

Bubblejet printer: similar technology to inkjet. Instead of firing ink onto the page after agitation with piezoelectric crystals, bubblejet printers burst bubbles of ink through a printhead onto the page after being heated by internal elements.

Laser printer: the most used office printer, giving high speeds and excellent quality. A page is first sent to the printer from your computer. It passes, through a *raster image processor* and then is converted to dots on a page. A device in the printer called an OPC is positively charged; then the laser hits the drum with the image of your page. Every place the laser hits the drum becomes negatively charged. Toner mixed with positively charged developer is attracted to the optical photoconductor, to which the image is then transferred. Negatively charged paper is then passed in front of the belt, and the image is transferred to the paper, which then passes through a fusing unit and out of the printer. In a color laser the image is split into 4 channels—CMYK (cyan, magenta, yellow and black), which are imaged onto the OPC individually before being transferred to the paper.

LED printer: similar to a laser but uses an LED array (a line of light-emitting diodes) instead of a laser unit. Color LED printers have four separate imaging units, one for each color. This gives much faster throughput of color documents, but black-and-white images are produced at same speed.

Multi-function printer: tend to be inkjet-based or copier-based products with the ability to print, copy, scan, and fax. Often it can perform these tasks simultaneously.

Dye sublimation printer: a continuous tone printer, with very high-quality output. Prints are made on photographic type paper. This printer is used for proofing, photo reproduction, and medical imaging. Every page costs the same to print regardless of what is on it. Printing cost is usually high.

Dot-matrix printer: impact printer that creates characters by striking pins against a ribbon onto the paper. Combinations of dots in different places create characters and graphics. This printer allows the use of multipart stationery, continuous stationery, and cut sheet paper.

Any printer may be networked to other computers in an office LAN to allow multiple users to print to the same printer.

103. Summarize what is required to (1) take intraoral pictures; (2) take still pictures of patients for cosmetic makeovers; and (3) store pictures of hard copy x-rays and paper documents.

1. An intraoral video camera and a video capture card with suitable connecting cables for RCA, S-video, or composite video.

2. A digital still camera. Specially modified digital cameras are available from Dine (www.dinecorp.com), Cygnus (Cygnus-technology.com), and others that add close up lenses to give an ideal full smile focal distance. Storage media and imaging software also are required.

3. A flat-bed scanner with a transparency adapter for x-rays. A semitransparent film, either a 35-mm slide or an x-ray, needs illumination from above to be copied by the scanner element, which is the reverse of coping a paper document. Most scanners are suitable, but the Epson 1680 (www.Epson.com) has a large full-bed transparency adapter that accommodates Panorex and Ceph films. A USB, Firewire, or SCSI cable input is suitable; the latter two are the fastest.

104. Explain ways to store large image files or any file data.

Extra hard drives are certainly an option. They are now available as external plugs in devices via USB 1 and 2 bus, or FireWire (www.iomega.com), up to 120 GB. Other options are a recordable CD (CD-R, CD-RW up to 700 MB) and the newer recordable DVDs (DVD-R, DVD-RW up to 4.7 GB). For smaller size and more portability Zip drives are excellent (Iomgea—250 MB)—and, of course, compact media (Compact Flash, Smart Media or the Memory Stick [Sony]). These devices are great for laptops with adapters for PCMCIA or CF slots.

105. What is the DICOM Standard?

DICOM stands for **d**igital **i**maging and **co**mmunication in **m**edicine. It is a set of protocols to transmit images and related files between computer devices. The standard is applicable to all image types used in dentistry and medicine, radiographs, photographs, and even CT scans. Adoption of these standards by venders of computer programs and peripheral devices ensures that image file formats are completely compatible with all computer applications; true interoperability will be the norm. Digital radiographs from any manufacturer's device, for example, will be compatible with all software applications, allowing diagnostic image transmissions among a host of clinical destinations. Thus, sending image attachments of x-rays or photos to insurance carriers for prior approval of treatment will be as seamless as routine e-mail.

BIBLIOGRAPHY

Internet searching tutorials
1. BrightPlanet's Guide to Effectively Searching the Internet. Available at <http://www.brightplanet.com/deepcontent/index.asp>.
2. The Complete Internet Guide and Web Tutorial. Available at <http://www.microsoft.com/insider/guide/intro.asp>.
3. An Extensive list of Internet Subject Directories, Search Engines, and Specialty Search Tools. Available at <http://library.albany.edu/internet/subject.html>.
4. Searching the Internet. Available at <http://library.albany.edu/internet/searchnet.html>.
5. UC Berkeley—Teaching Library Internet Workshops. Available at <http://www.lib.berkeley.edu/TeachingLib/Guides/Internet/FindInfo.html>.

Dental office management software comparison listings
1. Computer Networking. Available at <www.practicallynetworked.com> and <http://www.linksys.com/edu/>.
2. Computer Products and How To's. Available at .
3. Dental Practice Reports, January 2002, p 26.
4. Dentistry Today, September 2002, pp 124–139. Available at <www.dentistrytoad.com>.
5. Digital Photography. Available at <www.steves-digicams.com>.
6. FOLDOC: Free On-Line Dictionary of Computing. Available at <http://foldoc.doc.ic.ac.uk/foldoc/index.html>.
7. Glossary of Computer Terms. Available at Webopedia <www.webopedia.com>.

Dental informatics
1. Abby LM, Zimmerman JL: Dental Informatics:Integrating Technology into the Dental Environment, Springer-Verlag, New York, 1992.
2. Function and application of Dental CAD. CAM Int J Comput Dentistry 15(1), 2002. Available at <http://www.quintpub.com/>.
3. Schleyer T: Dental informatics. Dent Clin North Am 46: 3, 2002.

14. DENTAL PUBLIC HEALTH

Edward S. Peters, D.M.D., M.S.

If you do not have oral health, you're simply not healthy.
— C. Everett Koop, former U.S. Surgeon General

PUBLIC HEALTH PROMOTION

1. What is the definition of public health in its broadest sense?

In 1988 the Institute of Medicine defined public health as "what we, as a society, do collectively to assure the conditions for people to be healthy."

2. What are the three tenets of public health?

1. A problem exists.
2. Solutions to the problem exist.
3. The solutions to the problem are applied.

3. Public health efforts are usually directed toward acute problems such as infectious disease or chronic diseases such as cancer. What public health strategies are similar for these and most other diseases?

(1) Surveillance, (2) intervention, and (3) evaluation.

4. What constitutes a public health problem?

A public health problem usually fulfills two criteria of the public, government, or public health authorities:

1. A condition or situation that is a widespread actual or potential cause of morbidity or mortality, and
2. A perception exists that the condition is a public health problem.

5. Describe the current infection control recommendations.

Recommendations for infection control undergo frequent revision, and the reader is urged to refer to the most up-to-date source. For current recommendations, please check the Oral Health Program at the Centers for Disease Control and Prevention website: http://www.cdc.gov/nccdphp/oh/ichome.htm. The principles behind infection control involve **exposure control**, which refers to personal protective barriers such as gloves, masks, and eye protection. In addition, **heat sterilization** of all dental equipment, including handpieces, is required. Finally, the **handling and disposal** of all potentially infectious material must be properly performed. (See chapter 12.)

6. What are primary, secondary, and tertiary prevention?

Primary prevention involves health services that provide health promotion and protection with the goal of preventing the development of disease. Examples are community-based fluoridation for caries prevention and smoking cessation programs.

Secondary prevention includes services that are provided once the disease is present to prevent further progression. Such services include dental restorations and oral cancer screening.

Tertiary prevention services are provided when disease has advanced to the point where loss of function or life may occur. Definitive surgery or radiation therapy to treat oral cancer and extractions of diseased teeth to eliminate infection are examples.

7. What is health promotion?

Health promotion is a set of educational, economic, and environmental incentives to support behavioral changes that lead to better health.

8. How has health promotion been achieved in dentistry?

Examples of health-promoting activities include community fluoridation and sealant programs. On the individual level, health promotion is encouraged through oral hygiene procedures.

9. Give examples of community-based dental public health programs geared toward school children.

School-based fluoride delivery, dental screening, hygiene instruction, and sealant placement.

10. Before the implementation of any community-based program, the process of planning and evaluation is necessary. What are the basic steps involved in planning for a program?

Planning involves making choices to achieve specific objectives. Thus, a planner should review a list of alternative programs, assess the effectiveness of the program under consideration, examine the community to determine if the program is needed, and initiate the process to implement the program.

11. What skills must a person possess before managing dental public health programs?

The implementation of a public health program requires such skills as planning, marketing, communications, human resources management, financial management, and quality assurance.

12. Differentiate among need, demand, and utilization of oral health services.

Need can be defined as the quantity of dental treatment that expert opinion deems necessary for people to achieve the status of being dentally healthy. **Demand** for dental care is an expression by patients to receive dental treatment. **Utilization** is expressed as the proportion of the population that visits a dentist.

13. What factors influence the need and demand for oral health services in the U.S.?

Demographic and other variables influence the use of dental services. Such variables most notably include gender, age, socioeconomic status, race, ethnicity, geographic location, medical health, and presence of insurance. Women utilize more dental services than men, although the reasons are unclear. Dental visits are most frequent for patients in their late teenage years and early adulthood, with a gradual tapering of visits with increasing age. Socioeconomic status is directly related to the use of dental services. There are fewer dental visits in patients of lower socioeconomic status and in nonwhite or Hispanic populations.

14. The utilization of health care has been explained through behavioral models. One model demonstrates how variables influence the utilization of health care from the individual's perspective. What factors play a role in explaining a person's health care utilization?

1. **Predisposing factors**, such as (1) demographic variables (e.g., sex, age); (2) societal variables (e.g., education, job); and (3) health beliefs (e.g., how susceptible to disease the person believes that he or she is, how serious he or she believes the consequences of the disease to be).

2. **Enabling factors**, which allow the services to be used, such as personal income, community resources, and accessibility to health care.

3. **Need factors,** which determine how the services should be used (i.e., presence of disease).

15. What is the prevalence of smokeless tobacco use among adolescent males and females?

Surveys indicate that 40–60% of adolescent males have tried smokeless tobacco and that by 11th grade 5–35% report regular use. In contrast, less than 5% of adolescent females report using smokeless tobacco. It is important to note the wide geographic variability in the rates. The Northeast experiences the lowest usage, and the highest reported use is in the South.

16. What risks are associated with smokeless tobacco?

Smokeless tobacco increases the risk of developing oral cancer. It contains nicotine and is as strongly addictive as cigarettes. The use of smokeless tobacco leads to the development of leukoplakia in mucosal areas where the tobacco is placed. There is about a 5% chance of leuko-plakia becoming cancerous. Leukoplakia may resolve with early cessation of smokeless to-bacco use.

17. What is meant by the term "acidogenic"?

Particular foods have the ability to reduce the pH of plaque when consumed and are consid-ered to be acidogenic. The reduction in pH is considered a necessary condition for the develop-ment of caries. Such foods contain a high proportion of refined sugars (e.g., candy, soda).

18. Describe how the benefits of fluoride were first discovered.

In the early 1900s Dr. Frederick McKay, having recently graduated from dental school, moved to Colorado, where he observed an unusual blotching of tooth enamel in many of his pa-tients. This pattern was localized to communities that got their drinking water from artesian wells. He also observed that this blotching was associated with decreased caries activity. Eventually flu-oride was identified as the responsible agent. This finding led to fluoridation trials demonstrating that artificial fluoride prevents dental caries.

19. Water fluoridation is one of the few public health measures that saves more money than it costs. Why is water fluoridation so cost-effective?

Fluoridation is a low-cost and low-technology procedure that benefits an entire community. It requires no patient compliance and is therefore easy to administer. The major costs are associ-ated with the initial equipment purchase; later costs are for maintenance and fluoride supplies. It has been calculated that the direct annual costs for fluoridating American public water systems range $0.12–1.31 per person, with an average of $0.54 per person. For each dollar invested in flu-oridation, $80 in costs for dental treatment are avoided.

20. What are the major mechanisms of action for fluoride in caries inhibition?

1. The topical effect of constant infusion of a low concentration of fluoride into the oral cav-ity is thought to increase remineralization of enamel.

2. Fluoride inhibits glycolysis in which sugar is converted to acid by bacteria.

3. During tooth development, fluoride is incorporated into the developing enamel hydroxya-patite crystal, which reduces enamel solubility.

21. What percentage of the U.S. population is served by community systems providing op-timal levels of fluoridated water?

About 62–54% of the total U.S. population has an optimally fluoridated water supply.

22. What is the recommended level of fluoride in the water supply?

The U.S. Public Health Service sets the optimal fluoride level at 0.7 ppm.

23. At what policy level is the decision to fluoridate the water supply made?

Local governments make the decision. However, seven states have laws requiring water fluoridation.

24. A parent of a 6-year-old child asks about fluoride supplementation. The child weighs 20 kg and lives in a fluoride-deficient area with less than 0.3 ppm of fluoride ion in drinking water. What do you recommend?

You should prescribe sodium fluoride, 1-mg tablets, to be chewed and swallowed at bedtime.

25. What are the recommended fluoride supplementation dosages for children?

Tablets are available in doses of 1.0 mg and 0.5 mg for children and toddlers. For infants, supplemental fluoride is available as 0.125-mg drops.

Supplemental Fluoride Dosage Schedule

	CONCENTRATION OF FLUORIDE ION IN DRINKING WATER		
AGE	< 0.3	0.3–0.6	> 0.6 PPM
6 mo to 3 yr	0.25 mg	0	0
3–6 yr	0.50 mg	0.25 mg	0
6–16 yr	1 mg	0.50 mg	0

26. What are alternatives to systemic fluoride supplementation (i.e., tablets)?
 • Topically applied gels of 2.0% NaF, 0.4% SnF, 1.23% acidulated phosphate fluoride (APF)
 • Mouth rinses of 0.2% NaF weekly, 0.05% NaF daily, 0.1% SnF daily
 • Daily dentifrice

27. In prescribing fluoride supplementation, what tradeoffs must be considered?
 The benefit of caries reduction must be considered against the risk of fluorosis. Fluorosis occurs with the presence of excessive fluoride during tooth development and causes discoloration of tooth enamel. Affected teeth appear chalky white on eruption and later turn brown. This risk is especially important during the development of the incisors in the second to third years. To avoid this problem, you must assess the fluoride content of the drinking water before dispensing fluoride supplementation. The fluoride in water along with any supplemental fluoride must not exceed 1 ppm. If 1 ppm is exceeded, the probability that fluorosis may develop increases as the fluoride concentration increases.

28. Where is ingested fluoride absorbed?
 Eighty percent of absorption occurs in the upper gastrointestinal tract.

29. What are the manifestations of fluoride toxicity?
 The ingestion of 5 gm of fluoride or greater in an adult results in death within 2 hours if the person does not receive medical attention. In a child, ingestion of a single dose greater than 400 mg results in death due to poisoning in about 3 hours. Doses of 100–300 mg in children result in nausea and diarrhea.

30. How much fluoride is contained in an average 4.6-ounce tube of toothpaste?
 Either sodium monoflurophosphate or sodium fluoride toothpaste contains approximately 1.0 mg of fluoride per gram of paste. Therefore, a 4.6-oz tube of toothpaste contains 130 mg of fluoride. A level of 435 mg of fluoride consumed in a 3-hour period is considered fatal for a 3-year-old child. Therefore, only a little over 3 tubes of toothpaste need to be consumed to reach a fatal level.

31. What is the rationale behind the use of pit and fissure sealants in caries prevention?
 Occlusal surfaces, particularly fissures, have not experienced as rapid a decline in incidence of caries as proximal surfaces because fluoride's protective effect is confined to smooth surfaces only. It has been observed that sealing the fissures from the oral environment prevents the development of occlusal caries. Sealants should be part of an early preventive program for protecting permanent molars.

32. What proportion of U.S. children have received dental sealants?
 Less than 30% of U.S. children have received dental sealants. In addition, only half the states have school-based programs to extend this service to the neediest children.

33. Do dentists have an obligation to report child abuse?
 Yes. Dentists are morally, ethically, and legally obligated to report a suspected case of child abuse. Reports should be made to the local department of social services, although this may vary from state to state.

34. Where is the dentist's code of ethics found?

The American Dental Association (ADA) established a code of ethics that describes dentistry's responsibility to society. The code is published in the *Journal of the American Dental Association*. The code deals with issues of patient care, fees, practice guidelines, advertising, and referrals. The ADA Principles of Ethics and Code of Professional Conduct can be found at the ADA's website: http://www.ada.org/prat/code/ethics.html.

35. What does the ADA code of ethics state about the removal of dental amalgam to prevent mercury toxicity?

"The removal of amalgam restorations from the non-allergic patient for the alleged purpose of removing toxic substances from the body, when such treatment is performed solely at the recommendation or suggestion of the dentist, is improper and unethical."

36. How does the Americans with Disabilities Act affect dentists?

- Dentists cannot deny anyone care because of a disability.
- Offices must undergo architectural changes to allow access for the disabled.
- Employees are protected against dismissal due to a disability.
- Offices must accommodate disabled workers to perform jobs.

EPIDEMIOLOGY AND BIOSTATISTICS

37. Define epidemiology.

It is the study of the distribution and frequency of disease or injury in human populations and the factors that make groups susceptible to disease or injury.

38. Differentiate between incidence and prevalence.

Incidence is the number of *new* cases of disease occurring within a population during a given period. It is expressed as a rate: (cases)/(population)/(time).

Prevalence is the proportion of a population affected with a disease at a given point in time, i.e., (cases)/(population).

Example: A dentist counts the number of patients presenting to the office with newly diagnosed periodontal disease in a 6-month period. Ten of the 100 people who came to the office had periodontal disease. The incidence rate is calculated as 10/100 in 6 months, or 0.2 per year. The range for incidence rates is from zero to infinity. The prevalence of periodontal disease may be obtained by counting all patients with periodontal disease in the same period—that is, if 50 of the 100 patients have periodontal disease, the prevalence is 50%. Remember, incidence is a rate and requires a unit of time, whereas prevalence is a proportion and is expressed as a percentage of the population.

39. What is meant by test sensitivity and specificity? How are they calculated?

Frequently dentists wish to know if disease is present and may use some diagnostic test to arrive at an answer. In dentistry, the most frequent test is the radiograph. Dental radiographs are imperfect in that they do not distinguish all diseased from disease-free surfaces. Sensitivity and specificity are measures that describe how good the radiograph is in such differentiation. **Sensitivity** measures the proportion of persons with the disease who are correctly identified by a positive test (true-positive rate). **Specificity** measures the proportion of persons without disease who are correctly identified by a negative test (true-negative rate). Sensitivity and specificity are inversely proportional; as the specificity of a test increases, the sensitivity decreases. An ideal test would have both high specificity and sensitivity, yet tradeoffs can be made depending on the condition being tested. Sensitivity and specificity can be calculated from a 2 × 2 table as illustrated below. Sensitivity = TP/TP + FN; specificity = TN/FP + TN.

	With Disease	Without Disease
Test positive	True positive (TP)	False positive (FP)
Test negative	False negative (FN)	True negative (TN)

40. What is meant by positive predictive value (PPV)?
The PPV reflects the proportion of persons who have the disease, given that they test positive. It measures how well the test predicts the presence of a given disease. The PPV is calculated from a 2 × 2 table as follows:

$$PPV = TP/TP + FP$$

This calculation takes into account the prevalence of disease.

41. What does the p value represent?
The probability that the observed result or something more extreme occurred by chance alone. Therefore, a p value of 0.05 indicates that there is only a 5% likelihood that the result observed was due to chance alone. Traditionally, a p value of 0.05 is considered statistically significant. If the p value is > 0.05, chance cannot be ruled out as an explanation for the observed effect. It is important to remember that chance can never be ruled out absolutely as an explanation for the observed results. A statistically significant result indicates that chance is not likely.

42. What is relative risk? Odds ratio?
The **relative risk** measures the association between exposure and disease. It is expressed as a ratio of the rate of disease among exposed persons to the rate among unexposed persons. Relative risk estimates the strength or magnitude of an association. The calculation of relative risk requires incidence rates, provided by cohort studies.
The **odds ratio** provides an estimate of the relative risk in case-control studies; because disease has already occurred, the incidence of disease cannot be determined.

43. How do the mean, median, and mode differ?
The three terms are measures of central tendency and are used to provide a summary measure to characterize a group of people. The **mean** represents the average. It is calculated by adding together all of the observations and then dividing by the total number of measurements. The mean takes into account the magnitude of each observation and, as a result, is easily affected by extreme values. The **median** is defined as the middle-most measurement (50th percentile)—i.e., half the observations are below it and half are above. Therefore, the median is unaffected by extreme measures. The **mode** is the most frequently used observation.

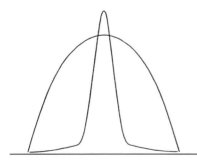

Two distributions with identical means, medians, and modes. (From Pagano M, Gauvreau K: Principles of Biostatistics. Boston, Harvard School of Public Health, 1991, with permission.)

44. Which of the following is most appropriate to test for differences between the means of two groups: ANOVA, *t*-test, or chi-square?
A *t*-test is used to compare the means between two groups. The ANOVA, or analysis of variance, compares the means in greater than two groups. The chi-square test is used to show differences in proportions.

45. Confidence intervals are often provided when data are reported. What do they indicate?

Confidence intervals (CI) represent the range within which the true magnitude of the effect lies with a certain degree of certainty. For example, a relative risk of 2.1 may be reported with a 95% CI (1.5, 2.9). This indicates that the study determined the relative risk to be 2.1 and that we are 95% certain that the true relative risk is not < 1.5 or > 2.9. If the 95% CI includes the null value (1.0), the result is not statistically significant.

46. Compare cross-sectional, case-control, and cohort studies.

Cross-sectional studies are a type of descriptive epidemiologic study in which the exposure and disease status of the population are determined at a given point. For example, the caries status of U.S. adults aged 45–65 in the year 1992 may be determined by a national dental survey and examination.

Case control and cohort studies are analytical epidemiologic studies. In **case-control studies** participants are selected on the basis of disease status. The "cases" are persons who have the disease of interest, and the control group consists of persons similar to the case group except that they do not have the disease of interest. Information about exposure status is then obtained from each group to assess whether an association exists between exposure and disease.

In cohort studies participants are selected on the basis of exposure status. Study participants must be free of the disease of interest at the time the study begins. Exposed and nonexposed participants are then followed over time to assess the association between exposure and specific diseases.

47. Which type of study—cohort, case-control, retrospective, or clinical trial—most closely resembles a true experiment?

In a clinical trial, the investigator allocates the participants to the exposure groups of interest and then follows the groups over time to observe how they differ in outcome. This method most closely resembles an experiment.

48. Discuss the importance of blinding and randomization in experimental studies.

Randomization and blinding are two methods of reducing bias in research studies. In a **randomized study** all participants have an equal likelihood of receiving the treatment of interest. For example, patients are randomly assigned to two groups, one of which receives a particular treatment and the other, placebo. Several techniques are available to ensure randomization of study participants. In a **double-blind study**, both the investigator observing the results and the participants are unaware of which individuals are assigned to which group. One means of achieving a blinded study is use of placebos.

49. Distinguish between split-mouth and crossover designs.

In **split-mouth studies**, different treatments are applied to different sections of the mouth. The effects of treatment must be localized to the region receiving the treatment. In **crossover studies**, patients serve as their own control and receive treatments in sequence—treatment A and then treatment B—and the disease course is compared between the two periods. The disease under investigation must be assumed to be stable during the period of treatment.

50. What is the difference between interexaminer and intraexaminer reliability?

The validity of an examination depends on the reliability of the examiner. Intraexaminer reliability refers to the ability of a single examiner to record the same findings in the same way over time. Interexaminer reliability refers to the ability of different examiners to record the same finding in the same way.

51. List and describe the most commonly used dental indices.

Measurements of dental caries are made with the **DMF index**. The DMF is an irreversible index and is used only with permanent teeth. *D* represents decayed teeth; *M*, missing teeth; and *F*, filled teeth. The DMF index can be applied to teeth (DMFT) or surfaces (DMFS). The DMFT score may range from 0 to 32, whereas the DMFS score may range from 0 to 160. The primary dentition uses the **def index**, where *d* represents decayed teeth; *e*, extracted teeth; and *f*, filled teeth.

Gingivitis is most commonly scored with the **gingival index** of LOE and Sillness. It grades the gingiva on the four surfaces of each tooth. Each area receives a score from 0 to 3, where 0 = normal gingiva; 1 = mild inflammation, no bleeding on probing; 2 = moderate inflammation; 3 = severe inflammation, ulceration, and spontaneous bleeding.

52. What is happening with the prevalence of caries in the United States?
The prevalence of caries has been declining in children during the 20th century. Results of the National Health and Nutrition Examination Surveys (NHANES) during the 1970s and 1980s show that the prevalence of caries has decreased significantly in the U.S. Elsewhere, the caries rate is also declining. A decline in adult caries is not as evident, because most adults grew up before the decline started. Fluoridation has received the most credit for the decline.

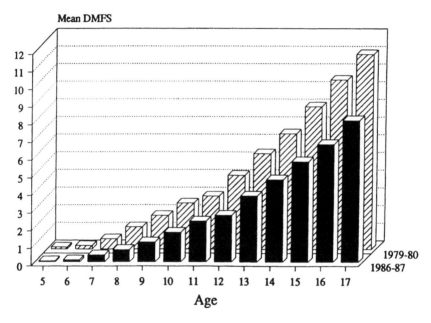

DMFS values for United States school children, aged 5–17 years, in 1979–1980 and 1986–1987. (From Burt BA, Eklund SA: Dentistry, Dental Practice and the Community. Philadelphia, W.B. Saunders, 1992, with permission).

53. In 1994 a *New York Times* article stated, "Half of today's schoolchildren have never had a cavity." Is this statement accurate?
The 50% estimate is overly optimistic because it ignores caries in the primary dentition. In fact, 50% of children have had caries by the time they are 8 years old. In addition, most of the research methods used to assess caries prevalence rely entirely on visual means and omit radiographs. As a result, most caries studies underestimate the true burden of disease. Eighty-five percent of American children experience decay by the time they are 17 years old. Low-income people exhibit more dental disease and more delay in treatment than those with higher incomes. (See figure, top of next page.)

54. What factors make a person susceptible to dental caries?
1. Host with susceptible tooth (mineral)
2. Agent—acid-producing bacteria (*S. mutans*)
3. Environment—dental plaque (sucrose)

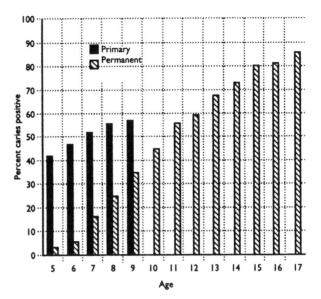

Percent of U.S. children with dental decay in primary and permanent teeth. (From the National Institute of Dental Research (NIDR) Survey, 1986–1987. Public Health Rep 110:524, 1995.)

55. What did the Vipeholm study reveal about the effect of diet on dental decay?

This study, conducted in a mental institution in Vipeholm, Sweden, is considered unethical and will not be repeated. The study divided patients into groups who received different doses of sugars. The sugar differed in amount, form, frequency, and whether it was consumed between meals. The most significant finding of the study was that the form and frequency of sugar consumption were most related to the occurrence of dental caries—that is, frequent consumption of sticky sugars increased the occurrence of dental caries.

56. What can you tell the parents of a toddler to aid in the prevention of caries?

Sugars are the most cariogenic foods, and the consumption of sugars between meals is associated with a marked increase in caries, whereas consumption of sugars with meals is associated with a much smaller increase. To prevent caries, avoid free sugars in bottle feeds, ensure optimal fluoride levels in water, and restrict intake of sugars.

57. Root caries is seen predominantly in what patient population?

The elderly. The rising incidence of root caries can be attributed to the aging of populations in industrialized societies and the fact that most adults are retaining more teeth. Increased gingival recession with exposure of root surfaces leads to the development of root caries.

58. What is the prevalence of periodontal disease?

Gingivitis and periodontitis are universally prevalent; in most countries more than 70% of all adults are afflicted. Some data suggest that there is no difference in the prevalence of periodontitis between developing and developed countries. More recent data obtained during the 1980s show that the prevalence of severe periodontitis ranges from 7–15%, regardless of a country's economic state, oral hygiene, or availability of dental care.

59. What is a common factor in both caries and periodontal disease?

The presence of dental plaque is a causative agent in both diseases.

60. How common are oral cancers?

Oral cancer accounted for 4–5% of all cancers diagnosed in the U.S. in 1997. Approximately one million new cancers are diagnosed in each year, and of these, about 40,000 are cancers of the lips, tongue, floor of the mouth, palate, gingiva, alveolar mucosa, buccal mucosa, and oropharynx. Oral cancer is twice as prevalent in males as in females. The age-adjusted annual incidence of oral cancer in white patients aged 65 or older was 20/100,000 in 1980.

61. What are the risk factors?

Studies of oral cancer have identified smoking and other forms of tobacco as the primary risk factors. In addition, alcohol consumption is a risk factor that may act as a promoter with tobacco. The combination of heavy smoking and alcohol consumption increases the risk of oral cancer 30-fold.

HEALTH POLICY

62. Differentiate between licensure and registration.

Licensure is granted through a government agency to those who meet specified qualifications to perform given activities or to claim a particular title. Registration is a listing of qualified individuals by a governmental or nongovernmental organization.

63. What are the types of supervision for allied dental personnel as defined by the ADA?

1. **Indirect:** The dentist diagnoses a condition, then authorizes the allied dental personnel to carry out treatment while the dentist remains in the office.

2. **Direct:** The dentist diagnoses a condition, authorizes treatment, and evaluates the outcome.

3. **General:** General supervision is defined by practice acts within each state and may require that the dentist be available but not necessarily on the premise or site where care is delivered.

64. What are the basic components of the dental care delivery system?

A delivery system is a means by which health care is provided to a patient and consists of four main components: (1) the organizational structure in which doctors and patients come together; (2) how health care is financed and paid for; (3) the supply of health care personnel; and (4) the physical structures involved in the delivery of care.

65. To what does quality assurance refer?

Quality assurance is the process of examining the physical structures, procedures, and outcome as they affect the delivery of health care. It consists of assessment to identify inadequacies, followed by implementation of improvements to correct the inadequacies and reassessment to determine if the improvements are effective.

66. Define structure, process, and outcome as they relate to quality assurance.

Structure refers to the layout and equipment of a facility. Included are items such as the building, equipment, and record forms. **Process** involves the services that the dentist and auxiliary personnel perform for patients and how skillfully they do so. **Outcome** is the change in health status that occurs as a result of the care delivered.

67. How do cost-benefit and cost-effectiveness analyses differ?

Cost-effectiveness and cost-benefit analyses are similar yet distinct techniques to help allocate resources to maximize objectives. **Cost-benefit analysis** requires that all costs and benefits be expressed in dollar terms to provide a measure of net benefit. **Cost-effectiveness analysis** allows alternative measures to value effectiveness. Objections to valuing life in terms of dollars led to the use of cases of disease prevented, life-years gained, or of quality-adjusted life-years. The result is a cost-effectiveness ratio that expresses the cost per unit of effectiveness.

68. What is adverse selection?

Adverse selection occurs when people at high risk for an illness are the predominant purchasers of insurance, especially when the risk for illness and the premium are based on a low-risk population. Thus, high-risk people are attracted to the insurance by its low rates, which allow them to avoid payments for a likely illness.

69. What is moral hazard?

Patients with insurance demand more medical care than patients who have to pay the cost themselves.

70. What is a community rating?

The premiums charged to all insurance subscribers are the same, regardless of individual risk. Regardless of who pays for medical care, the cost ultimately falls on the general public.

71. What are the different financing mechanisms for dental care?

Dentistry is financed mainly through fee-for-service self-pay; 56% of all dental expenses are paid out of pocket by the patient. Payment to the dentist by an organization other than the patient is called third-party payment. Third-party payers represented by private insurance pay about 33% of total dental expenses, followed by government-financed or public programs (i.e., Medicaid, Veterans Affairs).

72. What is capitation payment?

HMO premiums are usually made on a capitation basis—that is, HMO providers receive a given fee per enrollee, regardless of how much or little care is delivered.

73. Explain the differences among IPA, PPO, and HMO.

All three represent managed-care practices. Managed care refers to forms of insurance coverage in which utilization and service patterns are monitored by the insurer with the aim of containing costs. An HMO (health maintenance organization) is usually a self-contained staff-model practice in which no distinction is made between the providers of insurance and the providers of health care. HMO premiums are paid on a capitation basis. In contrast, IPA (independent practice association) and PPO (preferred provider organization) represent groups of doctors who practice in the community and are distinct from the insurance provider. However, the insurance agency contracts with the providers for discounted rates and may refer patients to these providers exclusively. If a patient elects to go to a different provider from the one recommended by the insurance company, the patient may face a financial penalty such as an additional charge.

74. How do managed-care arrangements differ from the traditional model of dental care?

Traditional medical and dental care has been paid on a fee-for-service basis. The patient chooses any provider in the community, and the insurance company usually pays a certain percentage of the charge. In the current era of cost-consciousness, many insurance companies are modifying or eliminating this model altogether. Fee-for-service usually provides no incentive for either the patient or provider to contain costs.

75. How do Medicaid and Medicare differ?

Medicare, an entitlement fund, was created to provide health insurance to people 65 years old and over, certain disabled groups, and people with certain kidney diseases. Medicare has two parts, an institutional or hospital portion (Part A) and a noninstitutional portion or physician-services (Part B). Part A has no premium, but Part B is supplemental and voluntarily purchased. Medicare does not provide dental care.

Medicaid is a means-tested program to provide health insurance to poor people eligible for welfare assistance programs. Medicaid covers both hospital and physician costs without a premium or copayment. Medicaid is required by federal law to provide dental services to children. However, adult dental services are optional, and the decision whether to provide dental care is determined at a state level.

76. Which agency administers Medicare funds?

The Health Care Financing Administration (HCFA), a federal agency, is responsible for funding Medicare. It determines how much providers will be paid and what services are covered.

77. How are the funds for Medicaid provided?

Medicaid is a joint federal and state program with federal guidelines that allow states some flexibility in what services are provided and who is eligible. The federal government provides states with matching dollars.

78. What percentage of the gross national product (GNP) is spent on health care?

In 1995, 13.1% of the GNP was spent on health care. The GNP represents the total production in the United States.

79. What percentage of all U.S. heath care expenditures is for dental care?

In 1990, the HCFA estimated that 4% ($46 of $988 billion) of all U.S. health care expenditures was for dental services. Approximately $44 billion came from private funds and $2 billion came from public funds, principally Medicaid.

BIBLIOGRAPHY

1. American Dental Association: Principles of Ethics and Code of Professional Conduct. Chicago, American Dental Association, 1992.
2. American Dental Association: Fluoridation Facts. Chicago, American Dental Association, 1993, 30 pp.
3. Antczak-Bouckoms A, Tulloch JFC, Bouckoms AJ, et al: Diagnostic Decision Making. Anesth Prog 37:161-165, 1990.
4. A quality assurance primer for dentistry. J Am Dent Assoc 117:239-242, 1988.
5. Burt BA, Eklund SA: Dentistry, Dental Practice and the Community. Philadelphia, W.B. Saunders, 1992.
6. Detels R, Holland WW, McEwen J, Omen GS: Textbook of Public Health, 3rd ed, vols 1,2,3. New York, Oxford University Press, 1997.
7. Dunning JM: Principles of Dental Public Health, 4th ed. Cambridge, MA, Harvard University Press, 1986.
8. Edelstein BL, Douglass CW: Dispelling the myth that 50 percent of U.S. schoolchildren have never had a cavity. Public Health Rep 110:522–530, 1995.
9. Feldstein PJ: Health Care Economics. Albany, Delmar, 1988.
10. Gift HC, Drury TF, Nowjack-Raymer RE, Selwitz RH: The state of the nation's oral health: Mid-decade assessment of Healthy People 2000. J Public Health Dent 56:84–91, 1996.
10. Hennekens CH, Buring JE: Epidemiology in Medicine. In Mayrent SL (ed). Boston, Little, Brown, 1987.
11. Jacobs P: The Economics of Health and Medical Care. Gaithersburg, MD, Aspen, 1991.
12. Jong A: Dental Public Health and Community Dentistry. St. Louis, Mosby, 1981.
13. Newburn E: Effectiveness of water fluoridation. J Public Health Dent 49:279-289, 1989.
14. Pagano M, Gauvreau K: Principles of Biostatistics. Boston, Harvard School of Public Health, 1991.
15. Public Health Focus: Fluoridation of community water systems. MMWR 1992; pp 372-375, 381.
16. Riordan PJ: Fluoride supplements in caries prevention: A literature review and proposal for a new dosage schedule. J Public Health Dent 53:174-189, 1993.
17. Ripa LW: A half century of community water fluoridation in the United States: Review and commentary. J Public Health Dent 53:17-44, 1993.
18. Rozier RG, Beck JD: Epidemiology of oral disease. Curr Opin Dent 1:308-315, 1991.
19. Silverman S: Oral Cancer. Atlanta, American Cancer Society, 1990.
20. Weinstein MC, Fineberg HV: Clinical Decision Analysis. Philadelphia, W.B. Saunders, 1980.
21. Weintraub JA, Douglass CW, Gillings DB: Biostatistics: Data Analysis for Dental Health Professionals. Chapel Hill, Cavco, 1985.

15. LEGAL ISSUES AND ETHICS

Elliot V. Feldbau, D.M.D., and Bernard Friedland, B.Ch.D., M.Sc., J.D.

LEGAL ISSUES

1. What general principles of law apply to dental practice?

United States law is outlined under principles of criminal and civil law; the latter is divided into contract and tort law. Most legal issues related to dental practice involve civil wrongs or torts; that is, wrongful acts or injuries, not involving breach of contract, for which an individual can bring a civil action for damages.

Malpractice is part of the law of **negligence,** which constitutes one kind of tort. A malpractice suit based on the law of negligence alleges that the dentist failed to employ the care and skill of the average qualified practitioner. It further alleges that the failure to employ the required care and skill was the "proximate cause" of the patient's injury. Malpractice is considered an unintentional tort. It is normally covered by dental malpractice insurance.

Informed consent cases used to be based on the theory of **assault and battery,** but today they are considered no differently from other malpractice cases.

Invasion of privacy, an intentional tort, results when a patient's image or name is used by a dentist for personal gain, such as in advertising. Discussing a patient by name without permission, with persons other than the clinical staff, also may be construed as a violation of the privacy implied by the doctor-patient relationship.

2. Under the law, how is the relationship between doctor and patient interpreted?

The law defines the doctor-patient relationship under the principles of contract law. The terms are usually implied but may be expressed. Upon accepting a patient for care, the dentist is obliged (1) to maintain confidentiality, (2) to complete care in a timely and professional manner, (3) to ensure that care is available in emergency situations or in the absence of the dentist, and (4) to be compensated for treatment by the patient. Of interest, the contract is termed binding at the earliest point of contact; that is, the moment of a telephone call to the dentist may be interpreted as the point of consummation of the contract, unless the dentist refuses to consider the caller for care or does not realize that the caller is a patient.

3. May a dentist dismiss a patient after beginning a treatment?

There are four ways to terminate the dentist-patient relationship: (1) the patient may inform the dentist that he or she no longer wishes to be cared for by the dentist; (2) the treatment has run its course; (3) the dentist and patient mutually agree that the patient will no longer be treated by the dentist; and (4) the dentist terminates the relationship. Perhaps an example best clarifies the second way. Suppose a patient is referred to an endodontist for treatment of tooth #9. Once the endodontist has completed treatment and any necessary follow-up, the dentist-patient relationship is terminated. In this case, the dentist is under no obligation to treat the patient at any time in the future. A possible exception may be if future treatment is needed for tooth #9. In cases involving ways (3) and (4), the dentist should avoid the risk of being liable for abandonment by notifying the patient of his or her decision in writing, by providing the telephone number of the local dental society that the patient may call for a referral, and by offering to provide emergency treatment for a reasonable (depending on the circumstances) period of time.

4. What is considered adequate informed consent?

A dentist must disclose to a patient the risks and benefits of a procedure, alternative treatments, and the risks and benefits of no treatment. Informed consent is not required in writing but may be helpful.

U.S. courts use one of two measures to determine whether the dentist satisfied the informed consent requirement. States are split approximately 50-50 on which standard to apply. One standard states that disclosure is adequate if the dentist has given the patient information that the "average qualified practitioner" would ordinarily provide under similar circumstances. The other standard requires a dentist to disclose to a patient in a reasonable manner all significant medical and dental information that the dentist possesses or reasonably should possess; the patient uses such information to decide to undergo or refuse a proposed procedure. The national trend is leaning towards this patient-centered approach.

5. When may the issue of informed consent be bypassed?

In an emergency consent is implied. Such an emergency exists when treatment cannot be postponed without jeopardizing the life or well-being of the patient and the patient is unable to grant consent because of physical impairment.

6. Who is responsible if a dental hygienist performs prophylactic treatment without proper premedication on a patient who develops subacute bacterial endocarditis after relating a history of rheumatic fever and heart valve replacement on his or her medical form?

Under the legal principle of "respondeat superior" ("let the master answer"), the employees of a dentist as well as the dentist may be sued for negligence (deviating from the standard of care) or other issues of malpractice or battery during the course of their employment.

7. Does a missed diagnosis or failure of treatment constitute negligence?

An incorrect diagnosis does not necessarily constitute negligence. Because of the many judgments involved in dental practice it is considered unrealistic to expect that a dentist be 100% correct. The plaintiff must demonstrate serious injury because of the dentist's failure to diagnose properly before there are grounds for negligence. Furthermore, it must be shown that the dentist failed to exercise the applicable standard of care. But injury alone is grounds to file a suit for negligence.

If the outcome of treatment is bad (e.g., a failed endodontic treatment due to a separated instrument), negligence is not necessarily supported if the appropriate standard of treatment is employed. However, if a dentist promises to effect a specific cure, to bring about a particular result, or to complete a procedure with no residual problems and fails to fulfill the promise, a lawsuit may be filed on the basis of breach of contract rather than negligence.

8. When should a patient be referred?

A patient should be referred under the following circumstances:

1. When there is a question of appropriate treatment;
2. When periodontal treatment not routinely performed by the general dentist is indicated;
3. When periodontal disease is advanced with severe bone loss;
4. When shared responsibility is desirable for complex multidisciplinary cases;
5. When complex care is required for medically compromised patients; and
6. When the patient is refractory to treatment or unstable with a well-documented history of previous treatment failures.

9. What are common reasons for patients to sue?

1. Lack of informed consent: a patient does not know the specific nature and/or complications of treatment.
2. Failure to refer: for example, treating advanced periodontal disease with only scalings.
3. Failure to treat or diagnose adequately.
4. Abandonment: if the patient was dismissed for nonpayment of services, the dentist must show that other avenues were tried, such as small claims court or collection agencies. The dentist should document the reason for the dismissal and make available a referral source and any necessary emergency care for a period of 60 days. Communications to the patient should be through a registered letter.
5. Guarantees by doctor or staff.

6. Poor patient rapport.
7. Lack of communication.
8. Poor recordkeeping.
9. Issues related to fee collection.

10. What is necessary to prove negligence?

Four elements are necessary to prove negligence and win a malpractice suit. The patient must establish that (1) a dentist-patient relationship existed (i.e., that the dentist owed the patient the care and skill of the average qualified practitioner), (2) the dentist breached his or her duty by failing to exercise the level of care and skill of the average qualified practitioner, (3) the patient suffered injury, and (4) a connection exists between the dentist's breach of duty and the patient's injury (causation).

11. What are grounds for revocation of a dental license?

Criminal convictions involving fraud and deception in prescribing drugs, gross immorality, or conviction of a felony under state law are grounds for revocation, usually by decision of the state licensing board. A license may also be revoked for a pattern of negligent care or for gross negligence.

12. What issues may constitute a defense against malpractice?

In a claim of malpractice or negligence, the patient must show that his or her injuries are directly associated with the dentist's wrongful acts or that standards of care were not followed. Failure to achieve successful treatment or to satisfy a patient with esthetic results does not necessarily constitute negligence.

"Contributory negligence" is a special phrase used in the law to describe what the plaintiff may have done to contribute to his or her own injury. Contributory negligence may occur if the patient does not comply with specific instructions regarding medications or home care.

13. What elements are contained in a complete dental record?
- Identification data
- Medical history, including updated antibiotic regimens for prophylaxis of subacute bacterial endocarditis, effects of medication on birth control pills, and medical consultations as needed
- Dental history
- Clinical examination
- Diagnosis and interpretation of radiographs
- Treatment plans
- Progress notes
- Consent forms for surgical procedures
- Completion notes

14. How should records be written and corrections be made?

All entries require ink or typed notes, not pencil, and errors must be lined out with a single line and initialed, with the substitute entry correcting the error. This procedure guards against any challenge to the reliability of record entries.

Practitioners who keep digital records (i.e., those who use a computer) should be especially careful. Because it is easy to go back and make changes, one is easily accused of making changes to the record to suit one's needs. Practitioners who use word-processing programs are well advised to take precautions so that they can prove when entries were made. Programs that record dates of entry are available but work on different principles. One program permits a person to make changes at any time, but an auditing program keeps track of when each and every keystroke was made. A different program requires one to type a word (e.g., "End") after an entry has been completed. Thereafter, the program does not permit one to go back into previous entries. Changes to the record must be made under a new entry, which should be labeled by the dentist to indicate that it is a modification of the record. Commonly, the word *Addendum* is used to label such an entry.

ETHICS

15. How is the practice of dentistry broadly governed?
The ethical rules and principles of professional conduct for the practice of dentistry are set forth in the American Dental Association's publication, *Principles of Ethics and Code of Professional Conduct,* which describes the role of the professional in the practice of dentistry.

16. What three ethical principles are outlined in the code?
1. Beneficence: being kind and/or doing good
2. Autonomy: respect of the patient's right of self-decision
3. Justice: the quality of being impartial and fair

17. How does the code define beneficence in the practice of dentistry?
The dentist is obliged:
1. To give the highest quality of service of which he or she is capable. This implies that professionals will maintain their level of knowledge by continued skill development.
2. To preserve healthy dentition unless it compromises the well-being of other teeth.
3. To participate in legal and public health-related matters.

18. Who is expected to be responsible for practices of preventive health maintenance?
The patient is expected to be responsible for his or her own preventive practices. The dentist is responsible for providing information and supportive care (e.g., recall and prophylaxis), but the patient has the ultimate responsibility to maintain oral health.

19. Outline the essential elements implied in the principle of autonomy.
The principle of autonomy requires respect for the patient's rights in the areas of confidentiality, informed consent for diagnostic and therapeutic services, and truthfulness to the patient. The dentist should work with patients to allow them to make autonomous decisions about their care. The dentist is obliged to provide services for which the patient contracts.

20. How does the dental profession serve justice, according to the code?
The individual dentist and the profession as a whole are obligated to be just and fair in the delivery of dental services. Self-regulation is a basic tenet of this obligation as well as calling attention to any social injustices in the allocation of societal resources to the delivery of dental health services.

21. A 29-year-old patient with poor oral hygiene and multiple caries requests full-mouth extractions and dentures. A complete examination reveals a basically sound periodontium and carious lesions that can be restored conservatively. What ethical principles apply to this basic case of neglect without advanced disease?
Respect for the patient's autonomy and requests is evaluated and judged against the duty of the dentist to provide the highest type of service of which he or she is capable. After full disclosure about long-term effects of edentulism, as well as the costs and benefits of saving teeth, the assessment of the patient's motivation is most important. Saving teeth that will only fall into disrepair through neglect and the patient's lack of commitment to maintain oral health must be considered carefully before a final treatment is elected or rejected.

22. A patient rejects the use of radiographs for examination of his teeth. How should this situation be handled, according to the code?
The dentist's only recourse is to use informed consent about the risks and benefits of an incomplete examination and the possible consequences of such a decision. The respect of the pa-

tient's right to choose (autonomy) prevails, even if it generates a negative obligation not to interfere with a patient's choice.

23. An adolescent presents with a suspected lesion of a sexually transmitted disease (STD) and asks that no one, especially his parents, be told. What are the ethical considerations?

The right of autonomy and respect for privacy are overturned by the public health law that requires the reporting of STDs to the health department. Public law is often the determinant in such situations.

24. A patient requests that all her amalgam restorations be replaced. Is this an ethical issue?

It is not unethical to replace amalgams on request. It is considered untruthful, and hence unethical, to make any claim that a patient's general health will be improved or that the patient will rid her body of toxins by replacing amalgam restorations. It is unethical to ascribe any disease to the use of dental amalgam, because no causal relationship has been proved, or to attempt to treat any systemic disease by the removal of dental amalgams.

25. What disciplinary penalties may be imposed on a dentist found guilty of unethical conduct?

1. **Censure:** a disciplinary sentence written to express severe criticism or disapproval for a particular type of conduct or act.

2. **Suspension:** a loss of membership privileges for a certain period with automatic reinstatement.

3. **Probation:** a specified period without the loss of rights in lieu of a suspended disciplinary penalty. A dentist on probation may be required to practice under the supervision of a dentist or other individual approved by the dental board.

4. **Revocation of license:** absolute severance from the profession.

26. For what acts may a dentist be charged with unethical conduct?

1. A guilty verdict for a criminal felony.
2. A guilty verdict for violating the bylaws or principles of the Code of Ethics.

27. To what guiding principle does the ADA's *Principles of Conduct and Code of Professional Ethics* ascribe?

Service to the public and quality of care are the two aspects of the dental profession's obligation to society elaborated in the code.

28. May a dentist refuse to care for certain patients?

It is unethical for a dentist to refuse to accept patients because of race, creed, color, sex, or national origin or because the patient has acquired immunodeficiency syndrome (AIDS) or is infected with the human immunodeficiency virus (HIV). Treatment decisions and referrals should be made on the same basis as they are made for any patient that the dentist treats. Such decisions should be based only on the need of a dentist for another dentist's skills, knowledge, equipment, or experience to serve best the patient's health needs.

29. May a dentist relate information about a patient's seropositivity for HIV to another dentist to whom he or she is referring the patient?

The laws that safeguard the confidentiality of a patient's record are not uniform throughout the United States with regard to HIV status. It may be prohibited to transfer this information without the written permission of the patient. As a rule, the treating dentist is advised to seek written permission from the patient before releasing any information to the consulting practitioner.

30. What is overbilling?

Overbilling is the misrepresentation of a fee as higher than in fact it is; for example, when a patient is charged one fee and an insurance company is billed a higher fee to benefit the patient's copayment.

31. May a dentist accept a copayment from a dental insurance company as payment in full for services and not request the patient's portion?

It is considered "overbilling" and hence unethical to collect only the third-party payment without full disclosure to the insurance company.

32. May a dentist charge different fees to different patients for the same services?

It is considered unethical to increase a fee to a patient because the patient has insurance. However, different treatment scenarios and conditions may prevail and dictate different fees, regardless of the form of payment.

33. Is it appropriate to advance treatment dates on insurance claims for a patient who otherwise would not be eligible for dental benefits?

It is considered false and misleading representation to the third-party payer to advance treatment dates for services not undertaken within the benefit period.

34. What are the standards for advertising by dentists?

Advertising is permitted as long as it is not false or misleading in any manner. Infringements of the standards involve statements that include inferences of specialty by a general dentist, use of unearned degrees as titles or nonhealth degrees to enhance prestige, or use of "HIV-negative health results" to attract patients without conveying information that clarifies the scientific significance of the statement.

35. How may specialization be expressed? What are the standard guidelines?

To allow the public to make an informed selection between the dentist who has completed accredited training beyond the dental degree and the dentist who has not, an announcement of specialization is permitted. The areas of ethical specialty recognized by the American Dental Association are dental public health, endodontics, oral pathology, oral surgery, orthodontics, pediatric dentistry, periodontics, prosthodontics, and oral and maxillofacial surgery. Any announcement should read "specialist in" or practice "limited to" the respective field. Dentists making such announcements must have met the educational requirements of the ADA for the specialty.

36. What are the stated guidelines for the name of a dental practice?

Because the name of a practice may be a selection factor on the patient's part, it must not be misleading in any manner. The name of a dentist no longer associated with the practice may be continued for a period of 1 year.

37. What does the code state about chemical dependency of dentists?

It is unethical for a dentist to practice while abusing alcohol or other chemical substances that impair ability. All dentists are obligated to urge impaired colleagues to seek treatment and to report firsthand evidence of abuse by a colleague to the professional assistance committee of a dental society. The professional assistance committee is obligated to report noncompliers to the appropriate regulatory boards for licensing review.

38. How are problems of interpretation of the *Principles of Ethics and Code of Professional Conduct* to be resolved?

Problems involving questions of ethics should be resolved by the local dental society. If resolutions cannot be achieved, an appeal to the ADA's Council on Ethics, Bylaws and Judicial Affairs is the next step.

BIBLIOGRAPHY

Law and Dental Practice
  1. Barsley RE, Herschaft EE: Dental malpractice. In Hardin JF (ed): Clark's Clinical Dentistry, vol. 5. Philadelphia, J.B. Lippincott, 1992, pp 1–26.
  2. Brackett RC, Poulsom RC: The law and the dental health practitioner. In Hardin JF (ed): Clark's Clinical Dentistry, vol. 5. Philadelphia, J.B. Lippincott, 1992, pp 1–42.

3. Pollack B: Risk management in dental office practice. In Hardin JF (ed): Clark's Clinical Dentistry, vol. 5. Philadelphia, J.B. Lippincott, 1992, pp 1–26.
4. Pollack B: Legal risks associated with implant dentistry. In Hardin JF (ed): Clark's Clinical Dentistry, vol. 5. Philadelphia, J.B. Lippincott, 1992, pp 1–8.
5. Pollack B: Legal risks associated with management of the temporomandibular joint. In Hardin JF (ed): Clark's Clinical Dentistry, vol. 5. Philadelphia, J.B. Lippincott, 1992, pp 1–11.
6. Risk Management Foundation of the Harvard Medical Institutions: Claims Management and the Legal Process. Cambridge, MA, 1994.

Ethics and Dentistry
7. American Dental Association: Principles of Ethics and Code of Professional Conduct, with official advisory opinions revised to May 1992. Chicago, American Dental Association, 1992.
8. Massachusetts Dental Society: Code of Ethics. Natick, MA, 1986.
9. McCullough LB: Ethical issues in dentistry. In Hardin JF (ed): Clark's Clinical Dentistry, vol. 1. Philadelphia, J.B. Lippincott, 1992, pp 1–17.
10. Ozar DT: AIDS, ethics, and dental care. In Hardin JF (ed): Clark's Clinical Dentistry, vol. 1. Philadelphia, J. B. Lippincott, 1992, pp 1–21.

INDEX

Page numbers in **boldface type** indicate complete chapters.